Ann L. Prior

J

M

*The Clinical Use
of Dreams*

The Clinical Use
of Dreams

WALTER BONIME, M.D.

foreword by MONTAGUE ULLMAN, M.D.

BASIC BOOKS, INC.   *Publishers*   NEW YORK

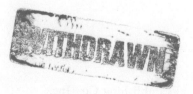

"A dream which is not explained is like a letter which has not been read."

TALMUD

Foreword

MONTAGUE ULLMAN, M.D.

Director, Department of Psychiatry
Maimonides Hospital of Brooklyn

The Clinical Use of Dreams is the first systematic and detailed clinical exposition of the analysis of dreams from a basically non-Freudian point of view. As such it has a certain timeliness as one surveys the current scene. Two significant contemporary movements are to be noted in regard to our knowledge of dreams, one experimental, physiological, and concerned with the process of dreaming itself, the other psychological, theoretical, clinical, and concerned primarily with dream meaning.

The first is of very recent origin and is rooted in the pioneering studies emanating first from the laboratories of the University of Chicago and later from a great many laboratories both in this country and abroad. The work relating the dreaming process to rather precise indicators—in the form of the electroencephalographic record and the occurrence of rapid eye movements—has initiated and intensified the study of physiological as well as psychological characteristics of cognitive activity during the various stages of sleep. We have learned a great deal about dreaming as a result of these studies. They have provided us with information concerning the onset, duration, and termination of periods of dreaming throughout the night, the patterning of such periods relative to the sleep cycle, the total dream time per night, the relationship of dreaming to stages of sleep as indicated by electroencephalographic data, the relation of direction of eye movement to the plane of movement occurring in the dream, the dream time of re-callers and non-recallers of dreams, the results of dream deprivation, the influence of drugs upon total dream time, the type of cognitive data elicited during periods of non-rapid eye movement, and numerous other correlates of the dreaming process. In short, these experiments have paved the way toward an intensive and realistic assay of the physiology and psychology of the sleeping human organism in a way that was never before possible. Currently, and probably for years to come, the implications of these findings for our theoretical approaches to under-standing the behavior of the waking organism will gradually come into focus and, hopefully, they may provide us with a more solid base upon which to build our conceptual schemes than the many conflicting and diverse points of view traditionally associated with the study of waking behavior. A mass of factual data is emerging which is bound to influence and perhaps drastically modify the speculative insights upon which dream theory has been built in the past.

The second movement referred to has had a longer incubation period. It began at the time the so-called culturalist movement took shape, when the confining strictures of classical psychoanalytic theory could no longer contain the curious and insightful explorations into the enormously complex array of relations and transactions subsumed under the designation of *therapeutic process*. The past two decades witnessed the evolving contributions of Horney, Fromm, Sullivan, and numerous others, all directed toward shedding additional light upon the complexi-ties of the interpersonal process, and all attempting to understand human behavior in the human context. Since this context is a social and cultural one, these efforts inevitably led to a deeper concern with the connection between individual behavior and the actual living condi-tions which go to make up the human environment. Although progress took place in bits and pieces, the change was, nevertheless, a revolu-tionary one. The basic issue was relatively simple. Should we accept the proposition that man, of all the known animal species, has a bio-logical endowment that inexorably and inevitably leads him down the path of suffering, neurosis, and global conflict? Or does it make more sense to assume that man, having created so many diverse possibilities for social life, has created some which are maladaptive at various stages of historical development? The latter proposition proclaims that the limiting factors in man's successful evolution as a social creature lie not in the biological equipment but in the imperfections of the social structures he has erected. The notion of imperfection implies not the existence of absolute perfection but the ability to progress toward a greater and greater relative perfection. In terms of behavioral consequences this means progress toward understanding and eliminating the causes of mental illness and the suffering associated with impaired or deviant personality formation. The young child is not inevitably destined to be victimized by his biological drives. He can be, and too often is, victimized by a culture that limits and fragments his maturational capacities. Is there a human being in the environment of the child who, by virtue of his own maturity, needs, and total life situation possesses the freedom to understand and care for this evolving human organism? This is one of the crucial factors which accounts for the presence or absence of suffering in the psychiatric sense. There are, of course, sources of potential suffering relating to genetic and congenital factors which are neither clearly understood nor generally agreed upon at the present time.

Inasmuch as every other organism has achieved a harmonious relationship with its environment, at least for a given time span, it seems foolish to assume that man is the exception and that his efforts to create a civilization that is truly human are doomed to failure because underneath it all he is only an animal. This basically appears to have been the thinking underlying the initial psychoanalytic formulations when the philosophical skeleton is dissected away from the rich clinical contributions. If, in fact, this endoskeleton is a mythological construct built up around the notion of instinct, then it has to be replaced by something of greater substance regardless of how ingeniously it held together the various tissues and organs of psychopathology and behavioral syndromes.

There are a number of illustrious thinkers whose work paved the way for the rich clinical exposition to be found in the pages to follow. The list is well known. There are two aspects of dream theory as expressed in contemporary thought that have their origin in the early divergent views of Jung and Adler. It was Jung who first attempted to grapple with the dream at a phenomenological level and who rejected wish-fulfillment as too confining a category for the range and versatility of the thought expressed by the dreamer. Despite the transcendental and religious overtones, his dream theory, insofar as it rejected the motive of disguise as well as the source of dream content in the residue of irrational childhood impulses, anticipates the work of Tauber and Green as well as the current existentialist writers. The dream is an experience in self-confrontation. Its intent is to reveal rather than conceal. The symbols exist not as subterfuges and disguises but as metaphorical referents.

Interestingly enough, there is much in Dr. Bonime's approach that is reminiscent of some of the early insights of Jung into the nature of the dream. Jung, in reaction to Freud's emphasis on the infantile and the irrational, felt compelled to stress the existence and importance of constructive forces in the dream. The dream has a compensatory and rectifying function. It depicts inner reality as it is and not as we perceive it to be. Distortion, censorship, and disguise become meaningless terms and the way is opened for a phenomenological understanding of the dream.

It was Adler who took the first steps in creating a social base for psychoanalytic theory. He rejected the notion of an unconscious, and with this the notion that the aim of the dream was to gratify desires. Paradoxically, he retained the notion of self-deception in dreams, but considered this within the broader context of the effort to preserve and re-enforce a particular life style rather than in the service of gratifying sexually motivated urges and desires. Abandoning the dichotomy between conscious and unconscious, Adler sought the key to the dream in the understanding of the life style and of the choices confronting an individual in a particular current life situation. For Adler, and for such later writers as Horney, Kelman, Robbins and Fromm, the dynamic meaning of the dream could be preserved without the concept of the unconscious as a reservoir of aggressive and libidinal impulses and as a subliminal stream continually attempting to force its way through the barriers of repression. The peculiarities of dream thought are to be understood as a particular mode of presentation of one's experience and not as the eruption of an unconscious mode of thought. The dream remains an expression of a unified personality structure. In defense of this position concerning the unconscious the following contemporary note is appropriate:

"The remaining question to be answered is, whether, for the explanation of the behavior of the patients, it is necessary to draw up the hypothesis of *the unconscious*. Surveying the preceding pages the reader must be struck by the absence of the word unconscious. Yet it is clear that numerous significations and relationships were discussed that are not clearly seen by man in general and very decidedly not by the patient. It is correct to say that surprisingly much of what happens in our life entirely escapes our notice and there is not the slightest objection to apply the *adjective* 'unconscious' to all that which escapes us. There is much therefore that is unconscious, nothing however that would lead us to assume 'an' unconscious (substantive), which would be supposed to exist as a second reality behind the phantoms of healthy and of neurotic life. There is but one reality: that of life as it is lived. 'The' *unconscious*, that 'part' of our personality therefore that, equipped with the most wonderful qualities, is supposed to be able to explain the problem of human life, is the product of a premature cessation of the psychological analysis of human existence." *

Referring to the genesis of his own thought, Dr. Bonime pays tribute to the works of Horney and Robbins. His contribution does follow most clearly in the tradition of Horney and Robbins. With the publication in 1937 of Horney's *The Neurotic Personality of Our Time* a refreshing new light was shed not only on psychoanalytic theory but on the behavior of man in the western world. Indeed, Dr. Bonime's book might be aptly subtitled "The Dream Life of the Neurotic Personality of Our Time." Like Horney before him, he writes about analytic data within the context of the actual lives that people lead. In his own words he is interpreting the behavior of people who have dreams rather than engaging in dream interpretation. The dialectic interplay between the social scene and the individual response is considered in its concreteness rather than as the presumptive antagonism of a given set of instincts. By implication the social scene moves and develops through its own set of integral laws which, though connected with human psychology—and, in fact, human biology—cannot be understood or explained by these factors alone. Society is not in its essence the structuralization of internal forces. Horney saw dreams as attempts at solutions of conflicting needs in the organized personality structure. Their analyses revealed self-defeating and contradictory value systems and modes of relatedness. Considering the hidden wish or the forbidden impulse as too constricted a framework, Horney herself, following in the tradition of Adler, saw in dreams a symbolic extension of the problems and adaptive maneuvers characteristic of the waking state. Bonime likewise devotes most of his efforts to uncovering the referents of the dream to the characterologic and social realities of the patient's life.

Horney concerned herself with the problem of how neurotic suffering derives from the social milieu. Although she was accused of being superficial, of by-passing genetic factors, and of operating within the realm of ego psychology, the fact remains that Horney's contribution shed a bright new light on psychoanalytic theory. She provided an enormous impetus to the development of the "culturist" approach and in all probability encouraged, within the orthodox camp itself, a greater recognition of ego psychology.

The teaching of Bernard S. Robbins centered about his concern with values, their social and cultural origins, and the manner in which

* Van Den Berg, J. H., "The Phenomenological Approach to Psychiatry." Springfield, Ill., Charles C Thomas, 1955, p. 83.

value systems were expressed in characterologic adaptations. To Robbins the term *unconscious* referred to those aspects of the individual's value system that remained expediently unknown at a conceptual level but which betrayed their presence in activity. Bonime, focusing more specifically on the competitive and cynical aspects of modern man, depicts the neurotic struggle of the individual to pursue one of two equally disastrous courses—either to rise above any vulnerability to social influence or to move into the social scene with techniques of domination. Perhaps alienation might be a more felicitous term to apply to modern man than competitiveness or cynicism. The latter qualities are certainly pervasive but by no means exhaust the repertoire of pathogenic adaptive maneuvers.

Robbins, employing a more discerning approach to the specific nature of the social milieu and the specific inequities wrought upon the individual, described psychopathology very much in terms of the dehumanization of man as the inevitable concomitant of the reduction of the humanist ethic to the business ethic. The repressive influences of civilization with which Freud was so preoccupied are not reducible to biological factors. They are given their just due but are not ensconced in a pessimistic certainty. There are no irreducible roadblocks to change traceable to biological needs or differences. At any given moment in history the prospects for human happiness and fulfillment may be relatively bleak, but the ultimate projection remains open-ended. It hinges not on the antithesis between man and the civilizing process he so desperately needs but on the question of man's capacity to arrive at a truly civilized state. When civilization stands in opposition to the human organism the culprit is not human biology but man's failure to arrive at as accurate a knowledge of the laws of social change and movement as he has of the laws of the exact sciences. What is true is that any aspect of one's biology, notably one's sexual potential and equipment, can be put to use as an adaptive response in a way that will ultimately result in a maladapted way of life. Our biology thus undergoes a social screening, but there is nothing intrinsically maladaptive or pathogenic about it. The disturbances come about when one's biological potential is misused in the service of solving interpersonal problems. Deprivation at a sensual, social, or maturational level throws the individual back on himself, so to speak, so that any aspect of his biological equipment can be pressed into the service of problem-solving. Freedom in connection with personality functioning becomes identical with the Hegelian concept of freedom generally—the notion of freedom as connected with the understanding of that which is necessary. Herein lies a clue to Dr. Bonime's emphasis on feeling. Felt reactions rooted in misconceptions and misunderstanding of social stimuli are inevitably associated with the absence of freedom. Technically this is referred to as the compulsivity associated with the operation of neurotic trends. The individual, unable to objectify a particular set of relations, is thus unable to change them; hence the activity displayed tends to be repetitive and stereotyped. The sense of freedom is identified not with the absence of the problem but with the ability, based on more rational perceptions, to cope with it. Therein is derived the sense of struggle, movement, and growth in contrast to rigidity, compulsivity, and stagnation. These abstract considerations are spelled out in their clinical concreteness throughout the book. The patient communicates, conceptualizes, and changes. Dream elements and the feelings they embody lead patient and therapist to the relevant data to be communicated. The dialectics of change are such that there is an initial fear of this freedom. The struggle between the reluctance to surrender the old and the adventure of the new accounts for the phenomenon of resistance. It is often difficult, always painful, and sometimes impossible to learn the technique of achieving freedom. It is important to emphasize that freedom, in any context, is always relative in character. Absolute freedom does not exist.

Although he employs a different terminology, there is much in the conceptual matrix of Bonime's thought that harks back to the early and important contributions of Harry Stack Sullivan. Sullivan regarded the dream, as he did the myth, as a relatively valid parataxic operation for the relief of insoluble problems of living. The impact of the dream lies not in what the dream elements should fit—i.e., their extrapolation to the syntaxic mode—but rather in what they obscurely deal with. In a more global sense, Bonime's emphasis on the interpersonal, interactional, and collaborative aspects of the therapeutic process is Sullivanian in character. Sullivan tended to link dreaming with the effort to satisfy unsatisfied needs by the covert operations and symbolic devices occurring in sleep. This concept of release paves the way for the linkage of the dream to suppressed impulses and for the notion of censorship. Here Bonime diverges from Sullivan's view. More in the tradition of Horney and Robbins, he explores the dream in the context of self-confrontation, which is the interplay between genuine awareness as well as neurotic techniques of avoidance. The dreamer is expressing who he is and what is happening to him at a given moment, despite the fact that this expression may be one-sided, distorted, or symbolically rationalized. In this way a rather sharp line can be drawn between those who view the dream primarily in terms of release and those who interpret its apparent subjectivity in its identity with waking behavior and consciousness. Put another way, the dream does not depict a need in its naked, released aspect, but in its identity to a behavioral component of the waking state. The identity is rarely obvious, for the simple reason that the dreamer is not primarily concerned with the obvious and clearly conceptualized aspects of behavior. The day residue and its attendant anxiety lead directly into an area of behavior that has not been mastered and where one's vulnerability has been exposed by the inroads of one's own experience.

Fromm relates the symbolic language of the dream to the question of activity. In his view the unconscious is an experience related to a special mode of life—that of non-activity. To transform this definition into a more accurate and positive form, one might consider that, rather than a state of non-activity existing during sleep, a kind of movement occurs which, although it differs qualitatively from the movement characterizing the waking state, is nonetheless a form of activity. I refer to the movement into and out of deeper sleep. Dreaming is associated with a form of consciousness which is relatively unstable, and which inevitably terminates in either a dissolution of consciousness itself—and, with that, a return to a deeper level of sleep—or the qualitative transformation of dream consciousness into another form, namely, waking consciousness. In either event there is an internal rearrangement or movement.

Now to consider the book itself. In the pages to follow, an analyst, experienced as a clinician and a teacher, has opened wide the doors of his own workshop, exposing to view a very systematic and comprehensive approach to the subject of dream interpretation. There, before us, even more important than the dreams themselves, are the dreamers as real people, the language they use, the problems they face, and the struggle they endure as they move from the realm of compulsive self-defeating neurotic activity to the realm of psychological freedom, maturity, and the enjoyment of life. The clinical material is so skillfully developed throughout the book that the patients spring to life in a manner most unusual in psychoanalytic writings. The author, insisting that rationality is a good thing, engages in a relentless pursuit of the irrational as revealed in dreams. To do this for a great number of dreams from many patients is no mean task, but the author succeeds very well. There are repeated references to earlier dreams and earlier analytic fragments. Although one might expect this to place an undue burden upon the reader, the opposite is indeed the case. The clinical pictures are so sharply etched that later references become readily integrated into the evolving picture of the analyses in progress. We emerge from the workshop enriched by the stimulating array of ideas, techniques, and experiences presented, and with an awareness of the stature of the author as a clinician, a theoretician, a therapist, a technician, and a tactician. The author's basic thesis, simply put, is that the irrational and the rational can be dissected apart by the intelligent application of the metaphor of the dream to the concrete life situation implicated in the dream.

Here I would like to insert a word of amplification of the author's prevailing emphasis on the importance of feelings in dreams and the assiduously applied techniques he describes for the ferreting out and utilization of the feelings that may accompany or be symbolized in a dream. With the particular emphasis placed on feelings the reader may assume that a dichotomy is implied between thought and feeling. This certainly is not the case. Rather we are confronted with an ineluctable unity in which two either identical or disparate reflections of reality are welded together. By the term *thought* we generally imply conscious processes signifying our concept of reality and our relationship to it. The word *emotion* seems to refer to the way this reality actually does feel, the actual meaning it has for ourselves. When the real meaning of an event and our conscious appraisal of the event are of one piece, then thought and feeling comprise a unified reaction. The difficulty arises only when our felt reactions are at odds with our conscious appraisal. This leads to the apparent dichotomy between thought and feeling. I say apparent because when this type of split occurs between thought and feeling, it is at a level where only the felt reactions register and where the attendant meaning is not clearly conceptualized, because of the operation of any one of a number of defensive maneuvers and because of unawareness arising from unfamiliarity or ignorance. Feelings, then, are always the personal residue of social interaction and are always personal interpretations of events involving the individual. Effective engagement with the social milieu is possible only when the attendant meaning of events can be accurately conceptualized. Feelings are a clue to meaning and meaning always involves thought processes regardless of the level at which such processes take place.

Dr. Bonime clearly states his bias toward the "culturalist" approach to psychoanalytic theory. The implications of this position in regard to dream interpretation are equally clear. Since it is not the intent of the author to present a theoretical treatise on psychoanalysis, a number of questions might arise in the minds of the reader who may be unfamiliar with some of the implications of this approach. What importance is attached to genetic material? How important is the actualization of earlier memories and experiences in the treatment situation? Are dream symbols handled too exclusively in their present reference? The author, while not explicitly developing his own point of view on these matters, does so implicitly and empirically by presenting sufficiently extensive segments of analyses-in-progress to suggest that keeping the focus in the present pays off in therapeutic dividends.

A more important potential objection arises around the question as to whether or not the author has abandoned the concept of unconscious mental processes and is thus dealing with dreams from outside the psychoanalytic frame of reference. Certainly he eschews the concept of "the unconscious." Any careful perusal, however, of the clinical material quickly reveals that the heart of the author's approach lies in his effort to transform unconscious aspects of behavior into conscious conceptualized form. It then becomes behavior about which communication is possible. The collaborative effort of the patient and therapist are directed toward a fuller exploration of this initial, perhaps minute, but accurate identification of a bit of behavior. What is substituted for orthodox notions of the unconscious as a topographical psychical area is a more realistic appraisal of total behavior and, specifically, a concern with those aspects of actual behavior which are unconscious—which are conceptualized in a distorted and inaccurate manner or are overlooked completely in the service of expedient neurotic needs.

This anchorage in behavior rather than primarily in the world of introspection has other important offshoots. It enables the author to take what others might regard as a "tougher" kind of interpretive approach. One either can identify the irrational behavior and its reflection in the dream, or one can not. In the former instance, such identification can always lead to exploration and newer knowledge. If one cannot make the identification, the dream remains uninterpreted. Proceeding this way one is never walking on eggs, fearful of coming up with too "deep" an interpretation. A so-called "deep" interpretation is really a pathologically shared autistic fantasy. The dream in everyone, including the sickest patient, always heralds a spark of readiness at least to confront an existing problem. The art of therapy is to recognize the problem in question and not to read into the dream "deeper" problems which are neither appropriate nor relevant. This does not lead to superficial interpretation. It leads to the theoretical position that there is at any given moment in the analytic process only one appropriate interpretation, and that is the one that sheds light on how the patient is coping with a particular problem at a particular time. Once the congruence between dream and reality is established, the interpretive potential has been realized and the terms "superficial" and "deep" pale into insignificance. Initial dreams are just as much the object of exhaustive interpretive activity as later ones. The only interpretation that is potentially traumatic to a patient is a wrong one, not a "deep" one.

In line with this, one may better understand two other dynamic principles underscored throughout the book. One is the emphasis on interpretive activity, the exploration of interpretive hypotheses rather than the giving of an interpretation. The other is the emphasis on collaborative effort by both patient and therapist that is necessary to arrive at an appropriate interpretation of a dream. The nature of the mutual interdependence of doctor and patient in the pursuit of dream meaning is made explicit; it is not simply acknowledged in a perfunctory way, or acknowledged theoretically but denied in practice by an arbitrary distribution of labor in which the associative groundwork is laid by the patient and the analyst as the architect puts the pieces together in accordance with his own theoretical blueprint. The communication system remains open at both ends. Associations and interpretive ideas come from both patient and analyst. There is freedom to pay more than lip service to the notion that universality among dream symbols does not exist. Interesting examples are given in support of this latter thesis.

A number of terms in everyday psychoanalytic parlance are subjected to a drastic critique. These include, in addition to the classical concepts of the Oedipus complex, castration, and penis envy, such concepts as guilt, dependency, and rejection. Guilt, for example, is considered as the anticipation of failure of a pathological interpersonal operation and not as the residue of an unconscious aggressive impulse. In the author's view, most of these pathological mechanisms derive fundamentally from the all-pervasive competitive quality that in our society characterizes the nature of human existence. Closely allied to this competitive matrix is the offshoot of cynicism and distrust concerning interpersonal transactions. Although the author's thesis is well illustrated by the clinical material at hand, this may be too one-sided a view of the sources and causes of human suffering as we witness this in the society about us. What is undoubtedly true is that the prevalence and degree of such distress is appalling and that it does in fact reach into the lives of almost every one of us. This fact alone should focus our attention on the value systems and institutions which exact so high a price in human suffering in exchange for the social gains they yield. Whether or not one agrees with these specific formulations concerning competitiveness and cynicism, what the author does demonstrate clearly and forcefully is the possibility of deriving dynamic and therapeutic import from dreams without the use of an esoteric mystique or, for that matter, a special jargon. Analyst and patient use the same language and continue to do so throughout the analysis. Just as the patient emerges in his human dimensions, so does the analyst. This exposure takes place not to superimpose or substitute one value system for another but to provide the patient with a fixed point of reference against which he can explore, identify, and test his own value and belief systems. There is also a give-and-take quality to the exchanges, which are skillfully directed by a therapist with a remarkable gift for the terse, pungent, and sharply appropriate turn of the phrase. Such expressions as "analytic brinkmanmanship," "therapeutic opportunism," "bargaining with insights," and "interpretive filibuster," sharply highlight clinical experiences common to all of us. A new and useful technical glossary emerges in the author's discussion of interpretive activity. Considered in detail are the artful dodges of patients in coming to grips with the dream. Evasions behind the use of "insulating terms" and "blurred communications" are examined in detail. Of particular interest and value is the author's consideration of the emergence of healthy trends as first noted in dreams, and of the sometime occurrence of emotional dissolution following sudden and profound movement toward health.

Symbolic or actual references to the analyst in the dream are considered as references to the analyst himself and not the analyst as a parental surrogate. Considering the therapeutic situation as an actual rather than a symbolic experience creates a setting in which the immediate exploration of the implication of irrational behavior can be explored *in statu nascendi*. Genetic factors in this context help to explain but not explain away and dilute the impact of such greater self-awareness. When this exploration is continued with regard for the patient and respect for the courage involved in self-exposure, massive and dramatic exchanges occur, deepening and intensifying the collaborative effort of patient and analyst.

Dream interpretation in analysis is, or should be, a skill passed on to the patient. The sequential treatment throughout the book of a number and diversity of dreams well illustrates the evolutionary stages of this process. A learning experience transpires, with the patient developing the needed skills out of the interpretive activity itself. There are no esoteric theoretical overtones remaining as a monopoly of the therapist alone. Eschewing polemics, the author effectively confronts us with a thoroughly worked out, therapeutically effective, clinical approach to dream interpretation. He has felicitously hewed to his original intent to produce a document about dream interpretation that would be of value to the practitioner. I know of no other book which tells the story of dreams in this context so well. Captured in the clinical episodes are the excitement, the interest, the creative experience, the sense of accomplishment, and the impetus to therapeutic involvement which are all so integrally associated with the art of dream interpretation. The dream presents a challenge to both patient and analyst and the rewards of mastery are richly exemplified. Dream analysis becomes an integral part not only of the therapeutic situation but of the daily life of the patient. He catches on to his own style of dreaming, enriching his grasp of the forces at work in his day-to-day living. It is amazing how real and credible the patients are as they emerge from what are in fact no more than brief, sharply etched vignettes of moments in their lives.

There is a further point that might be mentioned—namely, the question of doctrinal compliance, as described by Ehrenwald. This refers to the gradual occurrence of a certain congruence between the dream symbols appearing in the patient's dreams and the interpretive style of the analyst. Freudian patients after a while tend to dream in Freudian symbols, Jungian patients in Jungian symbols, and so on. There appears to be some validation of this in the present work. This is more than a matter of how to interpret a given symbol; it has to do with the kind of symbol used. In the present work the symbols tend to have very direct reference to various types of interpersonal processes rather than to castration fear, primal scene, and penis envy. On further reflection this fact is not at all surprising. Dream content is, and remains, a derivative of social experience. If the therapist plays a significant role in recasting the interpretation of the patient's experience in a different frame of reference, it might be expected that the new perspective would be reflected in the dreams in a manner that is congruent with the symbols used in this new and vital relationship.

Little is assumed or left to the imagination in Dr. Bonime's handling of clinical material. It is as if the analyst were in effect always saying: "Here is what I do. Here is what the patient does in return. This is the result which ensues." In this manner the clinical material speaks for itself. And in doing just this it will provide therapists of whatever persuasion a good deal to reflect upon, learn from, and perhaps emulate.

Preface

A GREAT DEAL OF FRUITFUL clinical work with dreams is at present going forward without recourse to classical psychoanalytic concepts. No organization of new approaches to the clinical use of dreams has, however, yet been available, and it is an objective of this book to make it so.

I address the volume primarily to the clinician—it is a practical book; but since theory and practice are inseparable, it has been necessary throughout to present the underlying dynamic concepts. Where these are in conflict with orthodox concepts, I have tried to avoid controversy, but occasionally, at points where the clinical inferences are crucial, it has been necessary to explain the contrast of views. This applies particularly to such areas as symbolism, sexuality, and transference.

I depart from traditional psychoanalytic views in that I regard personality as evolving fundamentally through interpersonal interaction; man's personality is not basically determined by the presence, nature, and vicissitudes of sexuality or any other instinct—on the contrary, his sexual behavior, like all other forms of behavior, reflects fundamentally his socially derived personality.

The implications of this orientation are crucial for all the forms and goals of therapy, and have particular bearing on the interpretation of symbolism. The meanings of dream symbols are most precisely discerned as specific for each dreamer, determined by his individual life experience.

All of the theoretical discussions, as well as the clinical work with dreams and other data, are predicated upon the concept of a continuum between sleeping and waking consciousness, and between awareness and unawareness. There is no employment of the construct of an "unconscious." Man has consciousness—the cumulative, dynamic, creative expression of his central nervous system. His consciousness functions in waking and sleeping states, with a great variety of processes and with a wide range of degrees of awareness. The correlation between dreams and waking behavior is the initial province of clinical work with dreams, and the application of the knowledge so gained to the healthy modification of personality can be the result.

Throughout, stress is laid upon feeling. Man in his evolution has developed a range of emotions, such as sadness, rejoicing, compassion, spite, and love, which express forms of experience outside the realm of instincts. Human emotions have conceptual and communicative implications which arise out of social interaction, and their identification and evaluation provide a focus of authenticity which is indispensable to the adequate understanding of both dream and waking data.

Finally, consistent with the fundamental premise that personality evolves through interpersonal experience and is modified through interpersonal experience, the element of collaboration is emphasized as central in the total analytic process.

It is hoped that this book will accomplish several purposes: that it will fulfill its primary objective of adding something to the analyst's comprehension and skill, and that it will thereby both advance and render more effective the clinical use of dream data; that in its non-confining approach it will stimulate professional communication about dreams in the broadening framework of new psychoanalytic thinking and practice, and that it will facilitate as well the combined enterprise of psychoanalysts with members of the other behavioral disciplines; and that it will ultimately make available to patients a more accessible, more productive tool—the active use of their dreams—for rational and healthily affective dealing with their irrationalities during and after the period of formal therapy.

The infinitely varied experience of a lifetime goes into writing any book, as it has gone into this book on dreams. Some of the professionally formative elements, apart from my debt to Freud and other creative workers in the field of human behavior, have in particular included my personal analysis, study and long teaching colleagueship with the late Bernard S. Robbins, early study and supervision with Karen Horney, and the many years during which the demands of psychoanalytic teaching * and clinical practice have provided continual growth stimulus from students and patients.

* This is as a faculty member of the eclectic postgraduate Comprehensive Course in Psychoanalysis of the New York Medical College, the first psychoanalytic training program to be established within a medical school.

The dedication of this volume is, nevertheless, to my wife. The resources of her craftsmanship as a writer and editor were available to me throughout the evolution of this book. There has been, as well, the stimulus of her rigorous thinking, the penetration and intensity of her inquiry into my ideas, and the perspicacity and authenticity of her own observations of human behavior. In the beginning, she needed also at times a high degree of emotional stamina to maintain clarity in the face of professionally patronizing rebuttals. There is hardly a concept or clinical fragment within the following pages which is not, because of our work together, more accessible to the reader.

I wish to express my gratitude also to my good friends, Doris and Francis Bartlett, gifted psychoanalytic therapists, who devoted vacation and other free time to the reading and the searching and invaluable criticism of portions of this manuscript; and to my faculty colleague and old friend, Montague Ullman, a leader in the field of dream investigation as well as a sensitive and skilled practicing psychoanalyst, who generously agreed to undertake the writing of a Foreword.

WALTER BONIME

A Note to My Patients

No individual is identifiable in this book. Some people are represented by a single dream or dream fragment, others by several. If you think you recognize a reference to yourself which you don't mind revealing, wait until completing a careful reading of the whole volume; there is the possibility that reference to the same material may occur in a later chapter with additional clinical comment or data with which you would not wish openly to be identified.

Acknowledgments

I want to express my appreciation to the following journals for permission to quote from some of my previously published papers: "Intellectual Insight, Changing Consciousness, and the Progression of Processes during Psychoanalysis," from *Comprehensive Psychiatry* (Vol. 2, No. 2, April 1961); "The Use of Dream Evidence of Evolving Health as a Therapeutic Tool," from *Psychiatry* (Vol. 21, No. 3, August 1958); The Pursuit of Anxiety-Laden Areas in Therapy of the Schizoid Patient," from *Psychiatry* (Vol. 22, No. 3, August 1959).

Contents

FOREWORD BY MONTAGUE ULLMAN, M.D.   vii

PREFACE   xxi

A NOTE TO MY PATIENTS   xxv

ACKNOWLEDGMENTS   xxvi

INTRODUCTION: A DYNAMIC CONCEPT OF THE DREAM IN
THE THERAPEUTIC SITUATION   1
    Recognizing the Elements of the Dream
    Associative Activity
    Interpretive Activity

1. SYMBOLISM IN DREAMS   31

2. FEELING IN DREAMS   49

3. INTRODUCTORY DREAMS   102

4. SEXUALITY IN DREAMS   129

5. ANXIETY IN DREAMS   157

6. RESISTANCE IN DREAMS   182

7. INTERPRETIVE ACTIVITY WITH DREAMS   229

8. EVIDENCE OF EVOLVING HEALTH IN DREAMS   253

9. OCCURRENCE OF THE ANALYST IN DREAMS   267

10. TERMINAL DREAMS   281

11. WORKING WITH DREAMS IN THE THERAPEUTIC SESSION 298

DREAM INDEX   331

GENERAL INDEX   335

The Clinical Use
of Dreams

INTRODUCTION: *A Dynamic Concept of the Dream in the Therapeutic Situation*

It is the purpose of this book to present, in an organized form, working hypotheses and derivative techniques for the utilization of dream data. The following pages will deal with the dream in the total life situation of the patient, in and out of therapy, with emphasis upon the interaction between patient and analyst while the two are occupied with the dream—this is the dynamic concept of the dream in the therapeutic situation.

The interchange between patient and analyst is the heart of the therapeutic endeavor. In this interchange, dreams are not only a rich source of data; they can also, because of their bizarre nature, become the best means of introducing the patient to the activity of free association, a seemingly abstruse aspect of a strange new experience. To the extent that the patient can, in the clinical use of dreams, be engaged from the outset in free association, he can then more readily be engaged in the basic mutuality of the total therapeutic process.

The greater the comprehension and skill the analyst develops in the clinical use of dreams, the greater also becomes the comprehension and skill of the patient in the use of his own dreams. As this occurs, the patient becomes better equipped for a rational approach to his problems during and after therapy.

What now follows is a pragmatic concept. It is an arbitrary structuralization devised to give more ready accessibility to the complex of factors involved in the therapeutic utilization of dream material. Formalized organization may be arbitrary without being rigid, and may give greater opportunity for correlating and integrating ongoing clinical experience as well as academic study. The schema to be presented will serve as a simple frame of reference in which individual aspects of dreams, and individual aspects of the activity of the analyst and patient in working with dream data, can be dealt with.

Any dream can, of course, be studied academically without reference to a therapeutic situation. A dream as part of the biographical data dealt with in therapy, however, becomes the focus of reciprocal therapeutic activity. The presentation of the dream and its clinical use engender many types of response in both patient and analyst. These will be examined in detail.

The proposed schema consists of three basic approaches. The first is the consideration of the dream through classification of its elements into four categories: action, individuals, surroundings, and feeling. The second approach is the consideration of associative activity. The third approach is the consideration of interpretive activity.

Recognizing the Elements of the Dream

ACTION

In everything with which both therapy and dreams are concerned, process is invariably present or inherent. The action of the dream (although not the action alone) symbolizes part of the total living process of the patient. Although only fragments of a dream may be preserved, or although the dream may be no more than a flash, a tableau, a sensation, a sound, a word or a pain, process is implied.

Throughout analysis the question is always present: What kinds of movement or movements describe the patient? Are these parallel, coordinated, or conflicting movements? What is the direction, the intensity? What is the nature of his thinking activity, his feeling activity, his behavior toward other people and behavior in response to them? Is pathology disappearing or merely moving into obscurity? Is new pathology developing or an old pathology moving into view? Is health evolving or is the patient struggling against change? Are both occurring? Is he working with the analyst or blocking him? Or is he involved in both processes? These are the problems of movement in therapy, and these are the processes that are reflected and may be emphasized by the action in dreams.

A few clinical examples will serve to illustrate the manner in which the action of the dream reflects significant aspects of the functioning of the personality.

In an anxiety dream which one patient experienced shortly after starting analysis, he is fearfully swimming away from a shark in a swimming pool. This dream reflects the patient's frantic efforts to get out of range of the analyst. The action in the dream is a desperate flight (Shark in Swimming Pool).[1] The activity in life is frightened evasion of another person's influence.

Another patient wakes up feeling that he has been dreaming, but recalls only the experience of pain in the crook of his elbow, which continues to ache after he awakens. He associates this pain with punishment from a teacher who made him stand in front of the class for an inordinate period holding heavy books without dropping them. The action here is less agitated than the swimmer's frantic activity of escape. This man faces therapy as if it were a painful, extended punishment. His dream action, reflected in the vestigial pain, corresponds to his interpersonal activity—in this case not to escape, but to endure.

The action of another patient's dream takes place in an elevator (Elevator Nightmare). She is inside the elevator while her little girl is caught between the door and the shaft. The child makes whimpering sounds and the corner of her dress shows inside the car. The mother behaves as though she does not know where her child is, trying to obliterate from her awareness the clear facts that point to her child's imminent destruction. Her activity in the dream, as in her life at that time, was that of self-blinding.

In another dream a patient digs a small irrigation channel in the garden, which in part represents her marital relationship (Irrigation Deluge). This action in the dream corresponds with efforts to enrich her marriage with more open and spontaneous feelings. But suddenly in the same dream a "deluge" rises up out of the channel and she runs away. A new and conflicting type of action, running away, appears in the dream, corresponding to her anxious evasion of spontaneous expression of emotion in her marriage.

A stubborn obstetrics intern fights against therapeutic progress, against the emergence of a new personality, and he dreams of himself in breech presentation (Breech Presentation). In the same dream, however, he reveals activity in the opposite direction, in the role of the intern making efforts to deliver. These conflicting negative and posi-

[1] A Dream Index at the back of the book lists all dreams alphabetically with the pages on which they are mentioned.

tive actions in the dream correspond to his balking and cooperative activities in the therapeutic situation.

Action, always present, is not always readily discerned in a dream. It may be obvious or implied, intense or subdued, single or multiple, appearing or fading. If activity is complex, its components may be parallel, re-enforcing, divergent, or conflicting. The activity of the dream reflects the functioning of the personality, the kinds of movements characterizing the thinking, feeling, and interpersonal relating of the dreamer in and out of therapy.

INDIVIDUALS

This category serves not only to identify the characters in dreams but also to identify specific personality characteristics. The individuals in dreams frequently represent significant attributes of people rather than the people themselves. The attribute may be the patient's or someone else's. The represented attributes may be (1) accurate perceptions essentially foreign to the patient's waking conceptualization; or (2) distorted perceptions about himself or others (often the analyst) of which the patient is unaware, or which he is unwilling to recognize.

Individuals in dreams are therefore frequently difficult to identify, and what they stand for is difficult to delineate. There may be multiple elements in the same dream pointing to the same person. In contrast, a single person, most often the dreamer himself, may appear in a single dream as several people, each representing a different attribute. The person in a dream may be quite clearly recognizable, yet be present only to serve as an attribute of the patient or of someone else. The *individual as an attribute* in dreams occurs in numerous instances to be mentioned in succeeding chapters (see, for example, Straight and Narrow, Bear Man, Bird of Prey).

Dream individuals appear in various forms: human, inanimate, animal, and synthetic combinations of these.

Following are some illustrations of the individual appearing in the dream in *human* form. Especially when multiple representations of the patient occur in a single dream, one aspect of the dreamer may readily be recognized while another, equally important in that context, may be lost. For example, in a crucial dream a patient was represented as three distinct individuals (Spilling His Guts).[2] One individual was clearly and unmodifiedly the patient; a second was a friend of his, a photographer; and a third was another friend who had committed suicide. Each symbolized a distinct attribute of the patient. In his dream he

2 Described in detail, pp. 299–302.

tried to get the suicidal individual out of the way while he, as the photographer, was trying to get a picture of himself. Thus, ambivalently, he was trying, as the photographer (a self-observant, analytic attribute), to get himself into focus and at the same time to eliminate from his awareness the almost suicidal intensity of his depression by getting his friend (a suicidal attribute) out of the picture. Later in the dream the photographer was injured, but the patient in his own semblance (the healthiest attribute) indicated a desire to get well by being profoundly intent upon the injured man's recovery. Three attributes of the patient appear in this dream, in the forms of three different individuals—his depressive, self-destructive tendency; his self-observant aspect; and his commitment to recovery.

At this juncture in the patient's life it was essential for him to recognize his suicidal tendency; but also, because of the very presence of this suicidal tendency, he needed to identify his positive capacities to observe himself and to accept his potential for recovery.

Multiple attributes symbolized by multiple individuals in a single dream can also be seen in the Breech Presentation dream referred to above. In this dream the patient is represented by three individuals: the pregnant mother, the delivering intern, and the infant. He shows his characteristic attribute of stubbornness by presenting his backside to the world; his attribute of suffering that results from this kind of activity (in the immediate context, his painful resistance in therapy) is symbolized by the mother in labor; and his healthier attribute, that of working to help a new personality to emerge in analysis—to overcome, that is, his habit of breech presentation—is symbolized by the intern. It was essential that the patient see not only his stubbornness and pain but also his constructive efforts.

In the dream Spilling His Guts, above, three attributes were represented by three clearly defined, recognizable individuals. In the Breech Presentation dream only the intern-individual was clearly identifiable as the patient. The mother-individual, although not clearly defined in the dream, and reversed in sex, "felt" like himself. The breech-baby-individual was connected with him by a complex of symbolic attributes: a changing, imminently emerging, and obstructive individual.

Individuals standing for attributes of the patient may, then, occur in a great variety of human forms: as the patient himself, as recognizable people, and as characters who are altered or fictitious.

The individual representing, in a dream, an attribute of the patient may also occur in *inanimate* forms. One woman dreamed about herself as a house (House Alterations). (Wherever any object represents an individual, it will be dealt with as an individual of the dream.) The structural defects in the house represented pathological attributes of herself. In the dream she was having alterations made, a symbolization of the therapeutic process. In the same dream the individual appeared also in human form; the patient was clearly present as herself, attending to the remodeling. In this form she manifested the attributes of impatience and superficiality of commitment.

A sadistic, accomplished scientist in one dream was represented in inanimate form as a metal robot, with the patient's attributes of coldness and methodical behavior.

An audio-engineer dreamed about a high-fidelity record player he had constructed (Blowing My Top). It worked perfectly except for a caplike cover that sporadically popped off. The individual of the dream —a hi-fi set—reflected in inanimate form two attributes: first, his emotional control, a perfectly regulated mechanism; and second, his tendency toward uncontrollable anger, toward "blowing his top." The patient was also represented in the dream in human form, clearly as himself.

In addition to the variety of human and inanimate representations of the dreamer's attributes, there are *animal* representations. A young man with a playful, somewhat winsome manner, combined with a penchant for covert malice, dreamed of a playful, romping puppy that had the head of a rat. With an uneasy feeling he watched, in his own human form, the romping of this creature. In this dream the individual appears both as the observer-patient and as the composite creature representing two of his attributes—puppyishness and ratlike malevolence. In a later dream the destructive attribute is represented alone, no longer puppyish nor with rodent proportions, but full-blown in the patient's clearer conceptualization: he is a large, crushing ape.

Sometimes even at a first interview a patient will present a dream in which a disturbing unrecognized attribute is represented by an animal. In such a first interview, a woman in her forties spoke of a repetitive dream that had disturbed her for years. In it, she is handling, like a lion tamer, a beautiful lioness (Recurrent Dreams of Lionesses). The beast moves magnificently, strongly, quietly, and under her direction. The individual of the dream was herself in two guises: in human form as a lion tamer and in animal form as a lioness. The beast represented several attributes she liked in herself (strength, beauty, grace) and it also represented a previously unidentified attribute—the desire to pounce. In her human form she was the incarnation of control.

The animal as a self-attribute was presented at the inception of treatment by a young man who recounted a dream in which he was trying to keep at bay, by staring it down, a closely hovering bird of prey (Bird of Prey). The setting of the dream was a college where he had once become engaged to a girl in order to get into bed with her. In his own likeness, he was one clearly defined individual in the dream, but he was there also in animal form—the bird of prey, representing an attribute of his personality, his predatory behavior.

In the preceding examples we have seen the individual in the dream representing an attribute of the dreamer in human form, in inanimate form, and finally in animal form.

The individual of the dream in all these forms may also represent personality attributes of others than the dreamer himself. These attributes may be—as may those of the patient—accurately or distortedly perceived or conceptualized. Our concern at this point is, however, not with the authenticity of the represented attribute, but merely with the observation of some clinical examples of dream individuals representing attributes of people other than the dreamer.

One of those most commonly represented in the patient's dreams is the analyst. (See Chapter 9.) He may appear as himself, emphasizing a particular attribute, real or illusory, as it exists in the conceptualization of the patient. The analyst is predominantly, however, dreamed of in altered form. He may appear distinctly as another real person in the patient's life, indicating, through the nature of that other relationship, an attribute the patient sees in the therapist. In one dream, a patient blocks the road for the analyst, who is moving along slowly in a car while the patient deliberately walks in front (Holding Him Back). The driver is in the guise of a friend who has, in reality, given the patient substantial help and who in the dream is good-natured about the patient's obstructing the way. The analyst's attributes, as seen by the patient, are good humor and friendliness, and are personified by a real person in the patient's life.

Another patient dreamed of the analyst in the form of a contemptuous uncle, his real uncle, looking down upon him as the patient went through the passionate activities of coitus (Contemptible Passion). The individual, the uncle, represented the attribute, contempt, which was the attitude the patient believed the therapist would have toward expressions of strong feeling on the couch.

Another patient saw the analyst as a repugnant middle-aged woman begging him to make love to her (Old Negro Prostitute). The attributes of abjectness and repulsiveness were conceptualized about the analyst and then embodied by the patient in human form in his dream.

Attributes of the analyst are frequently given human embodiment in a dream in the form of an individual epitomizing a generally acknowledged character type, such as a Nazi, a servant, a policeman, or a garrulous woman.

A dream that illustrates the analyst-individual in animal form is the previously mentioned Shark in Swimming Pool. In another dream the analyst is a poisonous dachshund (Poisonous Dachshund), and in still another, a woodpecker drilling from behind.

Wives, husbands, parents, children, friends, bosses—attributes of all these, as they exist in the dreamer's feelings and conceptualization, appear in human, animal, and inanimate forms. A woman chemist who had begun to realize that her lover was poisoning her life dreamed of being threatened by insidiously poisonous "cardiac glucosides"—her sweetheart, the individual in the dream, in inanimate form.

In another instance a wife's attribute appeared as the individual in the dream of her husband (who had given her little genuine affection), in the form of a bedraggled cat coming home to get some human warmth from him; her human attribute, her need for him, was represented in the animal form of feline behavior (Three Bedraggled Cats).

The various forms taken by the individuals representing attributes of the patient, the analyst, or others in the patient's life, will be copiously illustrated by the clinical material that follows throughout this volume.

SURROUNDINGS

The surroundings in the dream are significant to the extent that they make contributions to the identity and meaning of the other dream elements—action, individuals, and feeling. The surroundings include not only the places in which action occurs and where individuals are but also all the components of nature and all the products of civilization and any realistic or unrealistic synthesis or abstraction or fragment of them which is not identifiable in the dream as any of the other elements.

Items of his office surroundings often contribute to the identification of the analyst as the individual in the dream. The writer's office, for example, has been for years in a residential hotel; a hotel setting has often contributed to a patient's identification of me. The color of the office walls has helped to identify me as the individual. In one dream of a homosexual patient, a hot-dog stand on the street of my office helped to identify the patient's action (attempted sexual seduction) and the individual (myself) (Hot Dog). A wrought iron railing in my office appeared as an iron fence around a tiger, helping to identify the action (restraining) as well as the individual (the analyst). The rough-surfaced wall alongside the couch has served as a wall in a battle scene, contributing to the identification of the action (fighting) and of the individual (again, the analyst) (Battle Tactics).

The contributory role of surroundings may, of course, also be seen in dreams involving other than the analyst-patient relationship. The terrifying height and sheer face of a mountain wall as a part of the surroundings served in a patient's dream to accentuate anxiety, the feeling element. In addition, it identified by its form the wall of an excavation for a swimming pool that was under construction at the patient's suburban home. The pool project had become a source of tension between the patient and his wife. The wall thus pointed toward the marital milieu of the problem, toward the focal item (the pool), and in addition contributed through these factors to the identification of an individual (the wife) who otherwise appeared in the dream only in obscure form.

The preceding have been examples of the surroundings in the dream contributing to the identification of the individual, the action, and the feeling.

FEELING

An individual's ideas, behavior, and feelings are closely interrelated aspects of his total functioning. It is impossible fully to comprehend the nature of the person one is dealing with, the meaning of his thoughts and actions, without constant awareness of his concomitant feelings.

When intensive efforts are made by analysts and patients to detect, inspect, and evaluate every possible evidence of emotion in both waking life and dreams, information about the patient that is otherwise inaccessible comes to light. The associative activity concentrating around a discerned emotion can provide essential understanding of the meaning of related thinking and behavior that, approached by themselves, might remain hopelessly tangled in self-deception and confusion. This effort is facilitated and consummated often most notably by the pursuit of dreams. The clinical usefulness of dreams is, in fact, directly proportional to the attention paid to feelings in dreams.

The patient experiencing an emotion, awake or in dreams, is responding with his total personality, which has evolved through all his interactions, perceptions, thinking, and activity, in contact with the physical world and with other people, through his whole life history. His emotions, identified or not, both shape and are shaped by his conception of the environment in which he lives and continues to function.

Because of the complexity of personality, and of its reflection in dreams, a structuralization of the approaches to dream feeling can be helpful.

The element *feeling* in dreams can be seen in two distinct categories: *symbolized* and *experiential*. Symbolized feeling is the affective component not actually felt during the dream, but implied in the dream by aspects of any of the other elements—action, individuals, or surroundings. Experiential feeling, on the other hand, is the affective component experienced while dreaming.

Symbolized and experiential feeling may be present simultaneously, expressing the same or similar kinds of feelings, expressing entirely different though not incompatible kinds of feelings, or, finally, expressing feelings of a conflicting nature.

A further development of these ideas, with clinical examples, will be found at the beginning of Chapter 2, "Feeling in Dreams."

This concludes the consideration of the four elements that constitute the first of the three basic approaches to dreams. The second approach in the dynamic concept of the dream in the therapeutic situation is the *consideration of associative activity*.

Associative Activity

Detecting associations related to dreams or to any other biographical data is an activity participated in individually by both therapist and patient. The associations of both are valuable, and the mutual use of them is essential. Associative activity will therefore be considered in categories of the two participant individuals: the patient and the analyst.

ASSOCIATIVE ACTIVITY OF THE PATIENT: ASSOCIATIONS

For convenience, the associations themselves will first be considered separately from the associative activities in which they are involved. This separation will help to emphasize and clarify the *temporal* factor. While most associations tend to occur after the report of the dream in therapy, associations may also occur during and before the report.

It is a common and unquestionably important procedure for the therapist first to hear a dream and then to direct the patient to associate, but it is essential to bear in mind that, very often, crucial associations occur before the recall or presentation of the dream. All the material of any fraction of a session preceding the dream report may be significant associative material. Sometimes only part of the material constitutes associations. On other occasions one particular item suddenly brings a dream to mind and the patient states, "That reminds me of a dream." The item of data, whether conceptual, emotional, or even psychosomatic, that is being experienced at the very moment preceding the patient's recall of the dream, can be an important clue to the meaning of the dream.[3]

A second and more familiar group of associations are those that occur during the patient's telling of the dream. These may be recognized as associations and reported as such by the patient. On the other hand, they may appear to be digressions. The patient may stop reporting the dream and say, "I just thought of something," or he may, after a silence, simply start talking about another matter.[4] A patient who has become, on the other hand, more skillful and deliberate in the use of his dreams may state, in the course of reporting a dream, that he has had an association and may purposefully interrupt the reporting of the dream to describe the association. Another patient may abandon the dream at some point and state that "the whole thing is vague," or "doesn't make any sense" and that he wishes to talk about something "more important." All of these interruptions in the course of recounting a dream, and frequently even the deliberate digressions, represent associations and may offer important keys to interpretation.

A third category consists of associations of the patient which occur after he reports the dream. This is the commonest and the largest group. It is at this time that many patients begin to learn about associative activity and the use of dream material. The term "after the report of the dream" refers in general to the same clinical session in which the dream was reported. Actually, however, there is no temporal limit. Associations to a single dream may continue throughout therapy or even throughout life. The patient who continues to use the therapeutic tools he has gained may, following formal therapy, continue for many years to achieve new or sharper insight through the pursuit of further associations to old dreams.

There is a type of association succeeding the report of the dream that is often not regarded as an association at all. It may be called a *contextual association.*

After a dream has been interpreted, the whole dream (or an element) often becomes the symbol of a particular insight that has de-

[3] This phenomenon, with or without the verbal bridge (the patient himself does not always make the connection), is discussed as the "moment of association" in Chapter 7.

[4] Fight with an Antelope. See Chapter 3, p. 104.

veloped from it.[5] The dream thereafter comes to the patient's mind in later contexts. The new associative contexts may be of value in any of three ways. The circumstances in which the dream is remembered may serve to (1) substantiate the meaning already found in the dream, or (2) further illuminate the dream, or (3) illuminate the context itself through the recollection of an understood dream. Thus, even after a dream has been interpreted and has become meaningful, its recall, or the recall of symbolic elements in it, results in a new illumination either of the dream itself or of the context in which it is recalled.[6]

This concludes the discussion of the temporal categories of associations, and leads to the associative activity itself.

ASSOCIATIVE ACTIVITY OF THE PATIENT: ACTIVITY

The patient's associative activity can be conveniently considered to be made up of four kinds: (1) the occurrence of associations; (2) the search for associations; (3) their communication; and finally (4) the creative, conceptual processes transitional to interpretation.

Occurrence of associations refers to the whole complex of higher nervous activity involved in recall. There is often a marginal or focal flow of thought, mood, and memory connected with the dream which continues during the daily routines or other events of the patient's life following the dream and throughout the telling of the dream. The degree of concentration of these thoughts and memories related to the dream is probably in proportion to the pervasiveness or intensification of the problem expressed by the dream at that point in the patient's life or his analysis. It is likely that many of these fragmentary memories and thoughts, or a vague awareness or abstraction of them, would, if somehow captured in the course of waking consciousness, appear to be much like the dream. Part of any human being's response to his life's environment, social and physical, is made up of imagery and ideation derived from his total past experience. Whatever the associative process is in any normal phase of life, whatever resonances there are among stimuli and recorded experience, whatever interstimulating processes are at work, these processes take place also around any disturbed functioning of the personality. It is my feeling that most remembered dreams (apart from occasional creative or simple wish dreams) are expressions of disturbances in personality function. It is this probability that dictates the exceptional time and emphasis placed on dream data in the clinical effort. Associations to the dream come

---

[5] See Chapter 1, pp. 31, 32–33.
[6] Further developed in Chapters 7 and 9.

through processes occurring in relation to the same disturbances of the personality which cause the dream. In other words, when a dream is reported and examined by the patient, associations occur as processes related both to the dream and to the personality problems engendering it. Occurrence, then, is the first of the associative activities.

The occurrence of an association is something like the spontaneous creation of a simile. The individual is saying, in effect, "Something of what I am remembering is like something in the dream," or, "Something about my dream is like what I am thinking of now."

The conceptual aspects of the dream, or of the association, or of the link between them, are at first so often vague that associations might more appropriately be described as "emotional similes." It is as though the patient were to say, "Something about this part of the dream *feels* like what I'm thinking about now," or, "What I'm thinking about now gives me a feeling like the feeling I get from something in my dream."

However one may describe associations, their occurrence is the manifestation of highly complicated mnemonic, ideational, and emotional processes. These processes can be fostered in the therapeutic situation with or without the therapist's intervention, by the patient's *search for associations*.

The phrase "search for associations" may appear to violate the very essence of the concept of free association. Rejection of the idea of "searching for associations" as something opposed to the traditional "saying whatever comes" would be a quibble. "Saying whatever comes" requires the active effort of the patient in looking for what is coming to mind. This effort, as a matter of fact, was the essence of the method of free association at its origin. Freud, in first describing it, said very explicitly ". . . I dropped hypnosis, and asked only for concentration. . . ." [7] When the patient is saying whatever comes, he is already concentrating upon the search for memories, ideas, and sensations which are connected with his dream or with any element of it. Free association, whether connected with a dream or with any other occurrence, is the developing and maintaining of a condition of attention and concern in relation to some aspect of experience, and the capturing of all emergent thoughts, memories, emotions, and sensations.

Whenever an analyst asks what this or that element in a dream brings to mind, he is asking the patient to concentrate, to search for associations, to see what comes in the wake of the last thought or image or affect of a dream. The more fully committed the patient is to his

---

[7] J. Breuer and S. Freud, *Studies on Hysteria* (1925). New York: Basic Books, 1957, p. 109.

own responsibility for finding the data from which insight can be derived, the more intensively he will search for all feeling, thought, and
recall that he can capture and convert into communicable form.

The search involves the patient's readiness to acknowledge whatever comes as an association, as important data. If there is a silence in
the course of this activity, the analyst, asking "What are you thinking?"
is requesting the patient to seek sharper focus upon what may be only
vaguely present, or what has vaguely already passed through his mind.

The therapist, aware of the complexity of the activity within the
mind of the patient, seeks to engage the patient in capturing the content of that complex activity and sometimes in fostering the activity
in a more specific direction. The therapist is thereby encouraging the
patient's process of searching for associations.

Implicit in all the foregoing comment on the occurrence and the
search for associations has been a crucial problem of the therapeutic
situation—the *activity of communicating associations.* The requirement
of communication is not only a basis of the cooperative aspect of the
therapeutic process but also significantly influences the associative
search itself. Many thoughts occur to the patient in connection with
the dream, but the diligence with which he captures them, sharpens
their definition, looks for their precursors, and follows where they lead,
depends a great deal on the patient's feeling of freedom to communicate. A great deal more than he feels free to report will pass through
the mind of an individual who, for whatever reason, is noncooperative.
When a patient accepts responsibility for change, commits himself to
cooperation in therapy, and thereby frees himself to communicate, he
develops a greater capacity to associate.

The converse is also true. An unwillingness to communicate will
in the therapeutic setting tend to inhibit the occurrence of meaningful associations. Paradoxically, at certain times an ambivalence about
communication may lead to an abundance of associative and communicative activity, resulting in a confusion that prevents or obliterates
insight. This confusion of associative activity is a sort of involuntary
rescue from insight for the patient and a phenomenon that may conveniently be termed "psychosomatic confusion." [8]

The occurrence of, the search for, and the communication of associations will stimulate *processes transitional to interpretation.* All
associative activity is, to a degree, interpretive. The associations themselves are manifestations of the patient's involuntary correlation of his
immediate impressions with his past experience; they are manifesta-

[8] See Chapter 6, pp. 205–206.

tions of the beginnings of the process of understanding, of interpreting present stimuli by the criteria of past experience. These criteria from past experiences are frequently not illuminating, and the associations to a dream often do not illuminate but merely aggregate as a collection of items without apparent connection. The collecting of those items, however, the search for associations, is the beginning of a process. Every associative exploration is like Darwin's voyage on The Beagle, during which he collected specimens of all types and studied them for their relationships; many specimens were not immediately relatable, but none was discarded as irrelevant.

The collection of associations is the beginning of the attempt to understand. The communication of them is the tacit request for help in discovering and interpreting their relationship in a process ultimately reaching the level of full insight. When a patient reports a dream, or any other event he wishes to understand, his active search for and his faithful communication of associations constitute the processes of transition toward interpretation.

ASSOCIATIVE ACTIVITY OF THE ANALYST: ASSOCIATIONS

Associative processes are important also in the therapist's role, and the same necessity arises for the therapist to grope, to grasp at and recognize his own responses as he hears the patient's dreams and the patient's associations. The therapist's associations may parallel those of the patient, if they arise out of the patient's biography—but they may also be purely subjective.

The sources of the analyst's associations can for convenience be categorized. First, there is the knowledge he has acquired of the patient's biography. The life history of the patient includes, of course, not only the anamnestic data and the accounts of his life since the start of treatment but also the history of the relationship between the patient and the therapist. In the course of time, vast numbers of impressions of the patient's behavior impinge upon the analyst. There are the patient's mannerisms, inflections, gait, dress, and posture, his behavior on the telephone, his reactions to the personal behavior of the analyst, his dealings regarding vacations, his attitude toward bills and illness, and innumerable other interpersonal elements that become part of the store of immediate impressions about the patient. Any of these may suddenly come to mind on listening to a dream and to the patient's associative material.

A second source of the analyst's associations is his own life history. Elements of the patient's dreams or associations may stir the memory of personal experience, or may even bring back one of his own dreams, or remind him of a struggle with a similar problem in his own analysis.

The associative response of the therapist to the dream and to the associations of the patient is also of the nature of emotional simile. It is as though he were saying, "Something of what this individual is telling me is, or feels like, something from my own life." To be sure, this kind of association of the therapist is often not pertinent, due to the fragmentary state of what the patient is reporting, or to misunderstanding or lack of comprehension by the analyst. On the other hand, autobiographic "sympathetic vibration" stirred in the analyst's personal memory by what the patient says can be a valuable clue to the meaning of the patient's productions.

In addition to his own and the patient's biographies, the therapist's academic background and professional experience also form for him a third and extensive source of associations.

Before proceeding to the analyst's associative activity, a correlation may be made between the temporal categories of the associations of the patient and those of the analyst. Those of the therapist occur while the patient is recounting his dream and after it. He associates, as does the patient, in the same session and also in later sessions. The analyst may also have useful association to a patient's dream under a variety of circumstances after the patient has left the office. During the session of another patient, an associative correlation may illuminate the problem in the first patient's dream. An association may occur in an academic setting or at a psychiatric meeting or in the course of reading or discussing psychiatry. Such associations may also occur in any type of nonclinical or nonacademic setting, perhaps in a social situation in which some individual's behavior suddenly recalls an activity or affect of a patient as recently expressed by a dream. Associations may occur in the course of reading nonpsychiatric literature, seeing a play or a movie, or simply while observing people anywhere in any setting.

Furthermore, as with the patient, an interpreted, well-understood dream may itself occur to the therapist as an association in later sessions with that patient. The analyst, too, that is, may have contextual associations. An association in a new context may bring substantiation of the interpretation, further illumination of the dream or, by its occurrence as an association, it may illuminate the new context in which it occurs.

ASSOCIATIVE ACTIVITY OF THE ANALYST: ACTIVITY

The associative activity of the analyst corresponds in some ways with that of the patient, while in other ways it is specific to the analyst.

The *occurrence* of associations is the same sort of process in both, the stimulus being for the patient his own dream experience, for the therapist another's (the patient's) dream experience. With the occurrence of associations instituted, however, the therapist must engage in an activity which is different from that of the patient. The patient has the injunction to withhold nothing, the responsibility to communicate all that occurs to him. The analyst must do more than merely listen and plunge toward interpretation; he must be conscious that he, too, is having associations; he must recognize his associations.

The analyst's associations occur in the exceedingly complex context of his therapeutic role. He may at times be preoccupied with academic phenomenological considerations, distracted by personal problems, or in other ways responsive to factors having no relation to the patient. Unlike the patient, the analyst must differentiate these irrelevancies from his associations to the productions of the patient. Often he may rebuke himself for inattention, feeling that his thoughts are wandering. He may feel bored or impatient about the digressions and irrelevancies of the patient, and even justify his own subjective digressions. More frequently he will be so intently concentrating upon the productions of the patient that he will not be aware of his own marginal thoughts. During concentration, these marginal thoughts, as well as the unintentional digressions or the almost deliberate self-distractions of the analyst may constitute important associations to the dreams and to other aspects of the patient. The emotional accompaniment of these thoughts, or the fact that the analyst is bored, impatient, angry, anxious, or overly concerned, may be related to the therapist's associations to the patient's dream.

The whole subject of the emotional response of the analyst to the patient is an important one that has been extensively dealt with since the beginnings of psychoanalysis under the designation of *countertransference.*[9] Even in instances where it is to some degree pathological, the analyst's response may relate to something quite definable in the patient's dream and the behavior surrounding it. The significant point is that the therapist can find a valuable source of insight into his patient's dreams through the recognition of his own associations to these dreams.

The analyst has a fuller function, however, than to recognize merely those of his own associations that forcefully claim his attention. His spontaneous associations may be sporadic or inadequate. The patient's productions and behavior may be absorbing, or may deflect the

[9] See W. Bonime, "Liking and Disliking One's Patients," in A. Rifkin, ed., *Schizophrenia in Psychoanalytic Office Practice.* New York: Grune & Stratton, 1957.

therapist's attention in unproductive directions. Like the patient, the analyst must endeavor to search for his developing associations, and for those he may find by deliberate concentration on some item or element of the dream.

An activity connected with the analyst's associations, a part of the technique of therapy, is that of introducing his associations into the therapeutic session. The analyst's communication of an association may, for the patient, tend to have the weight of an interpretation, but it is not necessarily an interpretation. The association can be offered tentatively, just as it occurs, for whatever it may turn out to be worth.

A striking instance of this type of situation, though not related to a dream, occurred during a session in which a patient was maintaining silence while we were trying to look at a painful emotional reaction. I suggested that it would probably be more painful to evade it than to face it, and I encouraged her to try to verbalize her thoughts and feelings as best she could. She made an impatient remark that it was easy enough for the analyst to talk, and lapsed again into silence. I told her I appreciated the difficulty she had in facing and talking about her painful feeling, and indicated that we need not explore it completely in that session.

As I sat behind the couch waiting, I found myself thinking about an incident involving my four-year-old son. I had asked him to do something to which he had responded with an unequivocal "No." I had said, "All right, you don't have to." After a moment of silence he had replied, "I'm *still* not going to!"

I recounted my association. My patient was not amused, and informed me that she didn't want to hear any goddamn stories about my son. I told her I felt that it had come to my mind because I sensed that she was fighting me and that her stubbornness was something we ought to examine. The session began to be productive at that point, and an important problem, her stubbornness, was pursued fruitfully for some time after that. (The incident also impelled me to examine to what degree I had been placing unwarranted pressure on my patient—as well as on my son!)

The introduction of the therapist's associations to the patient's dream may have various effects. A too hasty or too emphatic introduction of such material may interrupt the associative activity of the patient. It may discourage his independent work on a dream because of some feeling that the analyst's omniscience is overwhelming. A pertinent association may, however, stimulate the patient's thoughts and feelings in a productive way. Also, the tentative offering of the analyst's association, especially when some item previously introduced by the analyst has been both proven and acknowledged to be worthless, may help the patient to sense his therapist's appropriate humility. This emphasizes for the patient the cooperative basis of psychoanalysis and thereby encourages a more intensive search for and communication of his own associations.

There remains to be considered the analyst's processes transitional to interpretation. A line of distinction between the various associative activities and interpretive activity cannot be sharply drawn. In the therapeutic situation, all associative activity has as its eventual objective interpretation and the achievement of insight. When, as the patient tells a dream, the therapist suddenly thinks of a person or an action, he is evolving a tentative interpretation, making what might be appropriately termed an associative hypothesis.

In a dream fully reported later (Spilling His Guts), the symbolized patient's fall from a platform linked up in the mind of the therapist with another figure in the dream who had years earlier committed suicide by jumping off a subway platform. The connection was re-enforced by the therapist's fresh awareness of the patient's current low spirits. That the patient, who revealed only a moderate gloom, was actually severely depressed, possibly fantasying suicide, was a speculative interpretation at that point in the process of formulation in the analyst's mind. Though it seemed to be only a cluster of associations, the linking up, the associative clustering, was an associative activity transitional to interpretation.

As indicated above, the introduction into the session of the analyst's associations is often taken by the patient as an interpretation. This cannot be fully affirmed nor entirely denied. The transition is taking place, and comes even closer to crystallization once it is formulated in words and then communicated.

As one considers the associative activities of both therapist and patient, it is useful to bear in mind that associative activities and interpretive activities, although they are not identical, do overlap. It is necessary and convenient to systematize them into separate categories, but it is important to be aware that both are basic aspects of a total effort, through biographical data, often brought to awareness through dreams, to understand the personality of the patient.

Interpretive Activity

The dream presented by the patient to the analyst becomes the focus of reciprocal activity. The study of the dream becomes an activity involving many types of reactions of both patient and analyst. If we

THE CLINICAL USE OF DREAMS

approach dream interpretation from this point of view, it will be found to fall conveniently into categories of the respective roles of therapist and patient. The interpretive activity of the analyst and the interpretive activity of the patient will be considered separately, in categories arranged in a developmental sequence roughly corresponding to their evolution during the therapeutic process. They are: (1) interpretation by the analyst alone early in therapy, and then later in therapy; and (2) interpretation by the patient in response to the analyst's stimulus, and the patient's own spontaneous interpretation.

All of these processes occur during therapy with a good deal of overlapping and variation in their relative proportions. Toward termination, interpretation by the analyst alone ceases. The patient needs less and less stimulus from the analyst, and is capable of increasingly valid, spontaneous, and independent interpretations.[10]

The designation of categories and their arrangement in a developmental progression is structured to facilitate the examination of a continuing process that is highly varied, intricately interwoven, and occurring in the complicated interpersonal relationship of patient and analyst.

INTERPRETIVE ACTIVITY BY THE ANALYST ALONE: EARLY IN THERAPY

The more exclusive interpretive activities of the analyst tend naturally to fall within the earlier period of analytic work. An important part of the therapeutic goal is the increasing involvement of the patient in the processes of his own therapy, and eventually the termination of his needs for professional assistance in these processes. In the early phase of analysis the patient is uninitiated in dream interpretation. He may know—as who can now escape knowing?—that dreams are significant and that their interpretation plays a part in therapy. He does not know, however, in what way this takes place.

It is commonly believed that interpretation is a function of the analyst alone. The beginning patient may understand that it is necessary for him to supply associations. Beyond that, however, he has little or no concept of the nature or even of the fact of his participation in the work of interpreting dreams. It therefore frequently rests with the analyst during the onset of therapy to suggest interpretive hypotheses (see Chapter 7). The more readily the interpretations are offered for what they truly are—hypotheses—the more readily is the patient likely to engage himself in the interpretive activity. The analyst, in other words, does not state a fact—he, in effect, raises a question. He offers

[10] The latter development is an important indication that the patient is confronting, exploring, and dealing with his problems realistically and independently; these activities are primary criteria for termination of therapy. See Chapter 10.

the patient not something to accept but "something to think about." This introduces the patient to the process of correlating dream material and associative material in a creative way, in a search for enlightenment about his behavior and feeling. It also encourages his venturing to verbalize tentative notions and interpretive hypotheses of his own.

When the therapist early "rings a bell" with his interpretation, the experience may cause in the patient a thrill or shock of recognition which impresses him with the value of the dream material. On the other hand, a too hasty introduction of an interpretation by the analyst, or a dogmatic presentation of it, or the presentation of an interpretation derived academically rather than out of the patient's specific biography, may discourage the patient's participation in interpretive activity.

Dream interpretation under some circumstances may unfortunately remain an activity exclusively of the analyst. The patient may be frightened, incredulous, or (equally deleterious) dazzled by the interpretation of the therapist. Any of these reactions, instead of encouraging his recognition of the usefulness of dreams in treatment, may drive the patient away, if not from offering dreams, then certainly from spontaneous participation in the clinical use of his dreams.

Unhappily, dreams offer a great arena for therapeutic exhibitionism. Whether the patient believes or rejects the interpretations made too consistently, too self-assuredly, and unilaterally by the therapist, he is sure to feel outside of the process of therapy. In response to the therapist's flare for interpretation, patients may feed dreams and readily accept interpretations, and thus unwittingly avoid involvement in their own treatment processes. They may manifest resistance in this way quite as effectively as by the withholding of dreams or the rejecting of interpretations.

In the early phases of treatment (and similarly during brief therapy or consultative interviews), it may be necessary for the therapist to interpret dreams unilaterally. This exclusiveness is a disadvantage, as is any other process in therapy that bars, attenuates, or fails to encourage the patient's active involvement in the search for insight and in the correlative efforts for change. Because the use of dreams is so foreign to him, any form of exclusion from interpretive activity tends to re-enforce his concept of psychoanalysis and other forms of psychotherapy as something which the therapist does, while the patient merely supplies the data. An interpretation made by the therapist alone, no matter how apparently astute, loses some value if it is introduced as *the* interpretation or flashed at the patient instead of being offered as an interpretive hypothesis in the framework of an appeal to the patient to approach the hypothesis and the dream with all his creative intellectual and affective capacities. From the onset, it is through the medium of fruitful therapeutic experience that the patient is encouraged and educated to enter actively into interpreting his dreams.

These views regarding the analyst's presentation of interpretations of dreams (views relating as well to interpretation of other biographical data) apply, of course, to all stages of analysis. They are expressed with particular emphasis attached to the onset of treatment, because it is then that the patient needs to be imbued with a sense of therapy as a cooperative process (see Chapter 3). The sooner this impinges, the sooner and more fully engaged are his own resources for bringing about change.

INTERPRETATION BY THE ANALYST ALONE: LATER IN THERAPY

Under certain circumstances, interpretation of dreams by the therapist exclusively has a legitimate place later in therapy. There are two categories of such circumstances. One when there is *limitation of time*, and the other when it is indicated *in the face of the patient's resistance.*

One circumstance involving limitation of time is the recall of a dream at the end of a session, when it may offer the opportunity to crystallize, to augment, or to focus (even as a question) the material of a whole therapeutic hour. There are times when a patient is working very productively, has a last-minute recollection of a dream, and can be counted on to carry on independently with interpretive activity after the session. The analyst's quick interpretive response at the end of a session may sometimes capture an insight or a question that offers a useful clue or forms a welcome stimulus to the patient, who leaves the session to work on his own.

Other similar situations are occasional sessions before weekends or before important events such as marriage, childbirth, or imminent crucial decisions. The analyst may also offer interpretations he has developed alone, when an interruption of the analysis is about to occur, as in the case of an actor, musician, or salesman going off on tour, or with patients who can see him only sporadically or infrequently, such as once a week. Finally, the analyst may sometimes engage in interpretive activity alone later in therapy when an unavoidable and premature discontinuance of treatment is imminent, as for a patient moving away, or entering college or the army.

The final category of circumstances in which the analyst, later in therapy, must engage alone in interpretive activity is in the face of the patient's resistance. In this situation the analyst may have great difficulty in reconciling his efforts to establish therapeutic cooperation with his decision to use his unilaterally conceived dream interpretation.

As in any circumstance, whether or not related to dreams, when the patient fights against insight while the therapist seeks to salvage significant data, results cannot be predicted. When the resistant patient withholds his substantiating associations, feelings, and interpretive hypotheses, he thereby re-enforces his logical grounds and combative self-assurance in repudiating the therapist's concept of the dream.

How much the persistence of the analyst leads to fruitful results, how much it is merely wasted effort, and to what degree it may drive the patient further away, depend on many factors. To discuss these factors fully would require volumes on psychodynamics and the dynamics of treatment. The general therapeutic principle involved, however, concerns the ill-defined question of "activity" and "passivity" on the part of the analyst.

One never forces an interpretation on a patient—in reality this cannot be done; mechanical acceptance, which may be forced is, of course, never the same as insight, which can occur only with the cooperative engagement of the patient.

The persistence of the therapist in introducing dream interpretations, while the patient is warding off the meaning of his life activity and its reflection in dreams, can nevertheless be advocated for several reasons. The analyst is aware that there exist some healthy elements in the patient, implicit in his coming to treatment. Since, furthermore, the present discussion relates temporally to a later stage in therapy, the patient's report of the dream is predicated upon some established relationship between the patient and the therapist. The patient reports his dream on the premise, experientially acquired in treatment, that the dream contains significant data. His reporting of the dream is at least minimal engagement: if he will not involve himself in interpretive activity, he is at least communicating the dream and listening to the analyst. The introduction, in the face of the patient's resistance, of a dream interpretation derived solely by the analyst, is an action addressed to these healthy elements in the patient.

In addition, if insight does not evolve, because of the patient's withdrawal from therapeutic effort, the established pathological behavior of the same nature will continue. More dreams, substantively related, will occur, presenting repeated opportunities to tackle the same problem. The continued interpretation of the patient's dreams and the ongoing correlations with his behavior may bring to the patient a consistent picture which generates a gradually increasing feeling of the validity of the analyst's hypothesis. The interpretations offered in the face of the patient's resistance, without insistence that they be accepted, can form a conceptual groundwork for the patient's later involvement in spontaneous therapeutic efforts.

In spite of all of the subtle forms of counteraction by the patient, if the therapy as a whole is eventually productive, the therapist's persistence in working with dream data as they arise will prove fruitful at a later time. A dream, if it has been dealt with in the life context out of which it was created, tends to be more meaningful when brought up at a future time than a dream unexplored because of a patient's lack of cooperation when it was first presented. It tends to be better remembered by both the patient and the analyst, because some clearer contemporary biographical connections were developed. An interpretive hypothesis, at the very least, establishes a common point of reference between patient and therapist, a communicative link. A link so developed may be tenuous, but it will be of value to whatever degree it is a mutually identifiable therapeutic experience.

In all situations in which the analyst interprets unilaterally, he is engaging in a compromise activity that has inherent limitations, and he does so with the hope that his initiative will not supplant but, on the contrary, will stimulate interpretive activity by the patient. During the course of stagnant, noncollaborative therapy, the persistent development by the therapist of interpretive hypotheses from the dream data may be utterly fruitless, but during such periods the analysis is likely to be in all other respects equally unsuccessful. The interpretive activity of the analyst alone is an important part of his therapeutic persistence in the face of the patient's total activity against healthy change. Sometimes the problems of the patient, as reflected in dreams, can be pursued relatively unilaterally for months, and then, after long delay, those of the therapist's comments and interpretive hypotheses that have had relevance and accuracy may at last become a common base of exploration.

In brief, interpretation of dreams in the face of the patient's resistance may be concurrently unproductive, that is, productive of results only later, if at all. The analyst's unilateral interpretation with the resistant patient may at times, however, be concurrently productive—that is, it may initiate a constructive response quite soon.

The kind of therapeutic development depends essentially upon the patient's basic approach to treatment. If the patient persists for long periods of weeks or months in fighting off the therapist's efforts, then the persistent interpretive activity, regardless of the richness of the dreams or the astuteness of the analyst, will produce no concurrent result. When, on the other hand, during certain periods the patient is intensely negativistic but is, nevertheless, basically reaching for health, his active resistance will not stand seriously in the way of his benefiting from the therapist's lone persistence in interpretive activity. Such activity will be productive of insight, will engage the patient within a brief time—possibly within the particular session, or within a few sessions (see Chapter 7).

The difference between the patients who fall into one or the other of these temporal categories of productivity arises from the relative balance, or perhaps more accurately the predominance of one or another group, of characterological qualities. In the concurrently unproductive situation (i.e., protracted period) the patients tend to be individuals who are so profoundly isolated, embattled, cynical, and frightened that they are predominantly incapable of engaging in intimate mutual effort. The patients in the face of whose resistance the analyst interprets with concurrently productive results are patients who, although they may have the same kinds of impediments to cooperation, are nevertheless predominantly capable of summoning the resolution and taking the risk of involvement in intimate interpersonal endeavor. Like most patients, they strive to maintain their personalities intact. They tend subjectively to experience change as a weakening (see Chapter 5), and therapeutic cooperation as a subjugation. They have, however, a predominant commitment to modify themselves, with the assistance of the therapist. It is with these patients that the analyst's interpretive activity in the face of resistance leads fairly readily to cooperative effort.

INTERPRETIVE ACTIVITY OF THE PATIENT

The interpretive activity of the patient can be considered in two classifications: (1) interpretation by the patient in response to the stimulus of the analyst; and (2) spontaneous interpretation by the patient.

A part of the goal of all psychoanalysis is to educate the patient in rational techniques for approaching his own irrationality. His use of dream data can be invaluable among the newly acquired tools. The patient learns in the course of treatment first to remember and present his dreams. Then he learns associative activity. And finally, in his efforts toward insight, he learns the activity of interpreting.

The ultimate goal in the use of dreams (as in the use of all other life data) is that the patient become independent of the analyst. In fact, the patient's spontaneous, independent, and productive dealing with his problems is one of the chief criteria for the termination of treatment. But he needs the help of the therapist for a long time.

One form of this help is specific stimulus to interpretation. Such stimulus may be, in varying degrees, direct or indirect. The analyst's associations may be the basis of a question or of a suggested direction for the patient's further consideration and exploration, and can serve as a stimulus to the patient's interpretive activity.

The patient's interpretation of his dream may come in response to a more direct stimulus from the analyst, even though the stimulus be less focal than the analyst's association. The patient may do a fine reportorial job with his dream, appending extensive associations, and yet need to be reminded to seek out the meaning. The analyst in such a circumstance may employ a direct stimulus such as, "What do you think the dream means?" or "What is there in this dream that you would rather not acknowledge?"

There are many variations, and these may be directed toward a particular element—toward the action, the individual, the surroundings, or the feelings—or toward what seems to be an underlying basic theme of the dream. The stimulus may be offered when the therapist has an association or a hunch; at other times the analyst may be frankly at sea about the dream, and, while prompting the patient toward further exploration, may also be seeking fruitful stimulus from the patient in order himself to be more useful. "Let's try to see what the dream means," or "Who do you think so-and-so is?" or "I don't think we've got to the heart of this dream" can all be honest, humble expressions, even though the patient frequently considers them leading questions, as at times they are. When this type of phrase is used, the analyst is taking the initiative regarding the patient's pursuit of insight from his dream. Eventually, the patient comes independently to use the same approaches, with or without their verbalization; he increasingly makes spontaneous efforts at interpretation of his dreams, and in all ways relies decreasingly, for the pursuit of insight, upon the stimulus of the analyst.

Although the patient increasingly relinquishes his requirement of the analyst's stimulus in order for him to investigate the difficult areas, cooperative activity in the pursuit of insight through the use of dreams and other biographical material does, of course, continue to the termination of psychoanalysis. In the actual work, regardless of the degree of progress, two heads still are better than one, especially when the patient has available the skill and collaboration of someone so well acquainted with him as his analyst. Even after the conclusion of formal therapy, he may, with others who are close to him, profitably avail himself of cooperation in the pursuit of insight for the remainder of his life.

Increased health is always manifested by increased initiative in the patient's rational approach to his problems. Increasing spontaneity in the patient's interpretive activity is, however, not necessarily evidence of increasing health. The overcoming of the patient's frequent confusion about the subtle, and not just the glaring, distinction between what is healthy and what is sick in any activity comprises a large portion of the total therapeutic endeavor. The patient must learn to recognize both the healthy and unhealthy aspects of all of his behavior, including his efforts in interpreting his dreams. This distinction is often difficult for both patient and analyst, because the patient's interpretive activity may be a manifestation of resistance even though it gives the appearance of astuteness and honesty. The healthy and unhealthy aspects can more clearly be considered separately; therefore, slightly suggestive of a developmental sequence, the *unhealthy* manifestations of the patient's interpretation of his dreams will be discussed first.

Whether in response to the analyst's stimulus or spontaneously communicating, the patient, though he appears to be engaged in associative and interpretive efforts, may actually be resisting insight. Such activity may be revealed in a variety of subtle forms. One form which is especially difficult to identify is sometimes manifested by a highly sensitive and communicative patient—his words describe him with exquisite accuracy, but his vision of himself is that of a glorified self-confronter rather than the neurotic individual his perceptive communication describes.

Seemingly insightful activity can be vitiated also by the patient's use of *insulating terms*. These are qualifiers that in effect deny the reality of emotion and thought, convert actual experience into mere hypothesis: instead of reporting anger or suspicion, for example, the patient says, "I guess I was mad," or "I suppose I thought she was lying."

Another form in which patients nullify the illuminating effect of effort is the dismissal of an occurring insight by attributing it to the analyst: "I suppose what you're thinking is . . ." Or the thoughts that come with conscientious concentration may be neutralized by transmuting them into negative constructions: the patient seeking to penetrate into some unaccountable behavior may, for example, finally come up with, "I couldn't possibly have been jealous."

It is sometimes difficult, too, to identify resistance in the patient who is concentratedly and extensively evaluating his feelings and be-havior, but who is actually maintaining an interpretive filibuster, ward-ing off any effective participation by the analyst.

There are also circumstances in which the patient hastens to find the proper attribution of his motive before the analyst can find it. The usefulness of his insight is attenuated in its effect on personality change, and serves predominantly to aggrandize the patient's competitive satis-factions.

Still another form of resistance operating obscurely within the patient's interpretive activity is the practice of interpreting and im-mediately rushing off to a new topic.

All the foregoing analytic maneuvers, more fully discussed in Chapter 7, are forms of participation by the patient in interpretive activity which is, regardless of the conceptual validity of its content, directed against acquiring insight.

In his efforts to recognize and to point out the pathological aspects of any seemingly healthy activity of the patient, in or out of therapy, the analyst takes a necessary, calculated risk. While the patient must not be permitted to fool himself, neither must he be permitted to be-come discouraged from making interpretive or other therapeutic ef-forts. In all of the above described unhealthy spontaneous interpretive activities of the patient, his response to the analyst's designation of his resistance maneuvers depends upon the patient's approach to therapy at the time. If the patient is basically struggling to become healthier, he will predominantly welcome the attention paid to these obstacles to his progress.

Finally, there are the *healthy* manifestations of the patient's spon-taneous interpretive activities. The bulk of this category has been im-plied in the discussion of the unhealthy manifestations, most of which are shared by the majority of patients. The course of analysis can be described in one sense as progress in the elimination of the obstacles to the productive use of dreams. (This is another variation of the defini-tion of analysis as the "overcoming of resistance.")

The substance of this category, the patient's healthy spontaneous interpretive activity, is in itself a major goal of psychoanalytic en-deavor. Fruitful independent analysis of one's dreams and fantasies becomes an acquired tool for rational self-observation, self-evaluation, and consequent modification of one's personality in the direction of greater realism and health. As stated earlier, the patient's regular, inde-pendent, and responsible use of this acquired approach to his problems constitutes an important criterion for termination of therapy.

The healthy manifestations of the patient's interpretive activity all bear evidence of genuine efforts to achieve an understanding of the reality about himself, regardless of the nature of that reality. The activity is not an academic exercise but a vital and intrinsic part of any patient's approach to living. In therapy the patient neither nullifies nor resents the assistance and intervention of the analyst. The patient seeks all the help he can get, but does not use such help as a substitute for his own efforts. He cultivates the associative process. He is not satisfied with a formulation, but is concerned beyond it with validation—the documentation from his living, past and present, within and outside the analytic situation.

The dynamic concept of the dream in the therapeutic situation has been developed for convenience and greater clarity in approaching the clinical use of dream data. Emphasis has been placed throughout upon process and reciprocity in the therapeutic endeavor, an emphasis which has been reflected in the very form of this section, through the constant juxtaposition of the activities of the patient and the analyst.

1. Symbolism in Dreams

T HE DISTINGUISHING QUALITY of dream symbols is their semantic specificity. They present themselves with exquisite individuality, arising out of the core of the patient's uniquely personal history and offering cognitive and emotional definitions of a specific plexus of his experience. They convey meaning with a vividness that would be impossible to achieve in verbal terms. The words "exploitative" or "predatory," for example, pale into mere academics for a patient whose use of people appears so much more meaningfully in his dream in the symbol of a hovering bird of prey (Bird of Prey). The specific symbol, *that* bird of prey, with all its context of feeling, association, and interpretation, becomes capable of mustering self-awareness concerning his personality problem of exploitativeness to a degree not achievable by any other form of conceptualization or communication. Not only is such a symbol pregnant with meaning in the therapeutic situation, but this meaning becomes expanded and enriched by its occurrence in new contexts during analysis.

For another patient, "resistance" is a very bookish word indeed to describe her resentful, passive role in analysis, as compared with her own vivid dream picture of a wrenching induced labor, which was painful and productive of nothing but a "bloody mess" (Induced Labor). Here was represented her determinedly passive resistance, her pain in the process, the consequent lack of therapeutic fruitfulness, and her associated hatred for the obstetrician-analyst. No other words could so well arouse her awareness of her own feelings and behavior as could the symbolic phrase "induced labor" after it was derived from her dream.

In the course of this patient's analysis, certain items from her dream life came to be recognizable abstractions from specific areas of her personality. For example, she developed through a dream another symbolized insight, crucial for all her interpersonal relationships and particularly important for a clear view of herself in many subsequent psychoanalytic hours. She dreamed she had shoplifted two or three cents' worth in some store, but felt it was not "really stealing" because she was willing to pay for it if discovered (Two or Three Cents' Worth). This self-exonerating rationalization was characteristically represented in her everyday life by her ready "I'm sorry" in frequent circumstances in which she victimized people. Through this "two or three cents' worth" dream, the nature of many of her actions became clear to her where before, instead of recognizing the central action, she had looked only at the extenuating behavior.

From the period of that dream onward, the phrase "two or three cents' worth" was a penetrating and expressive symbol for her deviousness. It had a sharpness and a specificity of meaning that could hardly have been conveyed by any terminology other than this symbolic derivative. Its primary value was, of course, its subjective function for the patient whenever it arose as an association. It served in addition, however, as a communication. Whenever it arose as an association of either the patient or the analyst, it would bring the patient's activity immediately into sharp and common focus.

Such interpreted derivatives from dreams become symbols for areas of experience and for particular ways of feeling and behaving. These understood personal symbols may be repeated in the same or modified forms in different dreams. More often they continue to recur as associations. They come to be significant terms of communication in the ongoing psychoanalytic process. The patient gradually builds up *a personal glossary of symbols* through his dreams.

Dream symbols arise out of the specific life history of each individual, and it is only from the individual's life history that we can derive the meaning of his dream symbols.

That, I believe, is the most important point that can be made in initiating a discussion of symbolism in dreams. There is no universal dictionary of dream symbols. We develop a definitive glossary of sym-

bols with each individual in the course of the analysis of his consciousness and practices.

The common cultural experience of different individuals may lead
independently to common symbols—nevertheless the meaning of a
symbol recurring in different individuals cannot be established by simple analogy with previous interpretations. It must be found independently and specifically from the life history in each case, and not from
any generality.

The repetition of symbolism by several individuals with a common
cultural background, although it may sometimes be suggestive, may
more often be misleading. The great variety of possibilities in symbolic
meaning can be inferred from the following hypothetical examples.
A patient dreaming about missing a bus may be dreaming about losing
an opportunity. This would be, for him, a dream charade or symbolic
dramatization of a common cliché—to "miss the bus"—derived from the
patient's membership in the culture or segment of it that uses this
idiom. The cliché "missing the bus" may, furthermore, because of a
common cultural background with the patient, occur also to the analyst,
and suggest a meaning. Such a connotation might be correct for a number of people living in the culture in which this phrase and its concept
are commonplace. It must nevertheless be determined what it means
to this patient to miss the bus, how it relates to his current existence
and to the problems discussed currently in therapy. Missing a bus
might relate not so much to losing an opportunity as to sabotaging an
opportunity, neurotically missing the bus to avoid reaching a point of
operation. A bus trip might relate to a specific incident in the patient's
life which was frightening or destructive. In that case missing the bus
might stand for escaping danger, or saving oneself by avoiding a dangerous enterprise.

Traveling on buses might for another individual represent spending money, and missing the bus could indicate penuriousness. For still
another, missing the bus might represent resistance, not getting to the
analyst, or not getting anywhere with him. Missing the bus in yet another person's dream could reveal an unwillingness to travel with ordinary people—could be concerned, that is, with snobbishness rather than
with losing an opportunity. If the patient happened to be a professor
of Elizabethan literature, the dream might bring to him the association
buss—to kiss—and might refer to his failure to kiss his wife, to his missing the *buss*. This would introduce a whole area of problems in his
marriage, perhaps related to the expression of affection.

When a universal dictionary of symbols is mechanically applied,
therapists may be seriously misled. They may miss, for any particular

patient, the unique significance of his symbols. One avoids this pitfall, when dealing with dreams or other material, by deriving from the individual himself the meaning of the data coming from him.

The dreamer sees his activity and attitudes in unintelligible symbolic representation, and does not recognize the reality about himself while dreaming. A dream represents an attitude or practice of which the individual is unaware, and which he is unwilling or reluctant to acknowledge when awake. On awakening he may recall the dream about himself. He still perceives, however, only the dream's symbolistic abstractions, which are meaningless when out of context.

Free association provides the relevant biographical context which can give the dream meaning. The associative context can lead to sharpness and concreteness of formulation about the reality of the individual. The abstraction, through a creative, associative, and correlating process, is shifted into a framework of understandable, communicable, usable conceptualization. Through the disciplined methodology of free association and interpretation, the individual can make this translation from the symbolic abstractions, and can be in a position then to correct the conceptual distortions of his waking consciousness and the concomitant distortions of his feelings, his attitudes, and his practices.

The subject of dream symbolism is integrally related to associative and interpretive activities, to the goals of therapy, and to all aspects of the personality and of treatment. In this chapter, however, the emphasis is on symbolism itself.

Dream symbols may be considered representational abstractions, comparable in some ways to metaphors and similes in speech. Symbols are subjective abstractions of qualities, characteristics, and concepts which might otherwise be communicated in the waking state by verbal analysis and formulation. When one speaks of similes or metaphors, one is referring to figures of speech whose essence lies in the isolated emphasis upon one or more particular features. When one says metaphorically that a man is a bull, one calls attention, according to the context, to his stolidity, massiveness, sexual potency, potential for anger, or possibly all of these features. If a man is called a fox, emphasis is often being laid upon his slyness. If a woman is called a cow, one is probably referring to a combination of qualities—stupidity and passivity, and sometimes to her nurturing qualities, instead or in addition. When a man's anger is described as "like an erupting volcano," attention is being focused upon the suddenness and violence of the anger. If he is said to act like a snake, it may be his sneakiness that is being emphasized.

It is always possible that the emphasis of a speaker, a writer, or a dreamer may be entirely clear and specific for him, while the emphasis that arises in the mind of the one to whom he is communicating may be quite different. In analysis such failures of communication are correctable. The determination of the specific emphasis of the dreamer is achieved through the joint associative and interpretive activities of the analyst and the patient.

It is also possible that the qualitative emphasis of a dream symbol is apprehended differently by analyst and patient, not through failure of communication but because of the patient's failure to recognize, in his waking state, the meaning of his own symbol. The correction of this situation, too, is the function of the associative and interpretive activities.

The dream symbol, instead of being a figure of speech, is the non-verbal, graphic representation of a quality or concept. Furthermore, the emotion or attitude of the individual dreamer in connection with that image corresponds to his feeling, most often unrecognized, about the special quality or concept it represents. Thus a snake in the dream may be the symbol—a pictorial simile or metaphor—for sneakiness; the dreamer regards someone as a "snake" and his feeling about sneakiness, perhaps fear or disgust, corresponds to his feeling about the individual represented by a snake. A cow might be a symbol for a particular woman's stupid, passive behavior, but the cow also connotes how the dreamer contemptuously, unconsciously, feels about the woman.

Such symbolic forms are ideational and affective reflections of what may be real qualities; or they may be reflections of the dreamer's distorted perceptions and conceptualizations. Whether accurate reflections or subjective distortions, the nature of the symbols is determined by the specific dreamer's total and unique history.

The individual's history teems with experiences. From the accumulating and interlocking myriad situations in his life, one seemingly insignificant object may come to represent for him the abstraction of a very important, clearly definable activity or quality. Thus a man who has seen a brutal kicking incident may dream of a shoe as a symbol of brutality. An experience in which chagrin was derived from wearing dirty shoes might lead to the occurrence of a shoe as an abstract pictorial symbol for the quality of humiliating embarrassment. A painful public exposure of an unpleasant personal quality in an individual might have resulted from the statement of a good friend, "If the shoe fits, wear it!" In his dream a shoe could be a symbol of chagrin, or of betrayal by a friend, or perhaps even a symbol of desire for revenge, if that emotion had been involved in the experience. It might also rep-

THE CLINICAL USE OF DREAMS

resent that quality in the dreamer which was specifically alluded to by the friend's "if the shoe fits" remark. Shoes by themselves have no universal symbolic meaning. The meaning of the shoe to the dreamer has a particularity derived from his life experience.

In order to illustrate further the wide variety of interpretive possibilities, it will be useful to examine a hypothetical demonstration of individualized symbolic meanings as they relate to a commonly abused "universal dream symbol"—the snake. Some of the *phallic* possibilities of the snake symbol will be considered first, and then the *nonphallic* dream snake will be considered.

If a woman were dreaming of a snake which associatively became established as a penis, it would still be necessary, if one is to achieve insight into her personality through her dream symbol, to establish the quality of experience with a penis which was symbolized by that snake. If she were a professional dancer largely preoccupied by a desire to be seductive, and if she had performed the dance of a snake charmer, then the penile snake could symbolize her desire to charm men or to control them by her sexual allure. The problem, however, would then be the characterological one of desire for control and manipulation. Such pathology, furthermore, would not be confined to the sexual sphere, but would be an aspect of her total personality, a determinant in her relations with men, women, and children, even though the penis symbol appeared to focus exclusively upon the manipulation of men.

If a woman had been made pregnant before a promised marriage by a man who later deserted her, the penile snake in her dream might represent the quality of deceit or poisonousness, or both, not only in men but also in any human being who offered intimacy. If she had had a puritanical upbringing and yet indulged in a sexual affair, the penile snake might represent hidden "sinful" desires or actual secret activities of a sexual nature. The possibilities, however, do not stop there. The violation of the sexual taboos of her puritanical upbringing could by subjective analogy refer to hidden "sinful" desires for the indulgence of other sensual modalities, as with food or perfumes. By still further extension, the snake could refer even to yearnings for other types of self-indulgence, self-gratification, even of nonsensual, esthetic, intellectual, or material nature. For a puritanically raised woman who had healthily rebelled, emancipated herself, and fulfilled not only her sexual desires but also her artistic and intellectual inclinations, that penile dream-snake might be a symbol for a healthy self-fulfillment in any of a variety of totally nonsexual spheres. In other words, by analogy with sexual emancipation, the snake, originating for this woman as a penis symbol, could come to be a broader symbol for self-emancipation.

In Clara Thompson's cultural framework of penis envy,[1] the penile snake might also refer to a desire for masculine status. When it is associated with the area of a particular woman dreamer's competitiveness with men, the penile snake can be a symbol, not for sex, but for her total problem of competitiveness.

The snake in another woman's dream might represent fear of sexual attack from men, or a related desire to castrate them in the manner of killing a snake. Or the penis might represent a pervasive contempt for men, a symbol of the attitude: "All men are pricks."

In all the preceding hypothetical examples the "universal" symbol for sex—snake—has been discussed in types of situations in which it was actually related to the phallus; in every case its significance for the patient was, as is repeatedly confirmed in psychoanalytic practice, of a characterological and not of an instinctual sexual nature.

In many patients, however, a dream snake may not in any manner refer to the phallus. A woman patient (this would be equally true of a man), during her childhood, while walking with other children, might have overcome her fear of being bitten by snakes by picking one up. For this patient, a snake in a dream could symbolize courage— a courage utterly unrelated to sexuality. If she had been laughed at on that walk because, unlike the other children, she had failed through fear to pick up the snake, a snake in her adult dream might symbolize humiliation.

Another woman, deceived by her closest female friend, might dream of the friend as a snake, with no penile implications whatever.

It is obvious at this point that the meanings of the dream symbols, as I view them, neither derive from a collective unconscious [2] nor conform to the requirements of a theory of a universal pattern of psychosexual ontology.[3]

[1] Clara Thompson, "Penis Envy in Women," *Psychiatry*, 6:123–125, 1943.

[2] C. G. Jung, *Psychology of the Unconscious.* New York: Dodd, Mead and Company, 1949.

[3] I have not found convincing the thesis that the dream necessarily represents a hidden wish, a wish that is moreover for fulfillment of hidden and unacceptable sexual demands; nor can I concur with Freud when he says: "When we have become familiar with the abundant use made of symbolism for representing sexual material in dreams, the question is bound to arise of whether many of these symbols do not occur with a *permanently fixed meaning, like the 'grammalogues' in shorthand;* and we shall feel tempted to draw up a new 'dream-book' on the decoding principle" (italics mine). S. Freud, *Interpretation of Dreams,* J. Strachey, translator and editor. New York: Basic Books, 1960, p. 351.

No one has satisfactorily explained the *dream work* which is the processing of our life problems—our unrecognized feelings, attitudes, and practices—into the affects and imagery of sleep. I speculate that the understanding of this will be related reciprocally to discoveries in the fields of the learning and the creative processes. In the meantime, it is possible to organize some empirical observations about symbols in dreams in such a way as to enhance the accessibility and clinical usefulness of dream data.

In the Introduction to this volume, three approaches to the dream were formalistically set forth, namely: (1) recognizing the elements of the dream; (2) associative activity; and (3) interpretive activity. The symbolism of dreams, as was suggested there, can be conveniently arranged and recognized under the subheadings of the first category— the *elements of the dream*. It will be remembered that the four elements are: action, individuals, surroundings, and feeling, and that feeling is separated into two categories—symbolized and experiential.[4]

A consideration of symbols involves the first three of the dream elements, and part of the fourth. In other words, actions, individuals, and surroundings, and all feeling except experiential feelings, are the subject matter of symbolism in dreams.

Any single symbolic component of the dream may have multiple reference. (This is what Freud discovered and described as *condensation*.) A single element may refer to a number of conceptually and affectively related items from the dreamer's life. For example, the individual in the dream may refer to a number of individuals in the patient's life.

A dream was reported by a homosexual young man just commencing analysis (Hot Dog). In it he was, with happy anticipation, waiting on line for a frankfurter on 34th Street. The frankfurter was a symbol of an individual of the dream. This individual (while specifically the analyst, whose office was on 34th Street) represented also a broad range of objects of seduction by the patient, frequently older men.

A woman in a dream may stand for many specific mistresses, and a woman may, in another dream, represent a number of women of authority in the patient's life—his mother, his aunt, his third-grade teacher, his music teacher, perhaps also his wife. She may be the aggregate, the abstraction, the condensation of all of these authoritative females in a series of similar experiences over the whole life span of the patient.

This intricate relatedness goes further. The individual of the

[4] For the distinction between symbolized and experiential feeling, see pp. 10, 50.

dream may symbolize not only a complex of persons, but also a series of interpersonal experiences over the whole life of the patient, and so may refer to *action*, too. If the authoritative woman of the hypothetical dream just suggested is connected in the patient's history with his own cowed and intimidated behavior, then this individual, just by her presence, may at the same time symbolize action in the dream.

To extend the concept of multiple reference to still another element, the individual may define or re-enforce also the *feeling* of the dream. If the emotional response of the patient to the authoritative woman who appeared in the dream has been for him a consistent one, such as resentment or fear, then the presence of this individual may of itself constitute a symbolized feeling. If the characteristic feeling of the patient in relation to such a woman happens also to be experienced in the course of dreaming, this would be an instance in which the symbol of the individual constituted also a symbolized feeling, which, in turn, re-enforced an experiential feeling. The hypothetical dream of the authoritative woman demonstrates the complicated kind of multiple reference which can be condensed within a single symbol. The dream woman is an abstraction of a great complex of separate people in the patient's life; as the individual of the dream, she also symbolizes two other elements—action and feeling.

In the dream of the homosexual patient referred to above, the hot dog not only designated the individual but also had reference to the action, fellatio, which was the patient's homoerotic behavior. Homoerotism itself, of course, stood for only the sexual component of the much more complex interpersonal activity of the homosexual, an important aspect of which is the activity of seducing. In this abbreviated illustration, then, there is symbolic multiple reference. The hot dog represents the analyst and also many other older men, and in addition refers to homoerotism and seduction, two forms of interpersonal action.

It is occasionally difficult to distinguish between *individuals* and *surroundings*. People may be present in a dream without signifying the individual. They may serve indifferently as part of a street setting; perhaps a Frenchman may help merely to identify a setting as France. A long-forgotten neighbor or schoolmate may primarily identify a period in the dreamer's life.

An enormous multiplicity of reference of each dream symbol always exists. This makes the recognition and interpretation of symbols challenging, confusing, and often therapeutically constructive.

Multiplicity of reference is a condensation of an extensive scatter of experience. The obverse condition also occurs. Multiple symbols may repeat or re-enforce a single meaning. (This is what Freud discovered and described as *overdetermination*.) In the Sickle dream the individual, the analyst, is indicated in three ways, involving all the elements of the dream. He is symbolized by the *surroundings,* in this case the second floor, where his office is located. He is symbolized by his *action,* that of looking from above at a reclining figure, the patient. He is symbolized as the *individual,* someone in a parental relationship to the patient. Finally, after the dream was interpreted, it became clear that the analyst was also indicated by the patient's *feeling,* in this case by dual experiential feelings in the dream, which included both fear of him and triumph at eluding him. These multiple symbolic indications may come from the same element, from all, or from any combination of the elements.

The relation of feeling to symbolism should logically constitute a portion of this chapter on symbolism in dreams. Feeling is, however, so important in dreams, in psychodynamics, and in therapy, that it has been developed, in relation to all these areas, in a chapter by itself (see Chapter 2).

Sexuality would also ordinarily be considered within a chapter on symbolism in dreams. Sexuality has, however, been treated only briefly in the present context and, like feeling, is dealt with more extensively in a separate chapter (see Chapter 4), but for different reasons. Sexuality occupies a central position in the controversial instinctual concepts of human psychodynamics, and the classical dream theory is both integrally and reciprocally related to these controversial concepts. A discussion of my own approach (or what, for want of a better term, may be referred to as a culturalist approach) to sexuality entails extensive exposition including many clinical illustrations, and therefore the consideration of sexual symbols and of sexuality in dream and waking life has been expanded in that separate chapter.

Individual symbolism, previously developed under the concept of *personal glossary* (see p. 32), involves consideration of some additional clinical phenomena. These are: (1) the repetition of symbols; (2) waking symbols; and (3) changing symbols. All of these phenomena can be more fully understood through an application of the significance of the personal glossary and, in turn, they extend the concept of the personal glossary.

REPETITION OF SYMBOLS

An individual's personality, unless it changes, is the basis for the persistence of a characteristic type of interpersonal experience. These experiences may be expressed in dreams by varying symbols. On the other hand, in the familiar phenomenon of repetitive dreams, people continue to reflect unresolved personality difficulties with the identical symbols. These recurrences form, for the present context, the category of repetition of symbols.

Usually, over a period of analysis while the patterns of the patient's way of living maintain some constancy, these patterns are expressed in many different kinds of dreams and with a great variety of symbolism. One patient's basic noncollaborative personality pattern was seen in various dreams in the forms of a fleeing bird, concealment of papers, destruction of data, passive resistance, and active combat. These symbolize her ways, active and passive, overt and concealed, of avoiding responsible cooperative activity. The interpersonal tactics and circumstances vary, and the symbols vary in accordance. The patient's basic problem of insularity and non-involvement remains constant; the theme is repetitive, but it is represented by diversified symbols.

The repetitive dream differs in that both the basic problem and its symbolic representation in the dream are repetitive. The patient reiterates, again and again, his symbolic statement of the core problem.

The Recurrent Dreams of Lionesses reappeared for years and were presented by the dreamer in her first analytic session. The lioness, she said, "I sometimes feared, generally tried to manipulate. The lioness was always very strong and beautiful. I always managed to keep her under control, but it took some very careful maneuvering." The lioness was a symbol of the patient's angry, destructive feelings. The dream represented in part her pride in her ability to control such feelings. It recurred because of the persistent, unsolved, dangerous personality problem, the continuing threat that these emotions would get out of hand.

Another patient had a repetitive dream reflecting his constant problem of seeking shrewdly to control, not a force within him, but the people around him. The dream expressed this symbolically in the form of his waving a wand to drive back menacing apes (The Wand and the Apes).

The repetition of identical symbols is not uncommon, but it is the less common form in which the patient recurrently reflects the same personality problem in dreams. Repetitive dreams have very commonly been associated with traumatic experiences and are practically a symptomatological constant in traumatic neuroses. The dramatic aspects of the trauma experience often deflect the observer from the existence and origins of the individual's difficulties before the incident that marked the onset of the clinical syndrome. A traumatic effect by itself cannot realistically be considered the sole cause of either the neurosis or the repetitive dream. The effects of the traumatic incident on the individual can be understood only within the context of the history of the individual. Closer examination may reveal the personality difficulties that pre-existed in the patient and for which the traumatic incident has become a vivid symbolization in itself.[5]

WAKING SYMBOLS

There are some symbols which resemble the patient's personal glossary of dream symbols, and which are derived not from dreams but from waking consciousness. They are included in this context because of their significant resemblances and relationships to dream symbols. Comparable to the items of a personal glossary of dream symbols, they are fragments of waking life that have the quality of condensing a broad span of experience and of representing insights in an economical and vivid form. Like dream symbols, they, too, become important terms of communication because of their power to evoke understanding in a profound conceptual and affective manner not equally achievable by ordinary language.

"Another olive" became for one patient the symbol of a type of interpersonal pathology that was the basis of much hostility, anxiety, and isolation. Two couples shared a summer cottage. The patient had quite unconscionably maneuvered the original plans, changing the geography and departure time in order to work in a few more analytic sessions, both before vacation and, by keeping closer to New York City, during vacation. All the changes in the original plans were negotiated with alternate pressure and contrition based upon the closeness of the friendship. When the four were finally ensconced in their vacation cottage and were gathered around the first meal, this woman at one point during the lunch, when the olive dish had been considerably reduced, asked in a mousey manner, "Does anyone mind if I take another olive?" This was the breaking point for the other wife, who attacked her mercilessly for the fraudulence of her self-effacement and for the pretense of undemandingness after all the inconveniences to which she had subjected everyone. The whole incident led in analysis to an intensive and productive examination of the patient's enormous demands on people, made behind the facade of a hesitant request for a crumb. "Another olive" became the precise, vivid symbol for this part of her personality.

"Another olive" was inherently related, furthermore, to the whole

5 This is discussed further in the author's paper, "Some Principles of Brief Psychotherapy," *Psychiatric Quarterly*, 27: 1–18, 1953.

complex constellation of her behavior and reactions. This involved her enormous demands, her manipulative techniques, her dissimulation and self-delusion, her anxiety over impending frustration, anxiety from the threat of exposing her hostility when frustrated, and anxiety over the threat of hostility from the objects of her manipulation. "Another olive," like many terms from personal glossaries of dream symbols, often led to an identification of any of these aspects of the patient's problems. The symbol sometimes arose as the patient's association, sometimes the analyst's. The olive, furthermore, would flash into the context of any part of the molecular complexity of the patient's problems. It might lead to insight, for example, as an association with an "inappropriate" anxiety. "Another olive," the waking symbol, made for ready affective and conceptual ingress to theretofore inexplicable feelings and behavior.

Another vivid waking symbol developed from a fleeting experience of an intensely sadistic man. His always covert cruelty often was practiced in the form of driving those closest to him nearly frantic with impotent concern. He would be miserable, demanding infinite solicitude, while remaining inconsolable in the face of endless efforts to comfort him. To persist with kind attention was futile, to discontinue was to expose oneself to accusations of insincerity. One day, in heavy but speeding traffic along a parkway, he saw a squirrel trapped on a narrow grass strip dividing lanes. The squirrel was dashing back and forth from one side of the island to the other, frantically seeking to make an effective effort in one direction or the other. The whole incident had a dramatic impact which carried it into the next analytic session. The patient, approaching and swiftly passing the squirrel, was suddenly overcome by such intense nausea that he nearly had to stop the car to vomit. The predicament of the squirrel was, as we had repeatedly seen in analysis, precisely the one into which he perpetually maneuvered people, and it was a behavior he was loathe to acknowledge. His revulsion was forcefully manifested psychosomatically. The squirrel became established as a symbol from the patient's waking life. It became a waking symbol which swiftly and sharply communicated between us his sadistic practice of entrapping people in situations in which their integrity or effectiveness appeared threatened, regardless of the course they chose.

The olive and the squirrel recurred, as do the waking symbols of many patients, in numerous contexts, serving to evoke and to communicate their respective insights with an inimitable expressiveness.

The consideration of waking symbolism has been included in this discussion of dream symbols because it may contribute to the understanding of symbolism in general and hence to that in dreams. Several factors are involved in this correlation. In the clinical example cited, the waking symbol "another olive" is clearly derived, like a dream symbol, from the uniquely individual life history of the patient. It is exquisitely specific in its connotation for her, and is readily communicable. It differs from the dream symbol in that the dream symbol arises involuntarily in the course of sleep; the waking symbol is consciously, voluntarily adopted in the course of therapy as a symbol of a specific aspect of the patient's personality.

Waking symbolism is actually a commonplace of everyday life, frequently manifested as some special term in the spontaneously arising private language of a marriage relationship, in peer groups, and elsewhere among people with shared experience. The choice of the single eloquent item from a complex constellation of activity, feeling, and response may be made with or without awareness. The exploration of the dynamics of this selectivity in expression and communication would extend into other areas of creativity, and into such fields as language and semantics.[6] Here the study of the creation of waking and dream symbols would tend to converge.

It was stated also at the outset of this chapter that this was the area, in the author's opinion, in which a fundamental understanding of the dream process would be likely to be found.

If one starts with the clinical example of the olive and begins to speculate how the olive symbol, which came out of the report of an incident, might appear in a dream instead, one is in a provocative position to ponder the dream process. In the waking session the patient and analyst chose the olive as an abstract condensation of a complicated experience and its meaning. Had the olive instead first appeared in a dream, then the patient would have elaborated out of it, as associations, all the experiential items that were telescoped into its creation as a symbol. In both situations the olive of the patient's experience is made into a symbol, a term pregnant with meaning, a rich vehicle of communication.

The introduction of waking symbolism in the context of dream symbolism thus raises questions concerning the processes of symbolization and dream formation. In the present text, which is oriented clinically, the most immediate justification for the emphasis on waking symbolism must rest with its therapeutic usefulness.

[6] For a provocative inquiry into symbolism, creativity, and esthetic communication, see Susanne K. Langer, *Philosophy in a New Key*, 3rd ed. Cambridge, Mass.: Harvard University Press, 1957.

CHANGING SYMBOLISM

An important aspect of dream symbols is the phenomenon of changing symbolism. This refers to a symbol's recurrence in a new dream in an altered form. Dreams reflect the attitudes, feelings, conceptualizations, and practices of the patient, and when these change in the course of treatment the symbols by which they are represented in dreams likewise show modifications. To the extent that these alterations of the same symbol take place in accordance with alterations of the personality during therapy, the symbol changes become important indicators of clinical progress.

Because the evolution of health as reflected in the analytic patient's dreams is of such clinical importance, a chapter has been devoted to it, and changing symbolism is there considered further (see Chapter 8).

Here, however, three cases can illustrate briefly the alteration of a dream symbol in accordance with changes in the patient's feelings and conceptualizations. The first is that of the young homosexual who dreamed of the hot dog. The hot dog represented, in an erotic framework, the analyst's penis, which the patient desired. In an interpersonal framework it also represented the analyst as a person, one whom the patient was hoping to seduce by flattery and by his analytic zeal and brilliance. Several years after this first dream, the patient had an anxiety dream in which he was followed by a dachshund, who was spraying a poisonous mist on him from behind (Poisonous Dachshund). The dachshund, the elongated German dog that frequently impersonates the frankfurter, was the new representation of the analyst (maintaining his position behind the patient). Instead, however, of being a passive agent (inanimate frankfurter) to be acted upon by the patient, as in the first dream, he was, though still considerably derogated, at least animate, very active, and exerting a profound influence upon the young man. For all the anxious resistance indicated by the dream, the altered symbol, having acquired activity and force, indicated a healthier awareness of the independence and influence of the analyst.

Another clinical example comes from a patient whose progress in her feeling about herself could be fruitfully followed in the alterations of a human symbol (in contrast with the categories of inanimate or animal symbol) of herself. The first sign that this infantilized and often militantly immature young woman was beginning to accept responsibility for her own life came in a dream in which she was shopping with a supermarket carriage on which was poised a baby, herself, whom she was happily taking care of (Supermarket Baby). In later dreams she was a ten-year-old prodigy being urged to develop (Prodigy). In a dream still later in therapy she was a young woman, sad and alone, toward whom she felt protective (Sad Young Lady). Toward the end of analysis she appeared in one dream in dual roles, one a helpless floundering "jerk" who was appealing for help to the other symbol of herself, a beautiful, mature, competent woman captain of a ship, who capably showed the jerk how to save himself (Captain-Woman). This dream in itself demonstrated a high degree of attained growth and acceptance of responsibility, but the retrospective glance over the increasing stages of maturity, the changing symbolism from infant to independent woman, considerably re-enforced the patient's awareness of her own developmental course.

A third demonstration of developmental process as revealed by the modification of a particular dream symbol is derived from a patient who saw herself in a dream as an emotionally impenetrable individual, in the form of a garden whose earth was a wooden floor (Wooden Earth). The gardener (analyst) could not get through the surface anywhere. The dream came during the third year of her analysis, when she had begun to make progress but had become temporarily resistant. (One of several instances occurring with her in the course of basically productive therapy.) A month later she dreamed again of being in a garden, but this time she herself was the gardener, and furthermore she was making spontaneous efforts to bring out her feelings. She was doing this by making an irrigation furrow in the earth into which water could flow from below. As she described it, "The earth was barren and it was perfectly natural to dig this little ditch because in the dream this would quite naturally bring water." One of the interesting symbolic ties to her dream of the month before was in the way she began to tell the dream: "The floor . . . [pause] . . . the earth didn't have enough water and I dug a trench with my hands." To be sure, she was nearly deluged by all the water that welled up in response to her efforts to get beneath the surface (Irrigation Deluge).

The difference between the hard surface of the Wooden Earth dream, which only the analyst was making efforts (unsuccessfully) to penetrate, and the earth which a month later the patient got into with her own efforts, represented a tangible change that was occurring during an important month in analysis. The change in the patient's feelings and conceptualizations about herself, her marriage, and her analysis was accompanied by changing behavior. The total evolutionary tendency in her emotion, philosophy, and activity was reflected by the illustrated modification of a specific symbol—the garden "floor."

SUMMARY AND CORRELATION WITH INTERPRETIVE ACTIVITY

Before concluding the consideration of symbolism in dreams, it will be useful to relate the points of emphasis to *interpretive activity*. The points have been: (1) the individuality of dream symbols—the specificity of meaning for the particular dreamer; (2) the consequent development of each patient's personal glossary of dream symbols; (3) the importance of recognizing dream symbolism as part of the broad field of symbolic processes, which includes the clinically useful category of waking symbolism; and lastly (4) emphasis was placed upon the reflection, in alterations of the symbol, of the patient's changes in feeling, conceptualization, and practice.

The patient's active role in the psychoanalytic process is nurtured by all these emphases upon the individuality of his symbols and the necessity for intensive, creative pursuit of their meanings.

The patient's increasing capacity, and progressive assumption of responsibility, for recognizing and rationally approaching his problems is a constant goal during psychoanalysis. In all the areas emphasized in this chapter, such an achievement is envisioned. The recognition of his problems often involves interpretive activity concerned with symbolic data. This is a process from which he may take refuge or even be deflected by an academic, dogmatic type of symbolic orientation.

Cooperativeness, in itself, is one of the most constructive developments of personality achieved in analysis, and is fostered in the patient-analyst mutual pursuit of the elusive meanings of symbols. The patient and analyst together must not only identify the symbols, but also engage in associative and interpretive activity together to find their meanings. The personal glossary established through this collaboration (and here, too, one must guard against a glib or academic use of a personal glossary) becomes a medium of vivid communication and of ready, incisive detection of many problems. This symbolic succinctness and vividness serves fruitfully in the repeated interpretations of many problems which, though once delineated, are often missed when they arise in new circumstances. The honest search for understanding often is rewarded by the associative occurrence of the familiar dream symbol where word formulations fail.

The patient's achievement of the use of his dream symbols helps him to use symbols from his waking life, in the better understanding of his feelings, attitudes, and behavior. A form of waking symbol not dealt with above, but worth mentioning in passing, is the *psychosomatic symbol*. Patients come to associate headaches, gut rumbling, and, of course, anxiety as the symbols of certain attitudes in particular circumstances. Some patients come to recognize the imminence of insight by yawning, some by anxiety, some by confusion. One patient learned to look for and recognize an otherwise unperceived anger at the analyst in the psychosomatic symbol of bladder urgency during the session.

The recognition of the changes in the symbols of his dreams helps to develop in the patient a sense of process in life, a recognition of his own potential for influencing these processes, and of his ability to change himself with the aid of honest self-observation. The patient who is helped by the interpretation of his dream symbols will be stimulated to engage in interpretive activity and to observe himself honestly in viewing other than dream data.

This chapter has been only an introduction to the nature of symbols and their role in the analytic process. A constant elaboration of the subject of symbolism develops inherently or explicitly throughout the considerations of the types and aspects of dreams that form the substance of all the succeeding chapters.

In all of these chapters, as in the present one, the emphasis will continue to be on the individuality of symbolic meanings and on the requisite mutuality of analyst-patient activity in the search for these meanings.

2. Feeling in Dreams

Probably the most significant expression of any individual's personality lies in his feelings. The effort to discover and to understand feelings is central throughout the therapeutic process. The detection of implicit or explicit emotion is also central in the consideration of a dream. Insight into the health and pathology of the patient is profoundly enhanced through the use of his dreams; this insight may, however, be lost if the affective element of each dream is not sufficiently pursued.

Feeling is an ingredient of all human behavior and conceptualization; yet, except in some of its more intense manifestations in waking or sleeping, it may be inaccurately or inadequately perceived in himself by the patient, or may not be perceived at all.

Access to the emotional life of an individual is gained through observation of multiple, partial, and often obscure reflections. An individual's activity, if understood, reflects his feelings. His conceptualizations also, as expressed in language and imagery, to some degree reflect his feeling responses to living.

Feelings, when detected and fully comprehended, are perhaps the most subtle, accurate, and comprehensive indicators of the total personality. As dream action helps us to recognize more clearly what it is an individual is doing or trying to do, dream feeling helps to reveal the

49

values and conceptualizations associated with these activities in the waking life of the dreamer.

What a man does, thinks, and feels are closely interwoven in every moment of his living. Because of this complexity of personality, and its reflection in dreams, a structuralization of the approaches to dream feeling was formulated in the Introduction (pp. 9–10). It will be remembered that feeling in dreams can be seen in two distinct categories: symbolized and experiential.

The distinction between symbolized and experiential feelings, besides being convenient for this discussion, is important for three further reasons in the understanding and clinical use of dreams. *First*, if both types of feeling are present in a dream experience, one type may capture the attention of therapist or patient as *the* feeling in the dream, when in actuality it is only *one* of the feelings of the dream. *Second*, unless vigilance is maintained toward the detection of a feeling, a patient having no memory of experiential feeling may totally neglect the symbolic evidence of feeling, responding on inquiry that he "felt nothing." In one dream, for example, feces on the leg, after what would ordinarily be considered a harrowing experience, betrayed associatively that a patient had really been "scared shitless," although she reported having experienced "no feeling" (Scared Shitless). *Third*, the distinction between symbolized and experiential affect is important to maintain because experiential affect is not inductive or interpretive—it is an immediate, undeniable datum. An experiential emotion never symbolizes anything. It is always an authentic response to something in the patient's life. In the case of a patient who denies having any feeling at all regarding some aspect of his life, experiential feeling in a dream, regardless of its nature, is irrefutable evidence of the existence of emotional response.

There are people who deny that they experience anger or love or anxiety or some other emotion. The life situation that is generating such feelings may remain obscure for some time. While symbolized feeling may not be able to convince such a patient of the existence of emotion in him, experiential feeling in a dream, subjectively identifiable, creates strong internal pressure for acknowledgment.

Some brief clinical illustrations will help to clarify the distinctions in dream feelings that have just been described.

Symbolized feeling was exemplified in the dream of the engineer whose *anger* was represented by a cap popping off the top of an otherwise carefully regulated machine (Blowing My Top). Another man, who looked for sexual solace with other women when he was angry at his wife, symbolized *anger* in a dream in which a small valve for letting off steam, like that on top of a boiler, was situated on the end of his erect penis (Statuesque Masturbation). The young woman cited above dreamed of finding feces on her leg as a symbolization of extreme *fear*. Another woman patient depicted *depression* in her dream by heavy "leaden feet" (Dragging Feet).

In each of these examples, the specific affect was not felt during the dream, but its presence was symbolized.

Anxiety is one of the most familiar affects felt during dreams, and numerous examples appear not only in the chapter on anxiety, but also throughout this volume. There is, however, an infinite range of experiential feelings in dreams. One woman in her dream defecated while talking with friends in a living room, and although she made great effort at concealment, left behind some of the feces as she walked out to clean herself (Shitty Behavior). She experienced during her dream a feeling of deep *shame*. Another patient, often plagued by social diffidence, in terminating a productive year of analysis had a dream in which she was called upon to express publicly some honest criticism of a group (Something To Tell). In the course of this activity in the dream, she felt *self-assurance*. The same patient in another dream was paying only the most perfunctory attention as some woman talked to her. She felt acute embarrassment at that point in the dream when her inattention left her unprepared to reply relevantly (Not Listening). One man looked out over fruitful green fields in his dream and experienced a "very contented feeling," but at the same time had a disturbing, conflicting, dissatisfied sensation that he described as a "discordant note" (Very Contented, But . . .). The homosexual patient mentioned earlier experienced *pleasant anticipation* in the dream in which he looked forward to seducing the analyst, but ended the dream experiencing a conflicting emotion, *disappointment* (Hot Dog).

New feelings emerge in the course of analysis as a result of new perception. The first detection and identification of such a new kind of affect often occurs by way of a dream.[1]

While separate illustrations have been presented of each of the two categories of dream affect, both types, as already indicated, may occur in the same dream. In the dream of the engineer with the hi-fi set (Blowing My Top), for example, he experienced *annoyance* as an affect during the dream. The popping cap was a symbolized feeling, anger (blowing his top, flipping his lid). The annoyance (occurring as experiential feeling) was his response to his own **failure** to achieve perfect

---

[1] This is illustrated by the patient with the Crazy Woman dream later in this chapter, and its sequential Shit Piles Up.

control. The anger reaction and the annoyance were present in the dream as symbolized and experiential feeling, respectively.

Similarly, the young woman who in her dream walked through danger without any experience of fear and found feces on her leg exemplified a clearly symbolized feeling (Scared Shitless). In the dream, however, she actually experienced some amusement in her mother's presence as she saw the feces, which was experiential feeling.

Another more subtle example of this dual occurrence is a dream in which, while the feeling is experienced, its intensity is symbolized. A woman experienced annoyance toward her mother and gave her a little get-away-from-me jab with the elbow; in response to the little jab, however, the mother flew across the room, landing in a heap on the floor (Annoyed with Mother). Some degree of hostility, annoyance, was experiential; the true intensity of her hostility, violent rage, was symbolized. Asking the patient about her feelings in the dream had elicited a mere retelling of her clear experiential feeling, namely that she was "annoyed." This patient's annoyance with her mother was no great problem or secret. Pursuit of the intense anger toward her mother, symbolized but not experienced in the dream, was, however, clinically productive.

There is always the danger of becoming clinically preoccupied with a single affect, either experiential or symbolized, and thereby not only losing a quantitative further illumination, but also possibly arriving at a qualitative interpretive distortion by not dealing with the relationship between the two feelings. One might have been led to think, for example, that the hi-fi engineer's experiential feeling of annoyance was related to technical perfectionism, had not the recognition of the symbolized temper revealed his preoccupation with control of anger (Blowing My Top).

The feces on the leg of the young woman (see p. 50) might have been attributed to a problem of infantilism. In conjunction with her experiential amusement when the feces were discovered in the presence of her mother, however, a more productive interpretive direction was possible, disclosing a serious tendency to disavow and laugh off anxiety.

The patient with the steam valve on his penis had the experiential feeling of *grandeur* in the dream, as he stood in statuesque proportions with a yard-long firm organ (Statuesque Masturbation). The steam valve might have been regarded as a symbol of super-charged libido, a mere elaboration of the experiential feeling of grandeur in the dream. Had the patient's report of his experiential feeling ended the investigation of feeling in the dream, there would have been lost the clinical value of a most significant item of symbolized feeling, hostility. This loss would have deprived patient and analyst of a very rich contribution to the development of awareness of the role of anger in the patient's sexual life.

Clearly, patients suffer not only from disturbed and distorted emotions, but also from misconceptions about the existence and nature of these emotions. These qualitative and conceptual distortions occur together, making the clinical exploration of emotion even more difficult.

The investigation of emotions may be productively pursued without recourse to instinctual psychodynamic concepts and their related concepts of the mechanisms of repression. In our culture certain types of emotional pathology are found clinically to be prevalent. Predominant among these are *cynicism* and *competitiveness*. The pervasiveness of these distortions is such that they have become vital elements of the milieu in which all consciousness develops. They must be recognized, then, not only as personality pathology, but also as significant and self-perpetuating cultural influences.[2]

A fruitful approach to the problem of affect in psychotherapy will be to begin by considering a common cultural phenomenon, the pathological reticence regarding the expression of emotions.

Denial of Feeling

Patients who have based an important sense of personal pride and strength on what they consider mastery of feelings (but which is usually the denial of feelings) can often begin to acquire some hint of the real nature and intensity of their feelings through the evidence of dreams. Both the emotions themselves and the patient's attitude toward his emotions are reflected in his dreams. Focusing on his deep fear of emotions in the affectively guarded and restrained individual, although it may produce anxiety, eventually helps to dissolve his barriers to acknowledging his feelings (Crazy Woman, see pp. 73–77).

Following is a series of briefly reviewed dreams of a physician initially reluctant to penetrate beyond the facade of calm and genial professional objectivity.

The patient's first dream in analysis was that of being in a very narrow passage (Edging Sideways). One wall was the back of a telephone switchboard. He could move along only by "edging sideways."

When asked what his feeling was in the dream, he replied with quiet finality, "I didn't have any feeling." I said to him that human

[2] Discussion of cynicism and competitiveness will be found, respectively, on pp. 64–86 and 86–95.

beings have some sort of feeling response in all their activities. He insisted that he had felt nothing, but he was willing to let his thoughts flow freely. In connection with the switchboard wall, he thought at once of "electrocardiograph." This reminded him that a friend had had a coronary attack, and that he himself had "worried a little" about such a possibility. I then asked him to try again to recall what emotions he felt while in the narrow passage in the dream. He replied matter-of-factly that he had had many dreams of being trapped in tunnels and narrow passages, and of being "scared as hell." He said, "They were real nightmares." For the third time I asked him to revive his brief dream of the night before, and to try to recall any feeling there might have been during it. "I had anxiety, all right," he said.

I then remarked on how reluctant he had been to recognize or to reveal this feeling. He answered that he had always been that way, and we concluded the session without interpretation, but on a note of emphasizing the importance of detecting, delineating, and reporting his feelings in the course of our work. The dream suggested that he felt cramped and anxious in a milieu of communication, the analysis. The narrowness of the corridor symbolized his "caught" feeling; the anxiety was experiential.

He came from his home in the suburbs to the next hour with another previous-night dream (The Poor Sprinkler). In it the sprinkler at the end of the hose on the front of the lawn had only a little water trickling out of it—very little pressure up front. He went to the back of the house and found water pouring out of the faucet under great pressure. The grounds around the back of his house were deeply flooded. In the dream he worried about how he could paint the back of the house, something he had planned before the flood. (The worry was experiential. The flood was symbolized emotion.)

Associatively he speculated that the trickle in front might be a phallic symbol meaning he was worried about being able to perform sexually. I suggested to him that the dream might be an expression of the nonemotional facade (front of the house) we had remarked on at the last session—his meager output of evidence of feeling. The high pressure and flood in back (behind the facade) might represent a flood of feeling that existed in contrast to what he let anyone see. This, he acknowledged with some contemplative nodding, seemed to fit him. (The high pressure at the back may also have had some psychosomatic relationship to a hemorrhoid condition which, as it later developed, was a problem.)

The night preceding his next session he had a severe anxiety dream (The Rocking Chair). He was on the porch of a hotel in front of which was a steep concrete slope, like a sea-wall. He sat in a rocking chair on which he had somehow arrived there. He sat in it to descend the slope, a feat that did not strike him as unusual or difficult. As soon as he started to descend, however, the rocker accelerated rapidly. He got out of the rocker for greater safety, but continued sliding down at a frightening rate, grasping at a few brittle twigs that grew out of the slope along the way. He felt terrified (E.F.) [3] in the dream and woke up in a panic. He was sure the dream had something to do with the talk about revealing his feelings, but he didn't know how it was all connected. I reminded him that my office was in a hotel. That brought an immediate association: the rocker reminded him of the calm, casual manner he had hoped to preserve through his analysis, his hope of "taking it easy," not getting upset in analysis (i.e., during his sojourn at a hotel). It was pointed out, by reference to the panic in the dream, how deeply he *feared* acknowledging and revealing his feelings. In addition, I suggested to him that his great *desire for casualness,* as symbolized by the rocker, was also an intense emotion.

Before the following hour he dreamed of speeding in his car and slowing down at a signal from a cop (Urinating in the Bottle). He resented (E.F.) having to slow down. (He interrupted with the association that the cop was the analyst. It was suggested that he wanted to breeze along through analysis and resented my slowing him down to a more careful pace, to examine his emotions.) After slowing, he proceeded to a house. He walked upstairs to the second floor to urinate. He had to urinate into a funnel that emptied into a bottle in the cellar below. The floor ended abruptly, revealing the cellar, as though the room were a balcony over the cellar. The neck of the funnel did not fit down in, but ended above the neck of the bottle. He thought this would make a bad smell, and was uncomfortable (E.F.) about it. (The bottle for collecting the urine had the peculiar shape of a vase that stands in direct view from the couch in my office. Like the room in the dream, my office is on the second floor and has a split-level arrangement between the waiting-room and the consultation room.) He thought interpretively that the dream had something to do with trying unsuccessfully to keep everything neatly contained. It was suggested to him that he was perhaps specifically trying to keep his feelings neatly contained, that this was impossible with the equipment in my office, and that his feelings would splash around and, because they were feelings, would make a bad smell (symbolized feeling—i.e.,

[3] Experiential feeling and symbolized feeling will be indicated in the text as follows: experiential feeling, E. F., and symbolized feeling, S. F.

urine = emotion). The importance of pursuing feelings, and the problem of his great constraint and unwillingness, were held in focus.

The next session dealt with a dream in which the patient was pushing a baby carriage while another man (associatively the analyst), who was more familiar with the district, acted as his guide (The Poor Guide). The patient began to push the carriage through a large puddle. The water became deeper and deeper, and he felt the guide didn't know his job.

I suggested that he felt like a baby for whom he had responsibility (a slight step forward—the job of getting into the realm of emotions was "his baby"). Perhaps he felt I didn't know my business if I insisted upon guiding him deeper into the area of his emotions.[4]

Two days later he came in, again with a dream of the night preceding the session (Burning Man).

"They were killing a man in a fireplace. He was lying there just the way I'm lying here. I felt they would stink up the place. They were going to get rid of the body by burning it up a little piece at a time. I felt if that's the way they were going to do it, if they were going to stink it up, well all right.

"The man was myself. He was lying on the fire just the way I'm lying here. This has to do with my withdrawing my emotions. Even in the dream! They were killing a guy. Even if it weren't I, I should have felt something. I just didn't allow myself to have any feeling. He was like a yogi, able to lie on a bed of nails or hot coals without feeling anything. I think this is what I've been doing with my wife. I've been afraid to allow myself to feel too much, for fear I'd be hurt too much."

I asked him what his feelings were in the dream. "I told you I tried to analyze my feelings in the dream. Even in the dream I suppressed my feelings. God damn it! I was detached—first thing when I woke up I tried to get my feelings."

I asked him what the setting of the dream was. "The fireplace in my own home," he said.

I said, "They were burning a man. Who were *they*?"

"They were vague. When I woke up I immediately thought *you* were the person, but it was they. There was a sense of *they*. There were no clear people, no figures. Maybe it was you and my wife."

"When you said, 'Let them stink it up,' you were expressing some sort of feeling toward the *they*."

[4] See the similar symbolism of Wading in Deeper, pp. 125–126.

"I guess it was anger [E. F.]—anger at you and my wife."

"The emotion of resignation was also in the dream, wasn't it?"

"I never thought of resignation [E. F.] as an emotion. I always thought of it as a withdrawal of emotion. They might kill me, but it would take a little time to get rid of me. This burning—it was as though my feelings were outside of me [S. F.]. I was not allowing myself to feel the pain, the emotions, the heat—I was externalizing it."

"You were pictorializing, symbolizing what you are experiencing here on my couch."

"The man lying on the logs in the fireplace was certainly in this couch position. But it was my own hearth, too. It was the pain I've had trying to avoid feelings when I'm with my wife, in order to be able to continue with her."

I said to him, "You know you cannot analyze while you remain detached. Let yourself feel the flame, feel your feelings, and say whatever comes to mind." (The patient's symbolized feeling was used specifically for immediacy in communication.)

He then spent ten minutes describing a domestic battle over a long-standing grievance. ". . . wife was mad as hell . . . I was goddamn mad. . . . She's been crabbing about that for fifteen years . . ."

I interrupted, saying, "For a solid ten minutes you've been describing this long-standing wrangle with your wife. You've mentioned repeatedly how you and your wife both get 'mad as hell' and you've recounted the whole situation with hardly a single inflection. You're standing apart from the feeling situation right here—this is very much like the dream."[5]

He added in the same colorless manner, "And when I sat opposite her at lunch after all that, I was sore as hell and didn't express a thing."

I said, "Describe what you felt, and the way you felt it while you sat at lunch feeling angry at your wife. What did you feel like saying? What would you have said if you had felt free to say anything, no holds barred?"

He laughed out loud. "All my life I've guarded my feelings. If I'd told my wife what I felt, she'd have been terribly hurt."

"I'm not telling you to start screaming angrily at people. I'm not telling you to start smashing things."

"It sounds to me as though you are." He was silent for a moment and then added, "I felt physically burned up—God damn it! I guess the dream wasn't too inappropriate!" Again silence, then, "Why should

[5] This is an example of validation of a dream; see pp. 229–230.

I be so goddamned mad at *you*, though? [Pause] Because you are making me acknowledge my feelings. All my life I've tried to be unemotional."

That was the end of the session. Before coming to the next session, this doctor-analysand dreamed of seeing an emergency case in a room which (again, like my office) was on the second floor of a hotel (Bleeding Patient). His patient was lying on a couch "like this one, and it was over here, like this one. This is a disturbed patient and I am told he gets excited and starts bleeding every time he is approached. I'm afraid [E. F.], and I think of the Thorazine in my bag to quiet him."

He immediately interpreted the dream. The patient of his dream becoming excited and bleeding was a representation of his disturbance and fear of injury when he "approached" himself in analysis as an emotional being.

Not only was the problem becoming clearer, but the patient was also making a forward step in treatment: he was recognizing, although with anxiety, his responsibility for dealing with the problem—in the dream, this was *his* patient.[6]

One brief additional dream that came two weeks after the Bleeding Patient dream will illustrate the movement in therapy achieved through the pursuit of affect in a man with a life-long commitment to denying emotion. In this dream the patient was one of three men in the front seat of his car (The Eliminator). The man at the wheel was a bit vague, but the patient knew it was himself; beside him was another vague figure who he knew was the analyst; the third man, seated at the other side of the analyst, was clearly himself.

"We were all talking about the way the car operated and you knew more about it than I did, and that annoyed me. After all, it was my car. The car had some equipment that was not basic; it was an extra; it was called an eliminator. You reached forward and removed it from the dashboard. I was angry [E. F.] when you took off the eliminator. When I woke up I knew the eliminator represented something to eliminate emotions."

During the course of the first two months the patient had made definite gains. From the initial denial of all feeling he had been brought to some awareness of the existence of his own feelings and of the need to confront them. This terrified him, as reflected in his nightmare of plunging dangerously down a concrete slope in front of a hotel to which he had come in a take-it-easy rocker. He was re-

---

[6] This was a greater step forward than in the Poor Guide, where the problem was "his baby." Here he is recognizing *pathology* more sharply and taking fuller responsibility for dealing with it.

vealed in the first three dreams as feeling alone in the analysis and threatened with destruction while trying to remain detached. After considerable confrontation with his feelings, after much dreaming and emotional turbulence, he progressed to the eliminator dream. In the latter he was no longer alone, nor was he taking it easy, nor was he threatened with destruction. He was at the wheel, responsible for his own progress. He was in the company of his analyst, whom he acknowledged (although grudgingly) to be better informed about the patient's structure and mechanisms. He tolerated the removal by the analyst of his apparatus for eliminating emotions. Although that action made him angry, certainly it did not lead to panic. He recognized in the dream that the eliminator was not basic equipment, but an extra that could be removed without jeopardy to his functioning. He had begun to face the basic problem of dealing with his emotional life, and in the course of facing this he became engaged in the psychoanalytic process, both independently and cooperatively. He had begun to seek out and to report his feelings spontaneously.

Denial of a Feeling's Intensity

The preceding survey of a dream-filled introductory phase of analysis was selected to illustrate the common problem of the patient's reluctance to discern, identify, and communicate affect.

Sometimes a dream reflects an already acknowledged feeling, but with an intensity so much greater than suspected that it is qualitatively a new feeling, and the understanding of it is a qualitatively new experience.

A young dentist, very proud of his composure, came to analysis specifically because of depressions. He never became overtly angry; he was conscientious professionally, gracious, generous, and had a remarkable sense of humor. To one of his early sessions he brought a dream which was at first totally incomprehensible (White Hot Car). He had already begun to explore himself, and knew that *some* anger was present in him. In the dream he was represented by a car into whose inner workings he peered. He had parked his car in a driveway between two houses.

"I saw that my car was smoking. It was quite hot and fumes were pouring out. I lifted the hood, I think, but nothing was amiss except that the car was giving off heat fumes. I replaced the hood and got into the car. There was no dashboard. The steering wheel was there, and the brake and clutch, but otherwise I could see the entire motor. I remembered a friend from my boyhood in the neighborhood who had told me that there is a valve that can be unscrewed when the car is too hot, to drain off the water. This valve was in the rear of the motor and I could see it. I unscrewed it but there was no need to drain it. The water was intact in the motor and was not hot. I replaced the cap and then suddenly saw that the metal of the engine was glowing. The heat was terrific. *The entire car was white hot.* [An excellent illustration of symbolized feeling—rage.] I got out and walked about to the front. From there I could see that there was a roaring blaze like a molten iron furnace. The car suddenly shrunk down to child's size and began to move backward by itself. I was suddenly frightened [E.F.] and shouted to those in the alley. They moved back out of the way. I expected that it would hit into the garage, but the garage faded away and the car, moving with tremendous speed, raced out onto a field toward a brick building in the distance. I could visualize the crash and explosion as it hit the building, similar to what a plane would do under similar circumstances, but it missed the building and disappeared around the corner onto a picnic ground where I knew children were grouped. I awaited screams and sounds of collision, but nothing happened and I awoke with a fright. My mouth was dry and my heart pounding."

The theme of this dream—"white-hot" fury and destructiveness (which he had previously described as "irritability" or "sometimes getting sore")—once discovered, carried through his whole analysis. It is introduced at this point to illustrate a misapprehension of the intensity of feeling.

Discrepancy Between the Individual's Emotion and His Concept of It

The practice of psychiatry involves in large measure problems of exploration and clarification in areas of the patient's consciousness in which his subjective picture of his emotional life deviates from the reality of his emotional life.

The coexistence of contradictory emotions is a common phenomenon which, although entirely compatible with health, is a frequent source of emotional distortion and obscuration. Every moment in the life of a human being, once he has begun to develop a conscious existence, is filled with a complication and a richness of feelings. The existence of contradictory emotions, if the individual is aware of them and is functioning in accordance with his knowledge of their presence (or even if he is unaware but is in a state of willingness to confront such contradictions), does not constitute pathology. When, however, two (for the sake of simplicity) contradictory emotions coexist and the individual is unaware of, and disposed against the recognition of, one of them, especially if it is the one which is predominantly motivating him, this situation may be taken as a definition of an unhealthy psychological state. The individual has some stake in not recognizing the dominant emotion. The feeling of which he is aware describes him in some way that to him represents a more defined self, greater strength, and better functioning. The contradictory feeling is unacceptable, and recognition of it would weaken and disintegrate his conception of his personality.

An individual in treatment often suffers from an incapacity to encompass consciously the simultaneous existence of opposite or in some way conflicting feelings. As he sees it, he can only be an all "this" or an all "that," black or white, strong or weak, loving or hating, remote or destroyed (as in the Burning Man dream, pp. 56–57).

A man says, "I love her, I don't know why I torture her so." He must regard himself as loving, even in the face of the evidence of his cruelty. If he regards himself as loving, he feels justified in demanding all benefits owed to a loving person. If he were to admit the existence of any hating, he feels he would have to believe there was no loving at all, and consequently neither the position nor the benefits of a loving person would be his.

Yet, if he sometimes tortures the "loved one," then he is clearly not a completely loving person. At least he is not loving at the moment when he tortures. In his acts of sadism, while some degree of affection may also exist, a desire to hurt is the motivating emotion. The moment he acknowledges that motivation, he must label himself all sadist, instead of all lover; therefore he maintains his conceptualization of his emotions by the formulation: "I love her, I don't know why I torture her." The reality is that this man's personality sometimes responds to this woman with a predominance of affection, sometimes with a predominance of desire to hurt. His behavior reflects the emotion predominating at the moment.

The recognition of the coexistence of contradictory emotions has far-reaching implications for therapy. It is important not only in detecting emotional pathology but also in detecting emotional health and in judging the course of the patient's progress.

In the clinical pursuit of affect, the analyst knows he must ultimately depend upon the patient for knowledge of the patient's emotions. Until the patient learns to observe them accurately and to report them honestly, the analyst's observations of emotions can be no more than hypothetical estimates. The patient, when questioned, may reply that he doesn't know what he feels, or that he feels "nothing." When he does report, and if his description is challenged, he may remonstrate that "*I* ought to know how I feel!" Even if the therapist is accurate in observing the patient's emotions, suggestions to the patient such as "You seem angry," or "You seem depressed," or "You seem relieved," do not become usable data until the patient subjectively discovers these feelings in himself.

The patient's mere statement of the fact that there is a discrepancy between his activity and his avowed feelings is also not sufficient. He may spontaneously pause before a discrepancy, stating, for example, "I don't know why I was so mean, I wasn't mad at him." It is not enough, either, for the patient to be deductive: "I told him to shut up, so I guess I must have been mad." The patient must contact his feelings; he must palpate them, sense them out, feel his feelings with his feelings.[7] With this kind of emphasis in the clinical setting, the patient learns from direct experience the important fact that many discrepancies exist between what he really feels and what he thinks he feels. He discovers that he often has profound feelings at moments when he thinks he feels nothing. The experiential acquisition of this knowledge is an invaluable gain for both the period of therapy and for all of life thereafter.

The example that follows, although it is not derived from a dream, illustrates the problem.

A bachelor in analysis reported a casual afternoon excursion with a young married couple. In the course of the afternoon, spent driving and stopping for a snack, the wife had repeatedly made derogatory remarks about her husband. The husband did not defend himself or retaliate. My patient explained in the course of the session that he had "felt very sorry" for the man who was the target of these constant, destructive, emasculating jibes, and had sprung to the husband's defense every time the wife attacked him. As he described the incidents of the afternoon, he emphasized his feeling of sympathy for the husband and some outrage toward the wife for her cruelty, for her "snipping off his balls."

Examination of the whole relationship revealed marked discrepancies between the patient's reported feelings and his actual feelings as well as the related behavior. It became clear that the patient's behavior had actually increased the pain which the husband suffered. Every time the wife made a derogatory remark, the young man intensified the humiliation of the husband by focusing attention on the remark. Secondly, by constantly springing to the defense of the husband, he

[7] This is discussed more fully in this chapter; see pp. 95–96.

provoked the wife into making further attacks upon her spouse. Thirdly, by being the exclusive source of defense, the young man was emphasizing the defenselessness of the husband. He had, throughout the afternoon, actually exacerbated rather than mitigated the painfulness of the husband's situation.

Not only was the patient's behavior inconsistent with genuine compassion, but his emotions too, when examined, were discovered to be quite different from those originally conceptualized and reported. Rather than wishing to ameliorate the situation, he acknowledged to himself and to me that he enjoyed aggravating it and watching the husband squirm. He felt, in addition, that the husband, because he put up with the wife's derogation, without defense or counterattack, was a fool and a weakling.

The patient, who thought he had been feeling and acting compassionately, had instead been indulging feelings of sadism and contempt.

A dream illustrating the same kind of discrepancy was experienced by a patient who had built up a financial debt to me and had expressed the profoundest conscientious desire to pay (Fruit Store Man). Before tackling the debt, however, he had a dream in which his wife answered the telephone and reported, "It's the man from the fruit store. He seems very excited. He wants his money." The patient replies, "What the hell is he yapping about! Tell him you'll send him a check. That'll shut him up. He can wait." The patient was shocked and chagrined to discover in the course of the session that the "fruit store man" was his analyst. The dream feelings of contempt and duplicity were in marked contrast to his concept of his own feelings of admiration for his doctor's generosity and conscientiousness regarding payment of the debt. Comparable discrepancies are illustrated in Hot Dog and in Contemptible Passion.

Family life is the arena of many discrepancies which have the most pathogenic influence on the developing personalities of children. The marriage contest often begins as soon as "the honeymoon is over." With the marriage under way, the husband may perform a number of ostensibly affectionate, solicitous acts toward his wife, which he would describe as an expression of his wanting her to be happy. In reality, he may be engaging in a softening-up process to establish his dominance in making decisions, having intercourse, and maintaining her generally in a subdued and uncomplaining role in the family and in their social life. When he is unsuccessful, he sulks, develops headaches, complains about small things, or exhibits occasional angry outbursts. The wife, in response, involves herself in adulatory and acquiescent activity, all of which she would describe (and believe it!) as manifestations of understanding and affection for her husband. A closer examination of her feelings would often reveal resentment over the subdued role she must maintain, contempt for his male pompousness, his nobility and "goodness," and often a gloating sense of power in her cleverness and ability to control her husband by responding in accordance with his own unexpressed vanity and tyranny. It is somewhat unlikely that the "primal scene" would ever deleteriously affect any child who had not already been deeply affected by all of these subtly hostile exchanges outside the bedroom between the mommy and the daddy who supposedly love each other.

The children in this kind of family milieu develop, unwittingly, techniques of acquiescence, bribery, and seduction which they think of as expressions of love for their parents. They are "good" in order to gain favors, to gain an ally in one parent or elude restrictions by the other, or to have advantages over siblings. When the child, with perhaps a further goal in mind, says, "I love you, Mommy," the designation as well as the behavior is readily endorsed by a parent whose experience of "love" in the first place has consisted in large measure of blandishments and return favors.

The blandishments and other maneuvers sometimes fail. In the pervasively manipulative, competitive struggle in which most people of our culture are involved throughout their lives, there is tension and anxiety resulting from the frustration of these strivings. On the other hand, when an individual succeeds without much struggle in prevailing over another, or succeeds after a great deal of struggle, he feels a surge of something which he mistakenly believes is affection or love. What he is often predominantly experiencing is a combination of relief, gratitude, and triumph, which are aspects of competitiveness (see p. 86). Associated with this is a desire to reward the other individual for making this success possible. The common professions of love under these conditions, especially by parents toward children whom they have handled, lead to confusion and to discrepancy between the conceptualization of emotions and their reality, in both the parents and the children. Carried to an extreme by parents, particularly if subtly done, this can be a most effective schizophrenogenic force.

This general type of parent-child relationship is, I think, the prototype for most affective discrepancies, and is the genetic and sustaining matrix of the distorting cultural influence—*cynicism*.

Cynicism

Cynicism may be defined as a disbelief in the existence of motivation that is genuinely affectionate or friendly. It denies the possibility of a primary concern for another's welfare, or of an unselfish, nonopportunistic desire to enhance the pleasure and fulfillment of another through helping him to exercise or increase his functions. Whether aware or unaware of his cynicism, a patient, because of it, misinterprets or fails to register many of his own responses in therapy, and this becomes a major obstacle in the clinical detection and evaluation of feelings.

The emotional and evaluative confusion starts early in the type of family life described above, where parents or other affectionally related people exploit the children for the fulfillment of their own "needs," [8] under the guise and with the self-delusion that this is love. The parents, themselves under pressure from their competitive culture, are driven not only to achieve some measure of success economically, professionally, and socially in the group, the neighborhood, and within the family but also to achieve success in fulfilling an image of dedicated and affectionate parenthood.

The developing child and adolescent, bound by his affectional and material needs to his parents, conforms to their plan of living, getting some form of approval and what seems to be affection in response. Regardless of the professions of solicitude, however, the child is somehow aware that his life is designed in many major respects in accordance with the parents' requirements, which may be meaningless to him, and the actual motivations of which may not even be clearly perceived by the parents. His deviations, his independent functioning, are subtly if not directly corrected by parental reactions of pain, disapproval, or coldness. Often some form of moral blackmail is exercised by word, grimace, or gesture indicating, "How can you do this to me?" The implication is, "After all my love, all my efforts and concern on your behalf, how can you be such an ingrate, so cruel?" To the extent that this kind of reciprocity exists, the growing individual is not involved in a truly affectional relationship, although all the forms of communication from the parent are implicitly designated as such. The affectional

---

[8] The term "needs" is placed in quotation marks here to distinguish it from the genuine human needs to give and to receive affection; the "needs" in this case are the *demands* of disturbed adults for control, for recognition as good parents, and for other pathological satisfactions.

bond as it is subtly combined with exploitative and manipulative practices constitutes probably the dominant factor in the growth of cynicism.

A child can be brought up to accept discipline, restrictions, and authority from his parents without feeling that these strictures negate their solicitude or their benevolent intentions toward him. Authority that is open, firm, even harsh at times, can be completely consistent with tenderness and affectional concern. The corrupting element is the use of techniques of control unrelated to the genuine emotional and other needs of the child, but practiced under the guise of parental love as though "for the child's own good."

The oversolicitous parent is a prime example. The child will not only feel the oppression and the restrictions of his parents upon himself —he will also see their comparable controlling, oversolicitous practices with others. Cumulatively, the experiences, observations, and accompanying emotions of the child will lead to a recognition, sometimes openly formulated, often never formulated, but tantamount to such a declaration as, "When anybody starts 'loving' you, watch out!"

In another family, a father, entirely decent in many respects, might cultivate logic and fairness in his parent-child relationship. If he is a skillful logician, and always gets the best of an argument with his less expert son or daughter, the child may grow up very cautious toward anyone who offers him the opportunity to sit down and discuss things "honestly and openly."

Another child may be governed by a seductive parent who is capable always of getting his way with the child by affectionate kidding or gentle suasion. The child may grow up with a profound mistrust of all good-humoredness and kindliness. To him they are techniques of manipulation.

In another family the child might be exposed to a parental martyr who demands, in return for self-sacrifice, the child's obedience and other less obvious types of conformity to the parent's will. Still other children grow up exposed to excessive generosity on the part of parents. They are overwhelmed with all that their hearts desire. In time they begin to recognize that while they have closets full of toys and months full of movies, the credit balance of claims for response is greatly in the parents' favor, and may involve a serious sacrifice of personal integrity, though the children would not, at the time, be able to formulate what is happening to them. These "cared for," "reasoned with," "gently guided," tirelessly served, and generously pampered children tend to grow up disbelieving and wary.

An example is a young doctor's description of his past and present relationship with his parents, particularly with his mother. The parents were endlessly concerned with his welfare, endlessly tending him.

"When I was a kid she always wanted me to come home from school and rest, not play. It was 'better' for me. When I went to the park with the fellows after school and didn't tell her, she would complain she didn't know where I was, and said I made a nervous wreck out of her. Even now, when I'm a doctor, twenty-eight years old, she acts the same. When I do something different from what she wants— like buying a suit by myself—I'm being 'mean' to her. Self-assertion is hostility! If I want to spend time in my own way, instead of visiting them, I'm trampling their feelings. Taking care of my own needs is being selfish and inconsiderate."

At the same time, while depriving him of adult respect, his parents were introducing him around for their own aggrandizement as "my son, the doctor." This man was able to "see through" everyone, and he established no close ties. Most of the time this patient's cynicism was more profound than he recognized or professed. At other times, however, he showed a recognition of and response to genuine feelings. The two contradictory attitudes produced in him a basic affective disorientation. Later, however, he established a good marriage with a genuinely warm and loving young woman. A prerequisite transition was the sharpening of his latent ability to distinguish between authentic warmth and the sterility of mere outward form, not only in others, but also in himself. The emotional sterility, disguised by the outward forms and expressions of solicitude in which he grew up with his parents, was dramatically symbolized in a dream a few months before his prospective marriage.[9]

A pathologically cautious young woman had been a child prodigy, psychologically whipped into excellence by her parents for "her own good." She became one who could well protect herself from the encouraging generosity of others, and could detect the pretense behind the kindness in anyone. She dreamed of the analyst as a kindly family doctor sitting by her bed, peering at her through eyeglasses that were curious because of a Y-shaped slit in the lenses (Token Kindness). This slit was characteristic of the New York City subway token, and revealed her estimate of the analyst, whom outwardly she had begun to trust, as manifesting only "token" kindness. The patient's coexistent, contradictory, trusting and cynically distrusting feelings are implicit in the symbolized feelings with which she endows the analyst through her dream: he has truly warm feelings—the kindly family doctor—or he offers a synthetic bedside manner—"token" kindness.

[9] See the dream of the Three Condoms, pp. 153–154.

The cynic's tendency toward blanket devaluation of all friendly activity cannot but result in misinterpretation of behavior. His emotions are then the responses to his misinterpretations. Upon witnessing generosity, for example, he may experience, instead of warmth, either contempt or admiration for what he regards as a clever investment in future favors. At the same time he may respond to the recipient of the generosity with scorn or pity for his being a sucker.

He may devalue any decent impulses of his own in the same manner. When he helps a friend, he may claim this is merely an investment in future favors, and subjectively blanket his feeling of genuine friendliness under a predominating enjoyment of his own shrewdness—he perceives the motivation for his behavior one-sidedly, and has therefore a distorted concept of his own emotions.[10]

The observation of cruelty, selfishness, manipulation, and exploitation would not by itself make an individual cynical. Destructive qualities and their associated practices do exist, and anyone unaware of them is self-deluded, strangely inexperienced, or a plain fool. The sensation of being used and manipulated, the observation that these maneuvers are performed behind a facade of decent qualities, the recognition that a promise of the satisfaction of a human affectional need may be only a bait—it is such experiences that provide people with the reality basis for doubting decent behavior when it is expressed toward them, asked of them, or observed in the relationships about them.

Cynicism, however, is not the observation that fraudulent solicitude exists; it is the interpretation of *all* friendliness as fundamentally self-seeking and consequently fraudulent. This kind of misinterpretation of constructive human motives does not result from just the frequent observation of fraudulence side by side with friendly and cooperative behavior. Cynicism develops to the extent that such fraudulence is a significant portion of the behavior of the people emotionally closest to the individual, especially in the early course of his life. It is reenforced by the child's engagement in the same practices.

In the developmental period, a far greater span of years for the human than for any other animal, the environment provides influences also for the growth of healthy consciousness. The physiological and social needs of the child may receive adequate attention from his closely associated seniors, particularly his parents, perhaps aunts and uncles, older siblings, friends, teachers, and neighbors. This help may come gladly, or at least willingly, with his welfare in mind. His parents' guidance may be genuinely aimed at encouraging the young person's

---

10 See coexistence of contradictory emotions, pp. 60–61.

capacity to function independently in the physical, intellectual, and social spheres.

The following passage will describe, somewhat diagrammatically, the evolution of healthy, constructive, positive behavior, feelings, and conceptualizations in a human being within an ideal family situation.

The early experiences of solicitude are associated not only with the sensations of touch, taste, and smell, but also with sounds, gestures, grimaces, and language. On the basis of these communications, the child begins to form his conceptualizations of the nature of relationships among people. He feels the pleasure of his elders in being with him, their specific concern for him, their fostering and delight in his enjoyment of his increasing capacity to function independently. All of this conveys to him the essence of what we call love in the human community. Because the institutions of man are such that solicitous activity cannot be practiced toward everyone, since this would expose one to exploitation in a great many situations, the child sees that the practices of love are usually confined to a relatively small circle. The practice of friendly, trusting, and cooperative behavior, he learns, extends more widely and with varying degrees of intensity toward others —a circle of friends, play, occupational, and interest groups, and the wider community. The capacity to become warmly attached to others grows richly within the immediate family. It is expressed as maternalism and paternalism toward the child. In the love relationship between wife and husband the most tender, empathic, joyous feelings and the fullest degree of cooperative experience develop. The child's response to this kind of behavior between his parents and toward him from both parents becomes the germ of his own capacity to be responsive, cooperative, and solicitous—to love. His early affectionate, cooperative feelings and practices appear first, and probably most strongly, toward the parents, and extend to include siblings, friends, and other adults. In the course of these experiences the young person's conceptualizations of the nature of the relationships among people continue to develop. Cynicism does not emerge in such an environment!

Ideal family situations, however, cannot in reality arise in this pure form among the members of our culture. What we find more commonly are the subtly corrupting developmental influences which produce the cynicism that is characteristic of our time. It is the covertness of the influences, the subtlety of the exploitative practices, that cause the evolving individual to become skeptical (aware or unaware) about the solicitous nature of many human activities.

Society harbors many actual dangers of deception and exploitation. The significant grown-ups in any family function in an adult world which realistically demands a capacity to work in a wary, insular, and self-interested fashion. The consequent distortions in the adult personality are perpetuated by his daily living and then operate even within the parent-child relationship. Actually there is, of course, safety for the parent from serious deception and exploitation by the child. But each of us has only one personality. The parent operates, in his relationship with the child, with at least some of the personality distortions that characterize his operations in the adult world. These distortions inevitably color the child's experiences with his parents and other adults, and through these experiences his own consciousness is formed: he develops ways of living, and he acquires the data which go into the formation of his conceptualizations about living. As he moves into the adult world, he in turn will become more deeply involved in the social currents which engendered the manipulative, competitive, and cynical elements in his parents' personalities.

A disbelief in the possibility of genuinely friendly and cooperative living is severely restrictive and distorting to the functional potential, and generates many of the problems that lead people to the psychoanalytic office. So often an individual may practice all of the outward forms of friendliness, but even in the midst of them may, through his disbelief in his own friendliness and that of others, remain isolated. He may react emotionally with feelings of emptiness, dissatisfaction, failure, anger, and depression. He may say, "I have everything, and yet I feel like a failure." The answer often lies in his having everything except what is essential for human happiness—intimacy. Meaningful intimacy, generosity, respect, admiration, enjoyment of his company by others, may all in some measure surround him, but he does not experience them because he does not believe they are real.

This disbelief leads to further distortions in his practices, for he then responds not to the genuine regard people may show toward him but to what he sees as their pretenses, adopted in order to gain some personal advantage. (Ironically, the very fact that one reward of friendliness is pleasure often serves as proof to the cynic that friendliness is offered from selfish motivation.) To the extent that his response to those genuinely friendly people is inappropriate, it elicits from them various kinds of unfulfilling emotional reactions and behavior. They may feel rebuffed and hurt, and become impatient and angry. He feels that he has given them a fair amount of himself, whereas actually he has withheld responsiveness, which he refused to show toward something he judged synthetic. He feels outraged, rejected, and still more of a failure because of their appropriate reactions to his behavior; and also he feels confirmed in his judgment that the friendly overture was insincere from the outset. As he goes along in life, this vicious cycle, or, more accurately, vicious progression, continues, and his cynicism is re-enforced. He deflects the possibilities of meaningful relationships, and he piles up evidence that there is nothing really decent in life. The individual loses the capacity to acknowledge genuine warmth in others, or to permit it in himself.

The young doctor who could "see through" all expressions of friendliness was the product of oversolicitous parents. Developmental distortions may also come about through deliberate affectional deprivation "for the child's own good."

The following case is that of a young woman whose profound disbelief in love or friendship developed during her childhood in a middle-class, economically stable family which fulfilled most of the outward routines of family life and child care. The concern of her parents, however, particularly her father, took the distorted form of demanding that she cultivate emotional restraint, insisting that this was the highest type of character development for her. This cruel use of his child in the cultivation and support of his own self-concept as an imperturbable Superman caused the patient to live without intimacy, warm physical contact, humor, tenderness, or even honest expression of anger. She grew up in the emotional contradiction between the implied solicitude of the nurturing family constellation and her parents' repudiation of the warmth and affection implicit in such care.

The case is presented as an illustration of a severely disabling cynicism, and as a demonstration of the clinical value of dreams in dealing with the pathological emotional reticence discussed earlier. The following dreams occurred when the patient had been more than two years in psychoanalysis, with sessions occurring twice a week.

During the previous five months she had been to a large extent concentrating upon her life-long problem of thwarting all friendliness in herself and in others. Until this recent period she had avoided investigating her childhood with any depth or conscientiousness because, she stated frankly, the prospect frightened her too much. During the five months preceding the dream, however, she had undertaken to recall and examine her childhood. This effort had brought to light the material about the emotional aridity in her family life, and particularly in her relationship with her father. She reported also her extreme competitiveness in school, through which she had maintained the position of the brightest child in her class. The patient had sought desperately to be teacher's pet because of the lack of recognition and sympathy at home, yet she felt that this academic prominence had isolated her from classmates and neighborhood children. She had no friends until the age of ten. At that time she often played with a little girl and a younger little boy. This small group held together for about four years, after which the patient's family moved to another town. She made no new friends, felt ugly, unimportant, and unwanted, and again strove to be bright in school.

Although she had had almost no dates until she went away to college, it was only in the course of this investigation in her twenty-fourth year that she dared to consider the idea that she had suffered during her adolescence from loneliness. She had little faith in her own friendliness toward people or in their friendliness toward her, although she was beginning to have experiences from time to time which tended to change these attitudes. This was particularly so in her relationship with her current roommate, toward whom she was becoming friendly and kind, even though she tried to suppress and conceal this by means of silliness or brusqueness.

The patient felt that everyone was like herself, resentful of the self-confidence and happiness of others. Therefore people would hate her if she appeared at ease or happy. To want friends was weakness, to have friends was to expose oneself to the jealousy of others. To be counted among somebody's friends was nothing, and made one the object of scorn; only to be the closest, the number-one friend (like teacher's pet), was acceptable to her as evidence of genuine friend-ship. In order to feel that she was liked, she must be instantly accepted as the best friend, even on first acquaintance. When she was not given this position, the other person was a hypocrite. Thus she had main-tained her painful isolation.

It had taken her much time in analysis to recognize her inordinate demand that she be the first in the affections of others, as the only alternative to immediately rejecting them.

At the time that this nightmare occurred, she was struggling, as she had struggled before, to get rid of her doubts about the friendliness of her analyst. She started the session by saying, "I can't bear to think you're really friendly, that you respect me—reason tells me yes, but I don't want it to be yes, emotionally. I want my armor, my cynical ar-mor. I'm afraid of the terrible misery that's going to happen if I take off my armor, the misery of loneliness, that for the first time in my life I've begun to experience.

"I told you that I was miserable as an adolescent. What the hell was it I said I felt? Oh, I told you it was feeling unimportant. I said I felt ugly. Being with people was agonizing. Each time it was nerve-wracking. When I was by myself, when I was alone, I guess I was lonely. I'll have to change my statement that *now* is the first time in my life that I felt lonely." This was a spontaneous focusing on feeling, which also led to sharper recognition of her adolescent feelings as having been the pangs of loneliness.

She had often reported her constraint with people, her uncertainty about what to say, how to say it, what to do, and whether her performance had been correct, adequate, appropriate. She had spoken of various techniques of being pleasant, destructive, or silly. All of her ways of getting along, she felt, had been synthetic, contrived.

She went on, "I'm not at all happy when I'm plying my neurotic ways of getting along with people. I really want to run away. Lately I've been trying to act like an adult, but I can't stand acting like an adult. It's true that when I act like an adult I don't feel degraded [as she would always feel when being silly or destructive]. But I feel so unimportant, and like nothing. When I act like an ass, then at least afterwards I feel good, because I've attracted attention and made people feel they're better than me."

At this point she said, "I had a dream." Her moment of association (see p. 11) with the dream came as she described her contrived behavior, her "acting like an ass."

"I am in this house [Crazy Woman]. *It's a nice house, by a park.* I'm alone in the house with this crazy woman. She's acting wild and unreasonable. I don't know exactly like what, something in an insane asylum. *It was a very nice house set in a park that was very nice.* She was very hostile and at the same time she wanted to hold me. I felt she wanted to hold me to crush me, to kill me. She hated me very much. I dropped my keys and she wouldn't let me look for them. I found them again and dropped them again, and because I had lost them I had to stay in this house with her. I wondered how others in the house could stand her. *I liked the house and wanted to stay,* but I was very afraid of her. [Coexistence of contradictory experiential feelings.] Then Marjorie came in [an acquaintance]. She was very different in the dream. In reality she is very meek, but in the dream she was very strong and confident. In the dream she is there because she is supposed to be a tenant in the house. I start to introduce her to the crazy woman but can't remember the crazy woman's name. I'm introducing Marjorie to her, but in my embarrassment [E. F.] at not being able to remember her name, I introduce the crazy woman as

Marjorie. I leave the house without my keys. I'd rather leave without the keys than stay. The situation is too horrible. My feelings were great horror, disgust, and fear of this crazy woman" (E.F.).

We had already extended the session beyond her time, and were not to meet for four days. I therefore offered some interpretive suggestions for her to consider before the next hour. I reminded her that she had started the hour by telling me of her fear of accepting me as being like a friend—a fear of getting close to me. I therefore suggested that the crazy woman might represent myself. She also had indicated that the house was a nice house by a park (my office is on Park Avenue) and that she liked the house. I suggested that having friendly feelings might be associated with the house in which she wanted to stay—that the house, in spite of all the horror she felt toward it, might also represent not just a nice house, but a nice way to live.

I also hypothesized that the Marjorie of the dream, who in reality was very meek but in the dream was strong and confident, might represent the patient. The change might represent her growing confidence, which was indicated in this very session by her greater trust in exposing her feelings.

Four days later the patient came in, lay down and started at once by saying, "The crazy woman in the dream was you. I've thought a lot about it, and I think it's right.

"I see normal emotions as being a raving maniac, because if I expressed mine, God knows what I'd do. I see everybody as having bad emotions basically.

"I'm sorry I brought up the subject and I want to talk about something else, so I suppose I should stay on the subject."

She then went on to describe her roommate, who had been sporadically a friend for several years. They had grown closer in the course of the past year, and finally took an apartment together. She said that her roommate was a "highly emotional person. We couldn't be more opposite. She's more than normal. She has so many emotions. That makes me anxious. I feel contemptuous of anybody expressing herself so freely. For years I've not only been a good friend to her, but I've also been a bad friend, by bringing out the worst in her. With that crazy woman, you, I've had a great fear of what I'm getting into. That's why I feel this way about you.

"The crazy woman in the dream hated me and wanted to trap me, to keep me there. It was a case of I could stay or I could go. If I go, I go without my keys, empty-handed. If I stay, I'd be trapped, caught, seduced, killed, all horrible possibilities. In the dream she put her arms around me, not in an embrace of liking me, but in a trap of getting me and crushing me with hatred. Her saying that I could go was also horrible: All right, go—I don't give a damn about you. But in the dream this damn woman was important to me." (Coexistence of contradictory experiential feelings.)

Since the interpretation that the crazy woman was the therapist had come from me, I thought it might be productive for her to think about other possibilities, even though the suggestion had remained with her, and had been to some extent fruitful. I therefore said, "Could the crazy woman have possibly been someone other than myself?" She replied immediately, "No person could be as important to me as you are."

She continued without interruption, "You suggested that Marjorie could be me. She is not only meek but also sort of grouchy. I'm usually one of two ways with people—either I'm aloof and grouchy, or silly and childish." (It will be recalled that the nightmare of the Crazy Woman had come up as an association just after she had described "acting like an ass," a synthetic technique of getting along with people.) I made no comment, and she continued, "I'm always ashamed of being silly, childish. To me *the way to be* [and she emphasized the last four words histrionically] is grouchy. That's the way I am in my mother's house, and it's the way I deprive her of me."

Here I interjected that both grouchiness and silliness were ways of keeping herself from people.

"Silly-childish is the way I am to attract attention, with people who are important to me. I'm never that way in my mother's house. There it's a tremendous effort to raise the slightest smile."

I said, "You speak of being silly-childish to attract attention. I think that you attract attention with grouchiness, too, but you only risk the grouchy technique with those you're sure of, those who won't turn you away for being grouchy."

"Whenever I have to see you," she responded, "the only way I'll meet you is with grouchiness."

I said, "You're sure of me."

She paused a little and then said, with a tone of dawning understanding, "This puts a whole new light on it, that I'm grouchy to attract attention! I hate people to be happy, and I think others are like me—I think people don't want me to look pleased, so I look grouchy, so as not to offend people. If I think people don't want me to be happy," . . . and then she stopped and groaned with shame. "Oh, this is terrible. I think terrible things of you, that you don't want me to have any pleasure, so when I see you I turn on grouchiness, for fear you'll resent my enjoyment. It's the next best thing to not existing. I think you don't want me to exist, and the next best thing to not existing is to be unhappy!

"So here in the dream Marjorie comes in grouchy. So I'm more secure being grouchy, and when I say grouchy, I don't mean complaining. I simply mean being funless."

"What were the keys in the dream?"

"I kept dropping them, so I had to stay. Wait a minute. I hope this isn't true. It means I don't work hard enough here. I keep dropping the keys."

I asked her if she meant keys to understanding.

"Yes. Free associating is a dangerous type of thinking, dropping into feeling, feeling lonely like shit. That's what I have to avoid."

Her next remark hypothesized a new interpretation for the crazy woman in her nightmare. *Maybe the crazy woman is just feeling in general*. Which is what I stand for, I think. If you leave, you give up the keys to understanding yourself, to changing yourself. If you stay, you're exposed to this crazy woman, to feeling, which you're afraid will destroy you."

At this point she had an association—a new acquaintance. "I like Barbara. I try very hard to be an adult so she'll be my friend, but I can't be with her without being a nervous wreck. I developed something new. I sort of stutter and get twisted up in my words, so I guess I'm determined to mess things up. It's another device. I can't stand being a woman and wanting a mature friend and acting in a mature way."

Referring again to the dream I said, "You feel that I hate you and want to destroy you because I keep asking you to express your feelings."

She answered at once, with great intensity, "You don't know what you're asking. You're asking me to do the most humiliating thing. It's as though you asked me to go to the toilet in front of you. No, it's even more humiliating than that. You can't help being contemptuous of a person you're asking to do things she feels most ashamed of."

It was the end of the session. I said, "I think you've been more profoundly affected by your father's attitudes than you know. You think that it's weak and contemptible to express emotions, and you feel this more deeply than you have ever been aware of, or ever expressed here."

She said, "But I've added something more to it: A person assumes too much importance if he expresses feelings. You assume you have the *right* to express your feelings, and if you do that, there's always a risk of being slapped down!" (This was probably the anxious basis for her stuttering when talking to Barbara.)

The patient came into the second session following the Crazy Woman dream and began by telling me that two nice things had happened, and that she felt good about both of them. Her roommate was engaged and had announced plans to be married. Secondly, her brother had been accepted by the engineering college of his choice.

I said that I felt her reactions, in contrast to previous feelings of jealousy, indicated a new capacity for spontaneous kindness. I added that I felt she was slowly changing. (This was the emergence of a new emotion—enjoyment of another's enhancement. It was probably, in part, a response to her cautious but growing perception of the analyst's enjoyment of her enhancement.)

She said, "You were just kind to me, and so I feel you must hate me now. People must hate after giving to others." Then she went on to say that there was something she was determined to talk about. Throughout the analysis, she declared, when describing situations, she had often left out specific details which she could not bring herself to tell me. She would speak in generalizations, instead. Today she was determined to tell everything, "the details and the conclusions."

"Maybe by telling you this it will be sort of practice in telling you very embarrassing things. I'll get used to the idea. I've been telling you things that are true, but they're not everything. They are conclusions and deductions from other things that I've never told you. 'Why should I tell him what isn't very important?' This is what I would say to myself. I would say, 'It is too embarrassing. It's hard enough to tell him the important part of it, the thing that is expressed in the incident. I don't have to tell him the embarrassing details.'

"But maybe I'm not able to deduce everything myself. So, instead of just conclusions, I'll give it all, straight."

At this point it appeared that she had gained some insight through the Crazy Woman dream into her irrational and fearful avoidance of feeling. She was about to trust me enough to express herself openly.

She said, "My mind is very preoccupied with shit. I use the word a lot to represent something disgusting. But saying it doesn't really mean anything. What I really hate to tell you is how much I'm preoccupied with shit. Last night, almost for the first time, it came up in a dream."

She explained that she and her roommate had a cat. She herself had not wanted the cat because of the expense, the bother, and the smell. But her roommate was eager to have one as a pet, and to keep the mice away. There was a disagreement about emptying the cat's sand box. The patient wanted it emptied every day, but her roommate was content to let it wait for a few days—so the patient emptied the box rather than put up with the smell.

In talking about the cat she said, "I've had a horror of pets based on two things. This is what I deserve. It's like some horrible people I've been stuck with. I've been nonhuman, and deserve only animal company, and so I don't want animals around to remind me of it."

Her second reason for horror of pets was her mother's almost hysterical fear of animals. "My mother has always warned me how they bite, scratch, stink up a place. They can't be trusted. Anything that is living and that has flesh is disgusting to her. She stayed over at our apartment on a weekend and had a terrific fear of this kitten. I didn't really think it was possible for a person to feel so afraid. She would freeze up when the kitten came near her."

The patient has already presented a considerable amount of association to the announced, but as yet unreported, dream.[11] She went on at this point to report the dream (Shit Piles Up).

"The shit piles up in the cat's sand box." Since her roommate won't clean it up, the patient won't either. "The shit piles up and smells and I'm disgusted and I feel hatred for the cat. I hate this animal that makes all this shit. I feel disgust and hatred. That's the whole dream." (Hatred and disgust are experiential feelings. Shit, as it develops below, is symbolized feeling: it is hostility, as well as the accompanying destructiveness. The cat is a good example of the patient in animal form.)

She went right on. "This is related to gas in the intestines. Sometimes I get it naturally, and sometimes psychosomatically. The thing that's increased recently and to a horrible extent is that I have a fear of farting, whether I have gas in me or not. I feel I have to have a constant, unrelenting guard on myself. I feel everybody else has to have some guard, like the feeling I've told you about, that everybody is full of badness. This is absolutely inseparable in my mind from being spontaneous. Showing emotions, this is absolutely inseparable from my fear of farting. This is the same as being destructive. But I'm confused. Why should I have a fear that I'm going to be destructive when I really am destructive?"

I said, "You do 'fart,' and you do destructive things. Of course you're destructive, but that's not all you are. You also do constructive things."

She continued, feeling her way with intensity and puzzlement,

11 This was the association before the report of the dream; see pp. 10–11.

"I have a great fear that if I'm spontaneous and express myself, I'll fart. It's not quite clear, because I know I also do some good things. But there's no such thing as goodness. That's superficial. The only *real* emotions are bad. If everyone were to be his real self, they would just be bad. They'd all fart.

"My fear of farting increases considerably in this office because you're encouraging me to be spontaneous, to express myself freely. So much is expressed through my bowels that I often have a slight diarrhea before or after coming here. But maybe that's good, better than having constipation, which would mean I'm holding back."

I remarked lightly, "That's a silver lining, all right," and she burst into hearty laughter, in which I joined her. After this moment or two of laughter I picked up the theme seriously again and said, "But now let's see whether it is true that if you let yourself be spontaneous, your feelings will be destructive, like farting in public. You started the hour by telling of two spontaneous, friendly, joyful feelings, one about your roommate's marriage, and the other about your brother's acceptance in engineering school."

She rebutted with an association of having baked a birthday cake for her roommate: but when her roommate was surprised and touched, and started to express her thanks and affection, the patient, constrained and frightened, turned the situation quickly into a total emotional non-sequitur by simply withdrawing and doing a silly jig. She could not tolerate the genuine warmth of her roommate's response. She ended the account saying, "I absolutely can't stand friendliness. It makes me so nervous."

"Why?"

"I don't want anything good, because I don't want to want these things. If I want them, I'll have frustration. That's something I'm just beginning to know, I'm just beginning to feel."

"That's like the loneliness that you're only now recognizing. You're only beginning to realize how much you want people, how much you want friendliness and warmth." (This was the emergence of new feeling, in part through perception of people as capable of genuine friendliness.)

"I always used to say to myself, 'What's unpleasant about frustration? So I won't have something. Who cares!' But I *can't* drop my armor. Before, I didn't know frustration could be painful. Now I know it is." The session ended there.

Ten days before, she had had the Crazy Woman nightmare, in which she had been horrified and disgusted at the prospect of getting close to feelings, which to her represented insanity, crazy destructiveness. Through our work with this nightmare, she had ventured closer to her friends and had risked a fuller communication of her feelings to me. She was ready to deal more courageously with the agonizing context of the succeeding dream, Shit Piles Up.

The patient had always been willing to acknowledge her destructiveness and her "shittiness" so long as these qualities were her "armor" and her strength. These same qualities now represented something different. Although there was no direct interpretive activity, the abundant associative activity before and after the telling of the dream suggests that, in the second dream, her "shittiness" represents not strength but the source of her newly acknowledged loneliness, and an obstacle to the satisfaction of a new desire—for friendship. Characteristic of evolving health, however, ambivalence was present, and there was not a total replacement of old strivings by the new. She had spoken of herself, like the cat, causing a stink, farting; she did this to stifle her *wanting*—"I don't want to want." In the dream, "shit piled up" and she refused to remove it. However, in the dream "I hate this animal that makes all this shit"; this is her recognition that her "shitty" practices are imposing upon her the frustration of her newly discovered friendliness and desire for people.

As she left, I said that I felt she had come a long way, and that it looked as though she was really beginning to feel like a member of the human race.

Three days later at her next session, she came in and started by saying, "I felt angry and upset when you said that I'm becoming a member of the human race. My fear of farting started only recently. It started when I began taking off my armor, and wanting people. Somehow I know that the more I pursue healthy goals, the more people like me and respond to me, the more I'm going to be destructive—that's why the fear of farting. That's why I have to have the hardest control, the greatest guard, on what I say. The healthier I become, the more I want to be destructive, and the tighter control I have to have on myself."

"Why?"

"I don't want to be healthy. The nicer a person is to me, the more I want to hit them on the head. If people aren't nice to me, it's much easier for me to be nice. I can't stand the feeling of people being nice to me. I don't want the feeling of wanting a friend."

"Why?"

"Because I don't want to get used to these luxuries, because they're not for me."

"At least it's clear now that you want friends," I said. "But what is this feeling that they're not for you?"

"First let me say one thing—guarding myself is the opposite of spontaneity. If I'm spontaneous, I'll shit things up like mad. Why aren't people for me? It's the opposite—I'm not for people."

This recalls to the analyst her feeling about hating pets—she feels she is not fit for human company.

"I suppose I could be for people. I try, but something stops me from being that good—something stops me from being a healthy me. The other thing always gets in the way. I automatically start out feeling contemptible, which isn't pleasant. I don't show the self-respect I should have. Every time I come here to talk about myself for fifty minutes, I'm so wretched you've no idea. Every sentence takes a monumental effort to get out, because I fear your contempt so for my talking about myself. So that's one thing that gets in the way, my not having self-respect.

"But this is just a little tangent. I have this very peculiar thing and I thought of it a little while back. It's not the whole why, but it's part of the why that I feel I'm not for people. It's my great discomfort when I'm taller than someone. [She is not at all above average height.] When I was a child it was a big thing. My parents and others were always comparing who was taller. We were always having to stand back to back, and it was taken for granted that whoever was bigger was better, so it stuck with me, the feeling that people must hate me if I'm taller than they are."

"That's probably connected," I said, "with the feeling that they'll hate you if you're taller in other ways than physical stature."

"That's right, that's right!" she said. "That's why I have to degrade myself, so people won't hate me! I'm thinking very clearly now. [This was the enjoyment of a new perception in the very areas she formerly dreaded to explore. A wide range of emotion was becoming, very slowly, tolerable, more readily accessible, and sometimes welcome.] I told you how terrifically competitive I was in school, and how none of my classmates had any use for me. There should have been a happy medium where I didn't have to be either too competitive or where I didn't have to degrade myself."

I asked if she had started to degrade herself when she was a child, so that her classmates wouldn't hate her for being smarter.

"Not while I was a child. I had to be smart for teacher's recognition. I got nothing at home, just criticism. I can't even remember getting dribbles of recognition at home.

"I didn't start this degrading business until I went to college and started to be more sociable after being isolated all through my high school years. When I was away at college, this was the first time in my life that I really *wanted* social life, so I had to think of devices of how I could get it."

I said, "Let's get back and look again at this feeling you have that you're going to shit things up. It seems to me that that feeling means a change from something that you're already doing. Why do you change?"

She answered at once and intensely, "Friendliness is not spontaneous. The desire is there, but I'm afraid. I can't do anything friendly spontaneously. Friendliness won't come out—only shit comes out."

"But," I reminded her, "you say the desire to be friendly is there. That desire *is* real and spontaneous."

"I can't stand the desire. From past experience spontaneity results in shitting things up. Now I want, and so now I can't stand to let shit come out."

"I understand. Now you have a great stake in being friendly, in having friendliness, and you don't want to shit it up."

"Yes. I have a big stake now. The trouble is I don't know whether what I'm going to do will be destructive or not."

"But you have recognized right here that something friendly *can* come out spontaneously. You do have spontaneous friendliness. Not everything that comes out will be shit."

"Yes, I see that I can have spontaneous friendliness. But now I have a new kind of trouble. I can't distinguish. I never knew that what I was saying was shitty and destructive until I thought about it later, and then I felt horrible. I'll just be making conversation, sometimes—after it comes out I see it's shitty. Maybe some day I'll reach the point where I don't have to watch so hard to see that shit doesn't come out. Maybe then it will be because I'm more conscious of my feelings. Maybe even when I think I'm being nice I'll be able to recognize my feelings of wanting to shit things up and be able to stop it. Maybe even I won't want to shit things up so much."

She then had an association of her roommate giving her a message from a mutual acquaintance. "Roberta sends her love." The patient said, "When my roommate told me this, I got into a panic. My English gets all mixed up. It's hard enough to receive such a message, but I couldn't say clearly what I wanted to say: 'Give my love to her.' Saying something like this makes me feel like an ass. I change the tense, or something. There is something wrong in my saying things like that, although nobody thinks that Roberta is a fool to say them. You see what happens when I try to be friendly?"

At this point I tried to formulate the difficulty. "There are really two problems. The first is that you want friends. You want to be friendly and to receive friendliness, and you are afraid of 'farting'—of 'shitting up' the situation instead. The second problem seems to be that you want to 'fart,' in order to stop the friendliness."

"That's what I told you. I want to shit it up."

"But why?"

"Because it's a luxury, it's not for me."

It was the end of the hour. I suggested to her that her concept that exchange of friendliness was "a luxury, not for her" might be a device for avoiding friendliness, but that this was not yet clear. I underscored, however, that there was at least a separation, and that she had two distinct feelings: one destructive and the other definitely constructive and warm, and that her warmth was not always contrived. There were clear evidences of spontaneous and genuine friendliness. (This is an example of the coexistence of contradictory emotions; see pp. 60–61.)

It will have been noted that in these two sessions following the Crazy Woman nightmare, the dreams were not pursued part by part, symbol for symbol. Instead, the crucial theme of the dream was sought for, in this case by the patient as intensively as by the therapist. Through this pursuit of the feeling of the dreams, a great deal of very fruitful progress was achieved.[12]

At the next session the patient came in after a weekend appearing more alive, happier, fresher, and looking more directly at me than she had ever done before. She lay down and started immediately, saying, "Last time I told you I was upset because at the end of the previous hour you said something optimistic, that thing about my joining the human race. I don't like optimism. If you're pessimistic, you can't be disappointed and may be surprised pleasantly. The idea of being disappointed makes optimism a torture. We were going to talk about my being upset and nervous when I have a success, or when people are nice to me." She went on to report that she had been hostess to a married couple from her place of work. It was the first time that she had ever cooked a full dinner, as opposed to hamburgers, hot dogs, or scrambled eggs. She had actually roasted a chicken. "It was great. I was complimented, and that made me a little nervous, but what made me extremely nervous was when I tested the food I cooked and it was delicious. It made me all tense. Yet I know I would have been unhappy if it turned out lousy."

I interrupted and asked, "Would you have been nervous if it were lousy?"

"No—that wouldn't have been the same thing at all. I'd have been

12 The pursuit of meaning through feeling: see further discussion in Chapter 7, p. 235.

unhappy, but not anxious. Also, never before when I tried cooking anything have I been so calm, enjoying it. This was a huge step. This made life easier, but I don't like it. I don't want to be like other people and do things that other people enjoy. That makes me fade away. I lose my identity. Anybody can cook. If I can say, 'Oh, I can't cook,' it makes me maybe less, but it makes me different from other people."

She went on to talk about her dreams. "I haven't tried to remember them. First I try, then I fall asleep and forget them."

I recalled to her that she had had some other fragments of dreams the night of the Crazy Woman dream, and asked if she remembered them.

She recalled a fragment. "I was going to marry Bob. He's the fellow in my office who I think is one of the nicest guys I've ever met. I said to him, 'I want to get married.' He said, 'You want to get married? How about me?' Then I thought to myself in the dream, 'My God, this is too wonderful to be true,' and I said to him, 'What do you mean?' and he answered, 'How about marrying me?' I went to pieces, I was so happy. I hugged him and said stupid things like, 'You're too good for me,' but I was deliriously happy. He wasn't as intense, although he was happy. I was so happy I could burst."

Then she spoke of another fragment of dream from that same night, in which she was near a strange building that was a telephone building, which she immediately interpreted as representing communication. She could not recall all the dream, but said it was near the park in which the Crazy Woman's house stood.

"The Crazy Woman's house was beautiful," she said. " 'Beautiful' is a word I don't want to say—but it was a beautiful park. I don't like to use words like 'beautiful' around you. 'Shit' I can say easily. I don't like to use words like 'beautiful' because I'm afraid I'll slip back into getting along by myself, giving up people. I'm very much afraid of the things that filled my life when I was alone, like enjoyment of art. I also think that because I think people are only posing when they use words like 'beautiful,' that you'll think I'm putting on an act. But I do feel things are beautiful. In my dream I'm touched by beauty, and this park which is Park Avenue is very beautiful."

This was a little more than two weeks after her nightmare about the Crazy-Woman-feelings which she thought would destroy her. She had already spoken of feeling friendly and wanting friendliness, and now she was speaking of genuine feelings of response to beauty.

She referred back to the successful Sunday dinner with friends. "I'm afraid of success. It's only temporary. They said they enjoyed my food, they enjoyed being over at my home that afternoon. Why shouldn't I believe them?"

"Why not?"

"I'm afraid. I've got to prepare for people hating me."

"Even if you don't 'fart'?" [13]

"I'm not afraid really of their hating me. I'm afraid of their not needing me. Oh!" And then she paused and groaned. "Why am I so pessimistic? My friend said she enjoyed it and said she wanted me to come to their house for dinner."

"I'm afraid that you're doomed to their friendship, unless you insist on 'farting,' doing something to spoil it, being silly or grouchy or childish, being sarcastic or unresponsive."

"I guess it may be just a matter of time. If I keep doing the right thing, the right things will happen, and so it will prove itself, that I can have a different kind of life."

"What do you mean by the 'right things'?"

"I mean if I'm friendly and don't fart, people will be friendly. I'll do my damnedest and hope.[14] But my damnedest isn't as good as a healthy person's behavior."

"Your damnedest is really very healthy—it isn't just a makeshift, the best you can do. It's healthy."

It was the end of the session. She said before leaving, "Let's get back to this joining-the-human-race business, because we haven't talked about all the reasons it made me upset." She had been rewarded with insight, confidence, and hope as a result of her courage in pursuing her feelings into frightening and operationally disorienting areas.[15] She concluded the hour with a spontaneously selected turbulent area for further exploration.

This brief passage, about two weeks, from the analysis of a patient indicates the value of stressing investigation of emotions, and demonstrates the extensive gains available in the affective area through pursuing dream material.

The patient's pathology was characterized by distortion in feelings and distortion in conceptualization of feelings. It was manifested as profound cynicism and reluctance to experience, identify, reveal, or communicate emotions, especially friendly emotions. Partly from work

[13] In the course of this session, "fart" became a part of her personal glossary, a psychosomatic symbol of a fear of spoiling good social relationships (see p. 42).

[14] This is an example of speculation; see p. 262.

[15] See the author's "The Pursuit of Anxiety-Laden Areas in Therapy of the Schizoid Patient," *Psychiatry*, 22: 239–244, 1959.

with the Crazy Woman nightmare and the Shit Piles Up dream, the young woman was helped to crystallize and make progress in overcoming all these affective problems.

Competitiveness

All the developmental interpersonal elements producing cynicism contribute to the evolution of the closely related affective personality distortion—competitiveness. Cynicism and competitiveness tend to produce and foster each other. The experiences of the growing child leading to his distrust of solicitude come from his detection, usually subjective and unformulated, of the use of him, the control and manipulation of him, and the overpowering of him, often under the guise of love. He develops, for the most part unawaredly, defensive and self-protective techniques for resisting these influences. Many a young individual, however, as his personality forms, goes beyond the point of self-protection. Vying with others to fend off their influence becomes itself an important basis of his sense of effective functioning. The child also imitates the manipulative techniques that are used on him, and when these succeed he has learned a way of relating and has experienced a feeling of personal power. When the manipulative techniques are the predominating pattern with the significant adults around him, interaction with other human beings becomes for him increasingly competitive. Competitiveness, the striving to prevail, in these mutual attempts to influence, becomes more and more a motivating force in his personality.

In order to operate successfully within this framework, the individual develops certain proficiencies regarding the use of emotions. He becomes skillful in his ability to *detect* and play upon the feelings of those about him. He learns, also, to *mask* his own feelings, for it would be competitively disadvantageous to expose them. And he learns to *simulate* feelings that may be tactically advantageous. All three of these ways of functioning distort both his affective life and his understanding of his feelings.

These interpersonal techniques, and the associated emotional distortions, appear in all of the patient's life situations, and also, of course, in the psychoanalytic relationship. Much resistance takes the form of the three above-mentioned tactical maneuvers. The patient tries to gauge the feelings of the analyst; he seeks to present emotions calculated to please, frighten, and otherwise disturb or divert the analyst. With exceedingly competitive and destructive patients, this kind of behavior may sometimes be deliberate. In most instances, however, the patient's efforts are altogether unrecognized by him, or are misapprehended.

Often the initial or principal clues to the existence of these hidden competitive feelings, with their concomitant tactics, are found in dreams. One intensely competitive patient, while professing his great efforts to express his emotions fully, had a dream that vividly portrayed the opposite. He was urinating (pouring out feelings) standing astride a large funnel-shaped toilet-opening in the floor (Pissing Dream). Below was a great pool of feces. An old woman (the analyst) opened a door behind the patient to enter the room. If the patient continued, he would be exposed in this very personal act. If, with his back to the old woman, he drew his spread-out legs together, he would conceal the stream of urine from the woman behind him, but he would slide feet first down the funnel into the fecal pool. In the dream he figured that the filth could later be washed off, and he chose to conceal the stream (his feelings) from the old woman, even though it meant his having to wade through feces (continue in the repulsive, humiliating kind of life he led).

This patient revealed all three of the competitive pathological uses of emotions. He shrewdly *detected* the "true" nature of the analyst—a snooping old hag; he consistently *masked* his feelings, refusing to trust the analyst; and in his relations with the analyst, in spite of repeated exposure, he continued his transparent *simulation* of anger, enthusiasm, compassion, his sycophantic admiration of the analyst and his charades of analytic zeal. The failure of these operations, and the associated sense of real failure in the analysis, were a constant source of feelings of self-degradation (sliding into feces), but his competitive determination to force the analyst to believe in his sincerity was so insistent that he managed usually to deceive himself. The self-deception re-enforced his determination, and somewhat ameliorated his sense of self-degradation and failure.

If people did not so pervasively strive for power over one another, using in their struggle even the forms of cooperative and solicitous behavior, cynicism would be far less prevalent. While much cynicism derives from the existence of competitive practices, it is equally true that pervasive cynical distrust in our culture fosters this competitiveness.

Competitiveness can and should be distinguished from simple and necessary competition. Competition is interpersonal activity ordered so as to elicit the highest effort from each, and under some conditions it is beneficial to all the participants. *Competitiveness is an aspect of per-*

sonality; it is characterized by a primary and often exclusive preoccupation with the victory as apart from the activity itself. The activity, with whatever potential benefits it may have, becomes meaningless without the victory.

The competitive individual casts all types of interpersonal exchange in the framework of competition, thereby losing the enrichment to be found in the mutual quality of the activity. For example, he creates an argument instead of a discussion, or he makes a conquest instead of a possible friendship. In tennis, a game of competition, there are numerous goals, among them to play well, to win more points than one's adversary, to win the set, to have as friendly a time and as much enjoyment as possible, to increase one's skill, and to better one's health. Many other social goals can be related to a game of tennis. The primary and sometimes exclusive goal of the competitive person, however, is that of triumph over the other contestant. The manner of winning, or the prize that is won, is of lesser consequence. A triumph may even be achieved by losing the game. For example, a young man might be determined to lose a game to his adversary in order to win in his competitive strife with his father, who wants him to be a good tennis player and who is paying for his lessons with a good coach. By losing the game, he becomes a victor over his father and the coach, who would then both be defeated in their efforts to have him achieve something which would bring them gratification.

It is sadly a common occurrence for people to sacrifice the achievement of valuable goals in life because of their competitiveness. Marital partners forfeit the achievement of many forms of mutual satisfaction because of their competitive strife. Parents lose many opportunities for good times with their children in their obsession with showing who is boss. Some young people flunk out of college in their competitive strife with parents or professors who look forward to real accomplishment, to the fruition of their parental or professorial hopes and efforts. These young people go from job to job, never succeeding, although their capabilities qualify them for excellent performances in many positions in which they fail. Their competitiveness may be expressed in unwillingness to let an employer benefit from their services, or in defeating his efforts to make them conform to a particular routine of work. Through losing jobs, they may disqualify themselves for marriage, and thereby defeat the aspirations of parents, sweetheart, potential parents-in-law, or friends who have their welfare at heart. One patient fought against her parents and succeeded against their wishes in becoming an actress. After years of struggle she brought her mother and father a thousand miles to the opening night of her first stellar role. It was a great success. They were converted to her career and very proud. At the beginning of the second performance, she lost her voice and didn't recover it for several years; she left the stage permanently, much to the parents' disappointment. She had proven them wrong to have opposed her, but could not bear their benefiting by their readiness to admit error. They had to pay double, while she sacrificed her career for the gratification of a vindictive triumph over them.

In the course of their development, competitive individuals have acquired techniques for resisting, and also for practicing both manipulation and exploitation. They have come to conceive of the relationships among people as consisting almost exclusively of these practices. One cynical and controlling patient finally achieved the concept of "genuine" friendship, bringing to his session the serious definition, "Friendship is mutual exploitation!"

The following clinical incident occurred during the analysis of a man a little over forty, a confirmed bachelor who had considerable money and a quiet, charming manner. This combination of assets had afforded him an endless supply of feminine company and sexual experience throughout his adult life. He had a long list of telephone numbers which he used at varying frequencies ranging from weeks to years. Women who did not give themselves to him sexually after an evening of expensive entertainment were crossed off his list.

When he was past forty he began to consider marriage. He was deliberately looking for a widow with children so that he could walk into a ready-made home and family situation. He made one after another conquest of this type, but ran away at each serious prospect of marriage. Then one young widow whom he liked very much let him know that he was not the kind of man she wished to marry, but that she would be happy to see him occasionally. They met a few times with this understanding. He told her that he appreciated her frankness. Shortly after their second date under the no-marriage arrangement, he had the following dream (Kept Calling Up).

"I called Pauline on the telephone night after night and kept begging her, pleading with her to let me come and see her for a little while, just once. She kept turning me down, saying there was no sense to it. Finally, after several nights of my begging her on the telephone, she said, 'All right, you can come over on Thursday night and sit with me for an hour.' I felt good about it. That was the end of the dream. I remembered the dream when I woke up this morning."

He immediately went on to say that the dream showed how much ". . . my security depends on people, especially women, accepting me. . . . I can't stand rejection."

There was a striking contrast between the woman's refusal, in the dream, to see him until he had begged and begged her, and the reality situation in which she made it quite clear that she liked his companionship and would gladly continue to see him. Had the patient, unknown to himself, wanted the woman desperately in marriage, the dream could have been a portrayal of that situation—but the desire for marriage did not at this time exist. The uncommitted arrangement actually satisfied him. In the dream, however, he continued to beg for, and finally got, something very much less than he already had in reality. This discrepancy was pointed out to him, and he recognized it. He added spontaneously that if this woman had shown any sign of being interested in marriage, he would have dropped her at once.

In exploring himself further, he became aware of his chagrin that she had dropped him "before I dropped her." His pleasurable achievement in the dream was exclusively that of "getting his own way."

With all his blandness of manner—his never letting any woman become too important to him, his book full of telephone numbers, his wallet full of money, his self-sufficiency, his easy-going carefree charm —the patient was activated by an absolute insistence upon having his own way with people, and particularly with women. He had always managed to be the one who turned down somebody else. In talking about the dream, he said, "I can't stand being rejected." However, the feeling experienced in the dream, when more accurately identified, was, "I can't stand not winning."

A correlation of his feeling of insecurity with those situations in which the advantage was not his, then developed productively. The criteria for his "security" (being in a position to prevail over, to reject, others) and his "insecurity" were copiously documented in many relationships with men and women. The insight furthermore clarified many psychosomatic disturbances, as well as their antidotal circumstances. He began to recognize that his essential interpersonal strategy, instead of being one of defending an insecure vulnerability, was one of subtle maneuvering for domination. In this case the term *competitive*, frequently before acknowledged by the patient as an accurate characterization of himself, was for the first time, through the dream, felt to be a significant and irrational element of his personality.

An admixture of competitiveness frequently pollutes relationships in which constructive, healthy, friendly, and cooperative goals exist.

A wife or husband may lose sexual interest that had been there a moment before, just because sexual initiative was taken by the partner. Competitively, it is more important to resist the influence of the other than to enjoy a sexual union. Sometimes a husband will sustain the pangs of sexual starvation or the humiliation of masturbation rather than do what feels to him like ceding a competitive victory to his wife by acknowledging her desirability, or by letting her make him the agent for the satisfaction of her needs. A man of this type will limit the enjoyment of a meal rather than yield to his wife the pleasure she would get from his admiration of her culinary skills.

The children of such a marriage are often mopey and bored, competitively braced against being seduced by a parent into enjoying some kind of mutual activity. Their attitude is: "Everybody is forever trying to get you to respond their way, for their pleasure." As they grow up, they cannot conceive of wanting to engage in an activity with another through which both can derive pleasure and benefit. The concept of pleasurable cooperation is foreign. Its emotional impact and developmental influence have never been experienced.

This kind of person will carry his competitiveness to absurd lengths, such as never laughing at the end of a joke because laughter is what the story-teller wants. The individual does not recognize his unwillingness to be influenced to laughter, but sees himself as above low humor or perhaps, more humbly, as a quiet type with slow or silent responses.

The feeling distortions resulting from competitiveness are frequently expressed in somatic symptoms. A wife or a husband who recoils from the sexual approach that was yearned for a moment earlier does not recognize the desire to frustrate or to resist the partner. The feeling is experienced somatically as an inexplicable loss of sexual appetite, and may be accompanied by expressions of regret, affection, and concern. The unidentified pathological attitude often takes the form of female frigidity and male impotence or premature ejaculation.[16] The conceptual distortion lies in the individual's belief that he desires to achieve sexual fulfillment both for himself, or herself, and for the partner.[17]

The classical circumstance of the jilted lover who makes the rendezvous for reconciliation and kills his sweetheart when she persists in rejecting him has been mentioned. Briefly, through his behavior he has

[16] See Three Condoms dream, Chapter 7, pp. 153–154.

[17] One frigid woman patient finally recalled quite explicitly that in high school, where her sexual life began, she had vowed to herself that "no man will ever make *me* respond!"

formulated the situation competitively as, "You think you can dispose of me? Never! I'll dispose of you."

On occasion, rebound marriage has the retaliatory purpose of proving how little the other's rejection meant. Retaliation may sometimes take the form of suicide or of alcoholism, associated with depression.[18] To look upon any kind of self-devastation as an evidence of intense love is a common, perhaps "romantic," failure to recognize an essentially punitive response to not having one's way. The suicide, often believing he loves so deeply he cannot exist without the beloved, nevertheless seeks to get even by blighting the beloved's life with an ineradicable guilt. The alcoholism of a rejected lover, too, is often mistaken as an expression of unhappy devotion, instead of being identified as competitive retribution—haunting the rejector with the painful specter of a shattered life.

A great deal of the relationship between men and women is openly competitive and a great deal of our humor is based upon this fact. Institutionally, men in our western culture have had the advantage over women. Women battle against this social inequity; the battle, however, seems in many cases to be not for equality but for their turn at domination. The reasonable struggle is also confused by women's efforts to maintain all of the special feminine prerogatives that were once their compensations for accepting a socially inferior role.

At the same time, men are fighting competitively to maintain their prerogatives as males. Petulant, sometimes outraged over the inroads that women are making and the concessions they are exacting, the men insidiously punish the women for the gains they have made. In the past, the men offered patronizing forms of gallantry in exchange for the women's accepting with grace their social inferiority. Now they tend not only to withdraw the gallantry, but to withdraw, as well, the common forms of respect, courtesy, and kindness. Many men consider themselves extremely enlightened in "allowing" women greater freedom. They, the men, are sacrificing their "natural" role of superiority in order to "give the ladies what they want." They experience inappropriate "generosity" in the place of honest acknowledgment of women's equal rights and ability.

A husband may be a very good-natured and generous fellow who "wants his wife to have everything." Yet, somehow, every time his wife makes a decision contrary to his wishes he becomes depressed. Nobody is sorrier than he is about his depression, but it happens every time her wishes prevail. In time the correlation is made by his wife. She learns

18 See W. Bonime, "Dynamics and Psychotherapy of Depression," in J. Masserman, ed., *Current Psychiatric Therapies*. New York: Grune and Stratton, 1962.

to avoid decisions which would make him depressed or "difficult." In a different kind of relationship, the decisions themselves might be quite acceptable to him, yet the husband might be obstructive, and in obscure and petty ways emotionally punitive, because his wife took the initiative. In either case, when the wife, either fondly or tactically, adapts her way of life to his irrationalities, he deludes himself by his good-natured acceptance of "her" plans into thinking he is easy to get along with and eager to please.

In and out of marriage, the distorting influence of competitiveness produces a wide range of pathological feelings, concepts, and activities between men and women, in forms which are disguised, misapprehended, or completely hidden. To the extent that this competitiveness exists, it thwarts the development of genuine love relationships.

The following is an illustration of a dream portrayal of unrecognized, although extreme, sadistic competitiveness between a woman and her husband. The woman, during seventeen years of her marriage, had been excessively acquiescent to her husband, but painfully uninspired by love, admiration, or responsiveness. Her sexual life had been utterly unsatisfactory except for a short and fulfilling extra-marital affair. In intercourse her husband was invariably premature, yet throughout the years he had been resentful of her for criticizing his performance, and had blamed her "lack of lovingness" for his inadequacy. It had been suggested to her in analysis that she might be partly responsible for maintaining his inadequacy, with all its unhappy consequences for her, because she gained some revengeful gratification from humiliating him. Intellectually she recognized this possibility, but she did not really believe she did anything to hurt him. She felt only how "awful" it all was for her.

The couple had a pet Siamese cat. The husband always, and sometimes openly, resented her affectionate attention to the cat; her caresses made him think of the affection never accorded to him. Compulsively, the wife would pet the animal in his presence. One day she brought in the following dream (Dog Eat Dog).

"I walked down a street and into a shop. Inside there were two dogs. One had his face half chewed off by the other. They had been together in there for a long time with no one feeding them, and one had started to eat the other's face. It seemed so awful to me." Without pause she continued, "I had another dream in which I was a cur slinking along. That was the dog that had eaten off the other's face."

"Dog eat dog," I said. She responded immediately, "That's David and me—I hurt him so in the argument the other night. He keeps after me to tell him 'my troubles' [instead of telling the analyst] and I tell him I can't. He said he almost left the house the other day when he saw me pet our cat—he never can stand it—if he keeps after me to tell him my troubles some time I'll blurt out about having a lover, and who he was. *I'd hate to do that.*"

I said, "I believe you want desperately to do just that—to make him 'lose face.'"

Her instantaneous association was, "He's so mean to me. We had dinner the other evening with another couple and he kept talking about my being no good in bed. I wanted to blurt it out right there, that I *am* good."

It had been a competitive necessity for her to regard herself as gentle and acquiescent, oppressed, scorned, patronized, and emotionally neglected, so that all the cruelty and exploitativeness in the relationship could be charged against her husband. In this session for the first time she felt the emotional impact of her desire to hurt him in retaliation, an excellent example of the *detection of a feeling*.

Similar competitive techniques operate widely among friends, behind a great variety of facades. An individual can be very amiable as long as his friends are adapting to him. Glumness and depression come upon him inexplicably, and he does not correlate these emotions with his not getting his own way. Much of his good-naturedness is a manipulative technique, and likewise his depressions. With geniality he seduces and rewards, with depression he warns or punishes. He covertly, sometimes sweetly, fights, attacks, undercuts, resists all, often while feeling blandly convinced that he is generous, supporting, tolerant, and genial.

Another type of competitive person attempts to prevail over others by techniques of helplessness (see Tiny Cobras, pp. 138–141). One timid, anxiety-ridden patient had a dream in which he sat on a platform borne on the shoulders of Egyptian slaves, ferociously whipping them all about him (Egyptian King). Analysis gradually revealed a fiercely competitive and tyrannical individual who used timidity as a whip to force others to serve him. He was intellectually highly endowed, academically well trained and experienced, but he was productive at a level far below his capacities. He suffered many panics associated with fantasies of his committing murder, while showing those about him a facade of vulnerability and lack of confidence. Nobody could defeat him by forcing him to grow up and assert himself openly. Instead, he enslaved others by his diffidence and inadequacy, thus maintaining a covert competitive victory in his prolonged contention with the world.

This type of timid person may, while he persuades himself that his feelings are only affection and gratitude, experience contempt for those who have been tricked into helping him. His hypocrisy is often sensed, although not clearly formulated, both by himself and by the object of the competitive practices, and re-enforces the cynicism of both.

In all interpersonal situations, whether among friends, marital partners, parents and children, or in other relationships in our culture, to the extent that competitive practices cast doubt upon the genuineness of solicitude, they foster an often unidentified philosophy of "every man is really for himself." This cynical credo, in a circular fashion, continues to breed still more competitiveness.

Technical Considerations and Suggestions

Competitiveness and cynicism have been discussed extensively because of their profound bearing as distorting factors upon the clinical problems for both patient and therapist of detecting, delineating, and evaluating feelings. We come now to some technical considerations and suggestions about the achievement and clarification of information about feelings. Some of the problems and the approaches to their solutions have been dealt with in the preceding discussions, and have been demonstrated in the clinical illustrations. Considerable further documentation will appear throughout this book. Explicit considerations of techniques will nevertheless usefully augment what is implicit in the previous and later discussions.

Since the clinical explorations for feeling in dreams and in other biographical material invariably overlap, the remainder of this chapter presents some techniques the analyst may use to help the patient achieve access to his feelings and to the means of communicating them, regardless of the nature or source of the affective data.

TALKING ABOUT FEELINGS WITHOUT FEELING

A patient's detachment from his own emotions in analysis is often difficult to convey to him. Some patients can describe their own feelings accurately, but as though they were discussing a rather interesting acquaintance. Many individuals are articulate, incisive, and explicit in making verbal distinctions, and this fluency is often a preoccupation that bars them from experiential awareness of the very emotions they are explaining. When they begin to understand the request—"to talk about your feelings with your feelings"—their productions sound less syntactical and more alive. Toward this end it is sometimes helpful to encourage the patient to use in analysis the kind of vocabulary, the intensity, and the inflection he uses with his most intimate family and his friends—to "be himself." When he refers to his "behind" or his "derrière," a question may elicit that during the actual incident he had said, "my ass." One learns that he talks of "taking a crap" to his friends, but of "defecating" or "moving his bowels" when he tells the analyst. He says to his wife, "Let's screw," but reports to the analyst that he "suggested to my wife that we have relations." He tells one of the "guys at the office" how "pissed off" he was at "that prick, Joe," but reports from the couch that he told "someone who works with me at the office that I was provoked at the supervisor." The patient who is doing this euphemistic editing is permitting something, perhaps his concern about the analyst's opinion of him, to block his view of himself. He can, if he is willing, be helped to get himself into focus by a suggestion from the analyst that he grope openly, forgetting considerations of style, using the first words that come to mind, and speaking in the language and inflections common to his informal relationships.

Although naturalistic expression may become a means toward a more immediate grasp and communication of emotions, it is of course no guarantee of achieving frankness, completeness, or ease in speaking. It is also wise for the analyst to bear in mind that a patient, even if he makes the most intense efforts and uses his personal vernacular, may speak haltingly because of his utterly honest search for words to tell exactly how he feels.[19]

BLURRING IN VERBAL COMMUNICATION

Fundamentally, if the patient by *any* means is being covert in his expression, he is interfering not only with the communication but also with the discovery of his feelings. A great many forms of obscuration are used in the communication of feelings. They are essentially resistance activities, yet may be overlooked as being merely speech mannerisms. Although the patient may be describing his feelings, it is necessary to point out to him that these blurring devices prevent the seemingly reported information from becoming established data.

Loose terminology is one such hazard. The patient may say he "feels funny" about something, or is "upset" or feels "peculiar." These terms can refer to such affects as anxiety, diffidence, suspicion, or anger. The patient has learned nothing about himself until he defines and

[19] A great deal of information regarding emotions is communicated nonverbally through inflections, grimaces, gestures, and bodily behavior. All of these are data to be gathered by both analyst and patient, and all are subject to valuable consensual validation.

communicates more specifically how he feels. The process may take time. Knowledge may come by association or may involve the recall of a dream. The important thing is that the search for clarification be instituted.

A conspiracy of silence sometimes occurs, perhaps a conspiracy of vagueness in which the analyst compounds the patient's unclarity by either insufficient interest or too much empathy. Such therapeutic pitfalls are still more likely with terminology that appears on the surface to be specific. Probably the fuzziest term in psychiatric practice is "guilty," which usually represents a constellation of feelings involving any combination of anxiety, contempt, gloating, compassion, chagrin, and other affects. "Guilty" often lends an aura of nobility (when the patient emphasizes contrition) or of pitiable vulnerability and diffidence (when the patient diverts attention to his helplessness against reprisals and other consequences). It is an omnibus word, often used by patients or psychiatrists, and mutually accepted without affording any actual useful data regarding the patient's emotions. When a patient uses the word "guilty," it is a sound practice to say something like, "Well, you have some kind of *uncomfortable* feeling. Let's try to see exactly what it is."

A similar procedure can be productively applied to the terms "insecure," "rejected," and frequently to "love." This consideration is relevant also to any vocabulary that the individual analyst may develop over the course of years. His too-familiar designations can easily become an evasive jargon for the patient, separating him from a clear, subjective picture of his own feelings, rather than encouraging a more direct search for them.

Another common form of blurred communication has been designated as *insulating terms*.[20] These qualifying words, phrases, and rhetorical devices, including negations and attenuations of the expressed feelings, and assigning of the feeling to the analyst's imagination, guard the patient from experiencing the full shock of recognition of his feelings. Here again it is important that the therapist does *not* supply the appropriate intensity empathically, in silence, accepting without comment the blurred communication of the patient.

By italicizing the blurred communication, the loose terminology, and insulation, and by directing the patient back to his feelings, one is likely to elicit angry accusations of "quibbling" from the elusive patient, whereas the patient who is honestly struggling to understand himself will welcome the assistance. Naturally, one does not seize upon every

[20] See Chapter 7, pp. 247–248; see also Introduction, p. 27.

instance, for there is danger then of stopping the flow of associations at a moment when fruitful material is being offered.

It is important, too, to evaluate and to respect the patient's frequently coexisting honesty and courage in pursuing his feelings. His full and direct confrontation of an emotion may not be possible until he has made more headway in dealing with his stake in evading it. Usually the initial exposure of a feeling opens the way to understanding the stake in concealment; and dealing with the stake in concealment leads reciprocally to greater capacity and greater desire to confront the emotion directly.

For the patient of the Crazy Woman dream, for example, part of her stake in refusing to experience the friendliness offered to her by others was the maintenance of her anesthesia against the feeling of loneliness in her lifelong and neurotically self-imposed isolation (pp. 79–80). When she became aware of the great variety of maneuvers by which she fenced off relationships that might awaken her appetite for friendship, she began to experience her loneliness. The loneliness, then, in turn helped her to delineate more sharply her isolating maneuvers, to overcome them gradually, and to begin to accept the friendliness offered by others.

USEFUL EXPLANATIONS AND ANALOGIES; WRITING DREAMS

Every patient can use some practical assistance in the struggle to perceive his feelings. Throughout the analysis he is enlarging his skills in the use of two important tools: free association, and dreams. Sometimes a simple suggestion or explanation may facilitate a patient's reaching into himself. It can be helpful for him to learn, for example, the relationship between emotions and free associations. A free association can be described as an emotional simile (see p. 13). The associative memory is of an experience (dream or waking) in which the emotional coloring is like that of the situation in focus at the moment. The feeling of the current situation may be completely undefined; the feeling in the association, however, may be quite clear, and may offer, if not a direct categorization, at least a significant clue. Also, the affective common denominator of several successive associations may gradually gain definition or increased emphasis.

Another simple working concept is that of sympathetic vibration. The patient may be offered the analogy that his feeling is like a tone, and that concentration upon it will tend to awaken other events with the same tone, the way a bell sets other bells to ringing. The other bells are, of course, the associations, memories of events with the same feelings. Or the feeling may be symbolized as a file folder—what comes out of that folder (all the associations while concentrating on the feeling) is connected in some way with that feeling.

In spite of possible drawbacks, *writing dreams* is a valuable practice. It may, like any other therapeutic activity of the patient, become a mechanical and consequently a resistance procedure. Even free association, however, can be used mechanically, and dreams can also be reported meaninglessly from memory. Many hours can be filled with dreams that are never put to use, if that is the patient's ultimate intention. Any one operation in psychoanalysis may be good or bad for the process, depending upon the spirit in which it is done.

A patient committed to self-understanding and to change may safely and profitably use any adjunctive procedure that appears to him or to the analyst to serve his purpose. The dream itself, associations, and especially the feeling in the dream, may be noted in full or by brief jotting, on awakening or at any time that he remembers them. The vividness of feeling, and also of actions, individuals, and surroundings, in a dream is often caught and preserved more sharply when written. It is a good practice to keep a pad and pencil beside the bed-lamp. Many valuable dreams have been salvaged by nocturnal recording. The signal fact to keep in the foreground for the patient is that the writing of a dream, and later the telling of it, is only the beginning of a process.

CAPTURING INITIAL REACTIONS

Eliciting accurate information about feelings often necessitates urging the patient to discipline himself to capture, by an intense degree of concentration, his initial reactions. The patient's immediate, spontaneous emotional response may be almost instantaneously edited and corrected, or replaced by a different, even contradictory, response. In circumstances where an individual has a stake—such as a self-concept or a role in the eyes of another—in having certain feelings, he often fails to register or mention the discrepant emotion. The wife, for example, who had the Dog Eat Dog dream (pp. 93–94), after recognizing the reality of her cruelty, still had to concentrate intensely to recall any of her initial "I'm glad" feeling when her husband "lost face." It had rapidly been replaced by her feeling "awful." Feeling "awful" was partly her not wanting to seem or feel like the dog (the bitch) she was in the dream. The feeling "awful" was also, in part, her experience of genuine compassion. Similarly, the cynical, frightened young woman of the Crazy Woman dream (pp. 73–77) had to concentrate intensely to recall her fleeting moments of trust and friendliness, which were rapidly replaced or submerged by hostile suspicion. The patient can learn to grasp a feeling despite its brevity. Analogy with lightning may help— lightning whose moment of illumination, no matter how brief, cannot be denied.

There are a variety of reasons why patients brush away their initial emotional reactions. Some patients "play it cool," in and out of analysis. Skill in imperviousness is a frequent source of pride, security, and sense of superiority. Others tend to whip up synthetic emotionality. Some resist the reporting of new kinds of emotion because of a competitive wish to deny that they have been influenced during the analysis, or merely because the analyst had previously speculated that such an emotion was probably there.

The new emotion may cause anxiety simply because it is unfamiliar. These new or unwelcome feelings may all be quickly replaced or submerged by more comfortable and familiar ones, and the initial feeling may not register sufficiently to be recalled without the most intense concentration on the part of the patient. It is sometimes possible to elicit this data by returning to the question of feeling with the inquiry, "Yes, but what was your *immediate* feeling? How did you feel the very first moment?"

PSYCHOSOMATIC CLUES

The psychosomatic avenue to knowledge of the emotions may also be made available to the patient. Many patients have grasped in a general way that physical symptoms may reflect the emotions and should be reported, but they need help in correlating symptoms with situations. Several patients, for example, have learned to look for anger in the presence of headache. One man was able to identify anger toward the analyst by the occurrence of urinary urgency during the session. On numerous occasions in the course of his analysis he had to leave the couch, returning from the lavatory usually more ready to tackle his problem. Three patients found that a yawn accompanying a formulation or emotional delineation—even on days following a good night's sleep—was actually a psychosomatic confirmation of insight. One woman used to develop a spasm of back pain with every intense resentment of a formulation. For her the symptom became a useful symbol of resistance, of "having her back up." The cardiac symptoms of anxiety, the rapid and thudding heartbeats, are the most commonly recognized. One patient's resentments were proclaimed by audible borborygmi. After she was able to accept the correlation, even mute intestinal tension became a useful signal to her. "Butterflies in the stomach," often occurring when an individual is in deadly competitive combat and worried about the outcome (see Fight with an Antelope, p. 104), are usually spontaneously recognized by patients as a somatic reflector of anxiety.

In general, using the somatic signal as a focal point for associative activity often leads to discoveries of emotions. After the signal has been established as a symbol of a specific group of feelings, it becomes possible for the patient to be more deliberate in his search for the feeling and its situational context. He may say to himself, "I've got a headache—what am I sore about?" The associations that spring to mind give him a clue, and then he begins to experience the feeling of anger he had not previously recognized as his response to the situation. (It is not uncommon for dreams, new or old, to be recalled in the course of such a somatically triggered associative search.)

The distinction between talk about feelings and direct contact with feelings is crucial throughout analysis, and demands close attention. The patient who does not deal directly with his feelings does not change. Those who maintain distance must be frequently confronted with the manner and degree of their distance. The degree of immediacy regarding emotions can usually be taken as a measure of the patient's commitment to the therapeutic effort.

By its relative size, this chapter indicates the importance of the realm of feelings in the pathology and therapy of psychoanalytic patients, and the importance of dreams as a source of information about their feelings. Some ideas, replacing classical concepts of instincts and their vicissitudes, have been set forth regarding the nature and sources of the emotional distortions most commonly found in people of our western culture. The reader will find that in the following, as in the preceding pages of this book, the question of the patient's feelings will seldom drop from sight.

3. Introductory Dreams

AN INDIVIDUAL ENTERING ANALYSIS approaches it with a concentration of concern, aware and unaware, on the aspects of his personality which are the foci of his interpersonal failures. His feelings and ways of behaving are immediately involved in the crucial relationship with the therapist; and they are always reflected in the patient's dreams.

The significance of introductory dreams in the therapeutic setting can best be demonstrated in the context of clinical material. The more important factors in the therapeutic value of utilizing introductory dreams may nevertheless be set forth in a series of formulations.

1. Introductory dreams offer the opportunity to induct the patient very early into intensive therapeutic activity.

2. The patient often reveals in his first dream one or more of his characteristic ways of relating to others, the dream frequently indicating this by reflecting how he relates to the analyst.

3. The dream becomes the basis of a new, therapeutically educative activity, particularly through initiating the patient in the use of *free association*.

4. Work with the first dream usually serves to introduce the patient to the intensive investigation of his feelings, a process which is to become a basic therapeutic orientation.

5. The analyst's offering of his contribution in the form of an interpretive hypothesis (see pp. 20–21) often constitutes the patient's first experience of analysis as a cooperative activity.

6. The work with the initial dream material also demonstrates to the patient the functional contribution of dreams to the total therapeutic process.

7. These approaches may then be applied by the patient to life experiences as well as dream material.

The foregoing formulations will be elaborated, first, in the discussion of work with several dreams of a single patient, occurring in the first few weeks of his analysis. In the second part of the chapter these concepts will be demonstrated through brief clinical presentations of the introductory dreams of different patients.

Following are the first dreams of a man in his early forties who came for help because of marital difficulties, in part related to occasional alcoholism. His wife, too, was in analysis, and the patient himself had had a brief period of approximately six months of sporadic sessions eight or nine years earlier with a different analyst.

The patient's manner was direct. He seemed determined to enter into the analytic situation whole-heartedly, ready both to express himself and to listen. A well-masked fear on coming to the first session was expressed at the second session. He conscientiously captured his associations in the course of listening or speaking. He did this, moreover, in a constructive way—that is, without using associations as an escape into circumstantial tangents.

He first reported dreams at his fourth session. He came in with an episodic dream of the preceding night and also with one that he had had soon after the second session and had forgotten to bring in at that time.

He said, "The dreams I had last night reminded me of the one I had last week after the second time I was here. This one from last week is about me and the cousin I told you about that I go out drinking with occasionally (Straight and Narrow). He and I were on a steep roof. We were both drunk. We weren't reeling, but we had been drinking. Someone else was there watching us. He was either on the ground or on the roof. My cousin and I were walking along the ridge with the roof going off at a steep angle on either side. I had a feeling of *terror* of falling off."

With no interruptions he went on, "I had some ideas about this dream. When I began this thing, this analysis, I set up a regimen for myself. I decided to set up some kind of discipline, a regimen . . . I decided to walk the straight and narrow. I was afraid of falling off.

When I get into trouble, it's always when I've been drinking. [Pause] The third figure was you."

Then he added somewhat academically that he had actually been up on the roof of his home in the suburbs doing some repairs, and stated that he had felt somewhat "skittish up there." He speculated objectively that the "skittish" incident may have had something to do with the rooftop dream, and said then that he would like to tell the dream he had had "last night." He had dreamed a great many things, he said, but two episodes in particular stood out.

"I was in a fight with an antelope (Fight with an Antelope). The antelope had an elaborate set of horns like a reindeer. These horns had many sharp points. I was anxious. I was nervous. I was damned uneasy about it. All these horns could pin you down. This fight was taking place on a stair landing. While I was fighting, I was wondering to myself, would it be cricket to grab those horns and make a sudden great twist and break his neck."

Interrupting himself, but without a moment's pause, he said, "I meant to ask you last time whether this session is one hour or forty-five minutes. While I was sitting outside today, I was planning to ask you about this and I had a fantasy of your getting into a rage and slugging me."

He then went on to discuss other fantasies he had had, at other times in his life, of being slugged. These fantasies had always involved being slugged by older, stronger, authoritative men.

He then reported another episode of the same dream. "My wife and I were in church [Faking It]. There were lots of candles around. The nave of the church was very narrow. It was time to kneel and we had a strange thing to kneel on, a sort of camp stool. My wife had one and I had one. My wife thought I didn't have one to kneel on but I said, 'Oh yes, it's here.'"

That was the end of the dream. I asked him what was the *feeling* in the dream. He replied at once, "As though I wondered if my wife would know what to do during the ceremony." And then, with the inflection of sudden recall, "Oh no—it was a question of whether *I* would know what to do. I was being watched from behind. I thought I was awfully clever because I could anticipate just what move to make, just what to do. I was faking it, but felt sure that the couple behind me, friends of mine, didn't know that I was faking it. I was catching on very rapidly to what the others were doing, when to stand up, when to kneel, and I did it all so fast that no one could detect that I was faking it."

As this dream-filled session in his second week terminated, I made some interpretive hypotheses.[1] The formulations were offered, not for acceptance, but to turn the patient's attention to a more probing examination of his feelings and behavior in this intimate interpersonal relationship. I suggested that the dream about the church ritual, as did the Straight and Narrow and the Antelope dreams, indicated uneasiness about my involvement in his life. In the Straight and Narrow, he felt anxiety about his ability to handle himself in a rigid regimen while under observation. In the Antelope, an immediate and direct competitive contest was threatening. Would the analyst "pin him down" or would the patient, with a shrewd movement, be able to "break his neck"? (He had associated the phrase "break his neck" with his impulse to confront me suddenly with my having, he thought, shaved fifteen minutes from his analytic hour.) Finally, in the church with its "narrow nave" (like the straight and narrow roof), he was again apparently dealing with the analyst not in a direct contest, as with the antelope symbol, but in an indirect contest, by a different kind of trickery—namely, by "faking it." He was planning to put on a shrewd, compliant, ritualistically accurate analytic performance for the benefit of the audience sitting behind him.

I emphasized to him that all of these attitudes represented his ways of dealing with people, including his analyst, and that it was necessary for us to watch for these elements in his behavior in the analytic relationship. I suggested that if he succeeded in repudiating me by means of his contempt for me, if he succeeded in deceiving me by a superficial but accurate ritual in a devotional atmosphere, if he tried to solve his problems by resolving to adhere to a straight and narrow regimen, that he would be preserving his personality difficulties intact. I said that I believed that he had some sincere motivations and honest activity; the aspects of his personality and behavior suggested by these introductory dreams, however, could interfere with the essential purpose of his being in analysis, namely, to examine, understand, and change his personality.

He came to the following session and said that after leaving the last hour he had been thinking about the specific friend who in the church dream was sitting in the pew behind him. This person, a friend at one time, had become mercenary as well as rich, and "he wouldn't

[1] The ready interpretive hypotheses here represent an example of a circumstance in which the analyst interprets alone (see description of dynamic concept, pp. 20–21). The patient was early in analysis. Although he had indicated an interest in and some limited capacity for using dream material, and had come in with an interpretation of the dream Straight and Narrow, he had not yet grasped the potential in dream data for acquiring new recognitions of his character.

stick his neck out five cents for me now." The patient recognized his distrust of me through this association.

He then went on directly to report another dream that he had had after leaving that last session, the session filled with dreams and interpretations: "There was a school sort of setting, but it was much fancier [The Toaster]. There was a conveyor belt, a sort of assembly line. The whole operation was one of dropping doughnuts into a large machine that was like a large toaster, very large. The doughnuts were dropped in and they popped up in the toaster as bread, that is, ordinary toast."

His feeling? "I felt very curious about the process."

This dream had in it a second episode in which he and a friend were in a school cafeteria getting some coffee. It was an unclear, shifting kind of situation in which his friend would now be on line with him getting coffee, or then would be behind the grating of the cashier's cage collecting money.

Was this friendship or a business deal? Continuing interpretive hypothesis, I again related this ambivalence to myself, associating the cashier's grating to the iron railing on the short stairway from my office to my waiting room, which is on a higher level. This piece of railing and the stairway were in sight throughout his sessions, as he lay on the couch. The piece of railing, with its series of upright bars, seemed to me also similar to the inner construction of a toaster. In the course of this identification of the analytic situation through elements of the *surroundings* (see pp. 8–9), I reminded him that the Fight with an Antelope took place on a stairway, and represented an unequivocal contest. In the cafeteria episode the analyst was not represented as an outright antagonist, nor exclusively as the money-taker. In the cafeteria the individual fluctuated between friend and cashier. That such an ambivalence existed already suggested some progress—it introduced the possibility of the analyst being the patient's friend. That idea, too, was offered.

Additional evidence of movement toward trust in me and confidence in the process of analysis came from pursuit of the Toaster dream and from the validating activity within the session and outside it. The patient reported that he disliked doughnuts but liked plain bread toast. I suggested to him that the Toaster dream might represent a healthy attitude toward me and the analysis: the doughnuts were perhaps the data—the dreams and other material which he brought to this school-like setting and which came out converted into something more appealing to him. The dream also suggested a healthy curiosity about the process, and perhaps even admiring amazement. This was in contrast to the other dreams.

He responded to the recognition of assets in his character by re-counting an experience that he had had after leaving the previous session. He said that he had made notes about the Antelope dream on the same piece of paper with a shopping list, and that he had continued seeing the word "antelope" as he went through two or three stores mak-ing purchases. He had almost asked a clerk for antelopes. It had crossed his mind that this would be a very charming story to tell to his analyst. He associated the fantasy, however, with two things: the sense of per-formance in the church ritual dream in which he was "faking it," and some discussion between us, during that and an earlier session, of his trying to charm and impress me. With this insight he vetoed in him-self the plan to tell the shopping incident as a charming story at the next analytic hour.

I took the opportunity to tell him that it was not enough merely to suppress the urge, but that it was important, as he had in fact done, always to recount even the occurrence of such an idea. The patient's impulse to impress me tended to validate the early interpretation of the church setting as the analytic setting. The interpretive hypothesis regarding the church dream—faking it in analysis—seemed to be bear-ing fruit. The patient was recognizing his desire to impress me. The recognition, veto, and report of the desire to perform for me indicated a tendency toward healthy change in the analytic relationship.

He started the next session with the statement that he had been "trying to be completely honest about my feelings." He recalled a fanatically religious old aunt during his childhood who had told him, "Somebody sees you, whatever you do." Then with some embarrass-ment he said that he actually had the feeling that I watched him com-ing to the office and leaving it by observing from my window. This "peculiar aberration," as he referred to it, might be regarded as tending to validate an aspect of his own interpretation of his first dream, The Straight and Narrow, in which a figure which he identified with the analyst was watching him as he was trying to maintain his balance within a restrictive self-discipline.

He went on directly to the expression of another attitude which tended to validate the interpretation of his competitiveness toward the analyst as manifested in the dream Fight with an Antelope. He said, "In a relationship like this, it's all one way. One guy gives everything and another guy listens. In every other relationship it's more give and take. I'm very curious about you." He was beginning to recognize his feelings and to talk about his problems more forthrightly.

The formulations about the patient's personality had been offered openly as tentative—as *interpretive hypotheses*. These hypotheses (which are not always derived initially from dreams but were in this case first highlighted by dreams) were presented at the outset, and thereby served to engage the patient in dealing with basic personality problems, and helped both the analyst and the patient to get right to work on a cooperative basis. The cooperative factor was particularly important with this man because in him there was so great an emphasis on the insular activity of making a good impression, even, if necessary, by "faking it."

While outstanding in certain patients, the attempt to make an impression of some sort on the analyst is present to a degree in all. Effort is required to orient the therapeutic relationship in the direction of the patient's discovering his personality, rather than presenting his illusion of it. On entering treatment, most patients, while looking for relief from pain, are also seeking to preserve the personality intact, to streamline the neurosis rather than to cure it. Irrationally sensing alteration of the personality as a threat to its integrity, patients tend to be both anxious and deceptive. Tendencies toward anxiety and deception notwithstanding, however, the very act of becoming engaged in examining basic personality problems and thus recognizing that these problems are not only identifiable but also may be soluble, can do more to fortify the individual and to encourage further self-exposure than it may do to shatter him and to encourage deception. Interpretive hypotheses derived from introductory dreams can thus move the therapy into a constructive course.[2]

The beginning work on dreams is for most patients the beginning of an education in the dynamic utilization of dream material. Many people who have some familiarity with the concept of dream interpretation do not, nevertheless, have any grasp of the process by which dream data can function as a tool in the modification of behavior. The patient who brought the above series of introductory dreams, for example, had had more than a literary skirmish with dream interpretation. He had had a brief psychotherapeutic experience about nine years earlier, and on the basis of it had "interpreted" his first dream. He had, however, no concept of relating the dream to the unhealthy aspects of his personality. He had performed what is so often falsely taken for interpretation—the mere identification of individuals or actions, mere symbol-labeling (the onlooker identified as analyst, the action as keeping sober).

Exploration through dreams of his personality began with the interpretive hypotheses that he had terror of not being able to handle

2 See also the series of introductory dreams in Chapter 2, pp. 53–59.

himself without help and of failing while under observation. Succeeding dreams introduced speculations on personality problems involving the patient's resentment, seductiveness, contempt, and competitiveness toward the analyst. This was fruitful, dynamic activity that began to develop in place of his going through the static ritual of identifying dream symbols.

An extension of this educative aspect of working on introductory dreams is the broader application by the patient to a great deal of other material of these new approaches. The newly introduced approaches to dream data are basically those of free association and the careful, honest search for full recognition of one's feelings.

The use of free association, in itself initially a somewhat bizarre thinking process, is more comfortably adopted and seems more appropriately applicable in the strange realm of dreams. Once it becomes fruitful, it begins to be a more acceptable intellectual tool, capable of wider application. The patient begins to appreciate the value of vagrant data—passing thoughts, impulses, sensations. Many patients not used to employing such data in seeking to understand themselves are initiated into the rational, intensive pursuit of a great deal of self-illuminating, previously disregarded material.

The discipline of freely associating, often first gained in the unfamiliar territory of dreams, can be extended to waking life, including the immediate as well as the remote past, somatic sensations, and fantasy. The patient comes to recognize, often primarily through his experience with dream material, the relevance of the irrelevant, the seriousness of the embarrassingly petty or the absurd. For example, the patient who dreamed of the Fight with an Antelope spoke of suddenly grabbing the antelope's horns and with a great twist breaking the animal's neck. While telling the dream he interrupted at that point (entirely unaware of the associative connection) to say that earlier, while in the waiting room, he had planned to challenge the analyst on whether the sessions were actually supposed to be forty-five minutes or whether he had been cheated out of fifteen minutes on each of the first few hours. The interpretive hypothesis was offered that the sudden thought while telling the dream was a pertinent datum—an *association*.

The lesson brought results. A few sessions later, still in the first few weeks of analysis, as the analyst, talking, leaned forward toward the couch, the patient, in response to an unwelcome formulation the analyst made, had a flashing impulse; it was a fantasy of swinging around and swiftly and dexterously poking his lighted cigarette into both of the analyst's eyeballs. After the analyst had proceeded another two or three sentences, the patient interrupted: *"I'd never have thought of capturing such a feeling and putting it into words,* but when you said something a few seconds ago this went through my mind." And he told the fantasy.

From the introductory work on his first few dreams, he had begun to approach vagrant thoughts (associations) as salvageable data; and he had learned also to apply this approach beyond the context of discussing dream material. He had applied it to an utterly subjective, fleeting, but no longer dismissable experience vis-à-vis the analyst.

These approaches to self-examination, often first encouraged and established by the analyst in working with introductory dreams, tend to foster not only cooperativeness but also a higher order of both concentration and honesty than the patient is likely to have achieved before. These new and essential attributes of the patient's role in therapy receive impetus from some special features of the analyst's approach. Particularly important among these is the analyst's intense concern about the careful delineation of feeling, which is a cardinal focusing area in the recall of every dream.

This patient became at least dimly conscious of a fairly wide range of emotions of which he had been essentially unaware. He discovered through the dreams of the first few sessions his *terror* at the possibility of failing in his mechanical self-discipline (Straight and Narrow), his *hostile desire* to render the analyst impotent (Fight with an Antelope), his *contempt* and *cockiness* in fooling the analyst (Faking It), and his *curiosity* (and possibly *amazed respect*) regarding the analyst's professional activity (The Toaster). The close search for feeling, prompted by the therapist, resulted early in the patient's own concern for clarity, honesty, and communication regarding his emotions. In the first few sessions after discussing the competitiveness of the Fight with an Antelope, he volunteered the recognition that he *felt subjugated* by having to tell about himself and not having an equal exchange from the analyst. He was also constructively impelled, when he experienced a wish to burn the analyst's eyeballs with a cigarette, toward "capturing such a feeling and putting it into words."

The precise capturing and description of feeling, and the ready report of vagrant thoughts, are processes through which the patient also develops his capacity to cooperate. The analyst, on his part, fosters in the patient intensity of self-inspection and honesty of expression, to some extent by the analyst's own humility in examining the productions of the patient. By being undogmatic, and presenting interpretive hypotheses in a frankly speculative fashion, he invites the patient to consider with him the possible inferences that may at each point be drawn regarding the patient's personality. The patient is stimulated by the mutuality of the process to intensify his search for contributory material.

For example, the concept that the antelope was the analyst and that the patient was fighting the analyst, was afraid of being pinned down by him, and was seeking to outwit and render him helpless— this was presented as a speculation and not as a definitive interpretation. The patient was not told, "This is what it means." He was told, "This is what these elements of the dream suggest." The patient was furthermore informed that the analyst neither knew nor understood him very well, and could be wrong in his hunches. Both patient and therapist would make mistakes in evaluating data.

Formulations of the analyst, no matter how accurate and astute they may be, cannot in their original form be facts which the patient can utilize; the establishment of facts through which the patient can understand and change his own personality must always come ultimately through direct, affective self-observation—not through formulation, but through subjective recognition. The patient's perception that the analyst, although experienced and skillful, does not pretend omniscience, and is quite as dependent upon the patient's collaboration as the patient is upon the analyst's, tends to cultivate the patient's self-respect, sense of equality, and sense of therapeutic responsibility. Where the therapist is willing to speak up without certainty and without demand for acceptance, the patient responsively often tends to be more forthright and courageous in expressing thoughts and feelings whose actual significances and manner of reception by the analyst are unpredictable.

The patient of this first series of introductory dreams reacted to the interpretations offered as hypotheses with early cooperation. He soon began to apply spontaneously to waking experience some of the directness of perception and communication he was acquiring in the pursuit of dream material. He identified and communicated his competitive feelings toward the analyst by voicing his objection to the self-exposure without reciprocal exposure, by expressing his desire to catch the analyst at cheating on session time, and by capturing and revealing his eyeball-burning fantasy that occurred while listening to the analyst.

In summary, these few early dreams from one patient have illustrated the nature of introductory dreams and their significance in therapy. Aspects of technique in the clinical use of introductory dreams have been examined. The delineation of feeling has been emphasized.

THE CLINICAL USE OF DREAMS

The foregoing approaches to introductory dreams in their clinical setting will now be illustrated through short presentations of a variety of early dreams from a number of different patients. The therapeutic activity is not fully elaborated, but in all of the ensuing clinical examples the indicated interpretive hypotheses were presented to the patient in the initial phases of therapy.[3]

Hot Dog

The bright young man of the Hot Dog dream discussed earlier had just been graduated from one of the country's leading universities. He came to analysis because, in the first place, he felt a lack of direction, and was taking a commonplace job in the business world instead of the postgraduate professional training his ability indicated; and secondly because he was a homosexual and was convinced that this was a sick way of life. I had been recommended to him by someone he respected. He came intimating that he had some preformed confidence in me; he expressed a profound wish to get help for his sickness and a desire to make his life more meaningful. After his third hour he reported his first dream.

"I am walking along 34th Street [the street of the therapist's office]. I come to a group of people waiting in line for hot dogs, especially good hot dogs. I feel, 'oh boy!' and I look forward to it. I find soon, though, that I am actually on a queue waiting for a bus. The discovery gives me *a feeling of disappointment*."

The patient's immediate association with the locale was the analyst's office. With the hot dog he associated penis, and with the bus he had the connections of "going somewhere, getting somewhere." He did not know how to evaluate the dream. He was confused by the thought of waiting for a hot dog (penis) when he was so eager to get into serious analysis. He pushed aside the confusion and stated his thought that the dream had "something to do with my being eager for analysis."

The interpretive hypothesis was offered that the dream exposed a discrepancy between his verbally expressed attitude and his predominating feeling, that it indicated a happy anticipation of seducing the analyst; this was represented in strictly homoerotic terms by his hoping to get the analyst's penis (hot dog), but in broader terms it signified his desire to make a personal conquest of the analyst. The recognition that

[3] It should be borne in mind while examining these dreams that this period of treatment, inception, is the one in which there occurs the greatest amount of interpretive activity by the analyst alone (see description of dynamic concept, pp. 20–22).

he was waiting in line for a bus, that is, to "get somewhere," was, by comparison with seducing the analyst, a *disappointment*. This was in marked contrast to his strongly protested desire to get help through psychoanalysis.

His dream was a simple but vivid one. He did not know its meaning, which could only be understood through the feelings involved in the dream—first anticipation, then disappointment. The dream reflected that the patient related to the analyst as he related to everyone—seductively. This was an approach diametrically opposed to the conditions necessary for analytic progress.

The importance of his attitude toward the analyst was indicated, along with the implications of the dream regarding his personality. The latter were offered as the analyst's hypotheses. For the mutual inquiry a double focus was established: first on the existence of a discrepancy between the patient's actual feelings toward therapy and his concept of those feelings; and second on his seductiveness, expressed through a pose of admiration and dedication, as a possibly generalized pattern of relating to people.

Annoyed with Mother

A middle-aged woman, the only one unmarried among several siblings, caught in a housekeeper role for her aging but not helpless parents, came to treatment because of a diffuse discontent. She compulsively confined herself to her role at home and could not develop interests, take vacations, do something that would be for herself alone. She came to her fourth hour stating, "I rarely dream," but bringing with her a dream she had bothered to recall because she had been told that dreams were important.

"I'm in the kitchen at home getting myself supper after coming home late. There are a few relatives standing around. Mother, who always makes a pretense of getting supper for someone, but bustles around ineffectually, is following my every step. I feel pressure from behind. In my *annoyance* I jab her with my elbow. I'm *surprised to find her hurled across the kitchen and to the floor.*"

The dream brought into focus two problems. The first was her hostility toward her mother. In her initial three sessions she had not mentioned any concern regarding the relationship with her mother, although this turned out to be a core problem in her life. Secondly, the dream raised the question concerning her subjective disavowal or minimization of her emotions. She recognized something of the *nature* of her feelings toward her mother, namely annoyance, but was totally unaware of the *intensity* of her feelings, so vividly dramatized by the dream.

In her family she was known as the "calm one," a designation applicable to her outer aspect and consonant with her conceptualization of herself. The dream brought up thoughts and emotions about herself and her mother that had seemed too petty to communicate. She perceived subjectively that she was not a "calm one." The interpretive hypothesis (that the dream indicated not a mere "annoyance" but a nearly homicidal rage toward her mother), while disturbing, activated her to look more directly at her feelings and actually led to the recall of many past dreams of anger at her mother.

In brief, this first dream (1) got her analysis off to dealing with a crucial relationship; (2) directed her attention to her previously unidentified angry feelings; and (3) awakened her to the recognition that her dreams were significant and could help her to understand herself.

Scared Shitless

A single young woman of twenty-one came from a distant state to work and to live alone in New York City. A year later, feeling almost hopelessly defeated following rejection by a boy friend, in great distress she looked for psychiatric help. Just before her first session she had a dream.

"I was on a street and there were bullets flying in both directions. I walked along in the midst of the bullets and I was not at all frightened. Suddenly the scene changed—not completely, but this street was a street along which there was a circus with a lot of little sideshows. I was with my mother. I looked down and there were feces on my leg. I was slightly amused and that was all."

There was a clear discrepancy in the dream between the depicted situation and the patient's lack of emotional reaction to it. It was possible to call this much to the patient's attention immediately, with the suggestion that the dream probably reflected a difficulty she had in recognizing and acknowledging some of her feelings. In a dream circumstance of extreme danger—bullets flying where she was walking—she was unruffled, "not at all frightened." Then, standing before her mother with feces on her thigh, her response was not one of mortification—she was "slightly amused."

The problem of affective discrepancy introduced through the dream was then correlated with the patient's behavior in the session. I called her attention to her smiles and chuckles that accompanied her description of the defeating experiences which had precipitated her

seeking help, and which she had openly presented as emotionally painful. From the bare situation in her initial dream, without any interpretation, it was possible to direct the patient's attention to an apparent
tendency toward the disavowal of feelings. With this as an example, it
was then possible to impress upon the patient the potential of dreams
for calling attention to broad, unrecognized personality problems.

So much alone would constitute a good start in treatment. Further-
ance of this introduction into the treatment process appeared possible,
however. The analyst suspected that contrary to the patient's feeling
"not at all frightened" among the flying bullets (the hostility of the
outside world?), she had perhaps revealed in the second part of the
dream, by the symbolic feces on her thigh, that she had in fact (in the
then-current wartime vernacular) been "scared shitless" in the life situation from which she entered analysis. This interpretive hypothesis was
extended. The speculation was offered that the patient's mother might
represent the analyst, and that the patient's amusement in the second
part of the dream might be like her chuckling and smiling to overcome
embarrassment at exposing to the analyst strong feeling, anxiety.

The hypothesis was carried further. The patient was called upon
to consider the possibility that she *felt*, in contrast to her studied composure, that the analysis itself was a dangerous situation.

Thus, in addition to the dream's focusing upon an important personality problem (her disguise of or blindness to her feelings), and calling the patient's attention at once to the usefulness of dreams, further
gains were introduced. She learned a little about the nature of interpretation and, even more important, about the nature of validation. The
latter was accomplished through the correlation of the action in her
dream (behaving with amusement in a mortifying interpersonal situation) with her waking activity (chuckling and smiling while exposing
painful personal difficulties to the analyst). She was introduced thereby
to the further concept that her behavior with the analyst could be significant in revealing the nature of her personality. She was invited into
the cooperative aspect of the therapeutic process when the analyst
offered his concept of her dream in the form of an *interpretive hypothesis* for her to consider and to pursue with him. (This last feature provided some reassurance for this "scared shitless" patient in the beginning of treatment.)

Bird of Prey

A young actor in his early twenties came to analysis because,
although he felt he was pleasant to people, he did not get along very

well socially and had no close friends. He had had mistresses, but no real love affairs.

In the initial interview it began to appear that, although outwardly always a gentleman and good-natured, he was condescending and scornful toward people, and was a skillful practitioner of sly, undermining wit. He felt far above the common male standards in his "considerateness" toward women, who nevertheless always turned out, somehow, to be difficult, rejecting, or inadequate for him. He spoke of a current sexually unconsummated attachment for an unhappily married young woman about whom he felt "very concerned." Speaking of her gave him even more surprise and confusion; his concern appeared to him strongly to refute the idea of himself as distant and disdainful which I had tentatively proposed. He was asked if he could recall any dreams, and he said at once that he had had one just before coming to this first session.

"I am seated on a grassy hillside with Roberta. On the slope below us I see twenty or thirty people. It's a pleasant, warm day and everyone seems to be enjoying himself strolling around playing and talking. The girl is someone of 'noble birth.' (She's a European girl whom I really tried to cultivate, but with little success.) I see a bird approaching. It hovers in mid-air directly above the group of people below us and, because of our elevation, it is just at my eye level. *The bird has a cold, cruel, inhuman eye that frightens me.* I think that its intention is to attack Roberta, not by moving but by becoming even more vivid and *frightening.* So I jump to my feet, seize some stones and begin throwing them at the bird to make it go away, but I don't think it's frightened. I think it stays, but at this moment I awoke."

He was puzzled by the dream, and particularly by the bird. He tried to connect the dream with his "concern" for the unhappy married woman with whom, at the moment, he was involved. The bird, he felt, represented some danger to this young woman, and his fear in the dream he ascribed to his protectiveness toward her.

The interpretive hypothesis was offered that the bird was not an outside force from which he was trying to protect her, but symbolized an *aspect of his own personality,* an attribute that it frightened him to observe. Perhaps *he* was something of a "bird of prey," like any of the wolfish ordinary men whom he scorned! He considered this possibility and was able to see some relevance in his immediate situation.

Then he suddenly remembered an involvement with a girl about two years earlier. "I became engaged to her just in order to get what I wanted. Of course this created a hell of a lot of anxiety." The possibility of danger then from that young girl's family, and in the present situation from the woman's husband, were realistic sources of fear. Anxiety, however, could be attributed to a different and additional jeopardy—the undermining of his picture of himself: the dream threatened to expose to him that he was not one of God's noblemen, a protector of women, above the common crowd, but instead a rather "cold, cruel, inhuman," predatory sort of bird.

He had the integrity to recognize that these were facts about his personality that he could not have discerned without outside help; the latter recognition in itself was a beginning corrective to his intellectual eliteness. In addition, the analyst was confronting the patient with a willing coworker who asserted no authority, made no pretense of transcendent knowledgeability, and was dependent for his role in the therapeutic progress upon the young man's cooperation. These therapeutic practices and attitudes fostered what healthy tendency he had toward revision of his snobbish personality.

With the concepts of the snob and the bird of prey, analysis moved at once into crucial personality problems.

Empty Suit

An efficient, intelligent woman of thirty-seven, a conscientious mother and a civic-live-wire type who had been married seventeen years to a successful free-lance journalist, came to analysis because she was depressed. She could not get along with her husband (who was my patient) and was losing the respect of her children. She had struggled a long while against accepting psychoanalysis for herself, but had finally come to a decision. Knowing that I sometimes treated both wife and husband, she wished to enter treatment with me. In the first two sessions she spoke of numerous disciplinary problems she encountered while trying to be reasonable and understanding with the children, a boy and girl both in high school. She spoke of protecting them from the physical and intellectual tyranny of her husband and of her endless "discussions" and arguments with him. She described how she had held the family together and provided her husband with moral support during a number of "black periods" when he was seriously worried about his professional capability.

She came to her third session with the following dream: "I was walking cautiously up in the rafters of a tremendous place like Madison Square Garden. There was sawdust below. There was a man with me. It was my husband, though it didn't look like him. He wasn't strong. I was leading. I was cautioning him not to step on this or that rafter. *Then he lost his balance*. I had been holding his hand, but at that point

I had let go. It was my responsibility to get us to safety, and I hadn't done it. I hadn't been cautious enough. He fell, and I looked down and it was *an empty suit lying in the form of a man* stretched out after a fall—like a crumpled body. The next moment I was beside him.

"Then I'm walking with him outside. I'm helping the man who was an empty suit. There was a black-haired, unscrupulous movie-villain type outside rubbing his hands together. *This is the enemy.* I was helping us to get away from the villain. He was trying to make us get into a coach, a sort of fancy old-fashioned carriage that was standing there. I kept steering us away."

This woman had conscientiously recounted the dream because she had been requested to report her dreams. It intrigued her because it was so vivid and yet so incomprehensible, and my deep interest in it seemed to bewilder her. Her only associations were those of giving her husband moral support when he was discouraged about his professional ability, and physical support during a long convalescence from a debilitating illness (hepatitis), a period in which he had also had a serious depression because of his general incapacitation.

This introductory dream has been presented for two chief reasons: (1) In this case the introduction of an interpretive hypothesis at the outset of therapy represented a clinical failure—the immediate effect was, in fact, apparently to retard progress in treatment. (2) The dream was tackled by the patient three years later when it was still vividly recalled by her. Her work with it at that time was extremely productive.

My interpretive hypothesis was strong medicine for her. It was suggested that she preferred to have her husband weak and that she resented his achieving strength with the help of someone else instead of continuing to need support from her; that she regarded him not as a man but as an empty suit, and felt concern for him only when he was in a state of collapse; that the villain was myself, who sought to lure them both away to the analyst's office (located on Park Avenue and perhaps representing the "carriage trade"), and that she wished to save them both from the influence of psychoanalysis. She hardly responded to the hypothetical formulation, except with subdued interest and puzzled disbelief. She worked poorly in treatment, going through long periods—months at a time—of depression, lack of therapeutic cooperation, and circumstantial complaining. She felt convinced that the analyst favored her husband, and she continually emphasized the evidence of her husband's strength and callousness. It had been a great shock to her, while she had felt so put upon by her husband, to hear the dream interpretation that she in any way sought to dominate him.

During the subsequent years of analysis the analyst's original interpretive hypothesis was referred to in the contexts in which it appeared to be validated by her behavior and feelings. In spite of the initial intensification of resistance, and the risk of its resurgence in response to later reintroductions of the original formulation, it remained my feeling that direct dealing with the problem presented by the dream was the rational therapeutic choice.[4]

Three years later, the slow and painful accumulation of evidence of her quietly disguised competitiveness, tyranny, and contempt for many people, for men especially, and for her husband more especially, had brought her to a new approach to this introductory dream. She recalled the dream of the Empty Suit vividly, with details she had not at first reported, and accompanied by associations and interpretive readiness that made the dream a rich source of spontaneous insight. (Some of the details and associations were too specific to be included here.) Some of the previously unreported material of the dream, however, was that the coach was "gold, and like a hearse."

"I got us into a shadow where there was a little chance to hide. It was my chance to save us, save my husband. I was scared, too. The villain was going to get us. I was mostly worried about my husband, because I was in command of my faculties and he was dazed. It might look like Cinderella's coach or a queen's coach, but it's nothing but a hearse. It may look good for a lot of other people, but it's no good for us. I felt he should have some kind of treatment less intensive than psychoanalysis, so he could be weak and need me. Psychoanalysis is no good because it will make him strong, and he'll hurt me—well men, strong men, hurt. Not needing me to take care of him will make me weak. I was going to marry a sweet guy and that big strong bastard forced me to break off and marry him. When he started analysis, I thought, 'Dr. B. will make him strong and he'll push me around.' The only time I could have any affection for him was when he was depressed and physically completely depleted by hepatitis."

At this point, three years after the dream, her honest and courageous approach to it (in addition to the crystallized insight from it) was a measure of her progress. Hindsight regarding the patient's resources and pathology might have dictated a more gradual induction into the examination of this dream. Such insight is, of course, unavailable when introductory dreams occur; nevertheless, the sins of diffident omission in the pursuit of dream data seem to outweigh those of commission. While this tough interpretation of a first dream conceivably accentuated this patient's resistance to the analytic process in the initial

[4] See Chapter 6. See also, the author's "The Pursuit of Anxiety-Laden Areas in Therapy of the Schizoid Patient," *Psychiatry, 22:* 239–244, 1959.

stage, it brought about acceleration in a later period. She was able to attack then a new important question: how much of her husband's intolerable behavior might be a response to her own unrecognized covert efforts to make or to keep him weak?

Contemptible Passion

A young psychiatrist came to analysis as part of his psychoanalytic training. He had known me for some time as a student in my classes and had formed an opinion of me. In his first session he spoke of his deep respect both for my psychoanalytic views and my apparent warmth and "humanness." It was these personal qualities particularly that he stressed as having influenced his choice of me as his training analyst. The night before his first hour he had the following dream.

"A young man was on a couch 'screwing.' He was going through awkward, violent movements. You couldn't see the woman. Next to the couch there was a chair on a sort of high platform, a little like a referee's seat at a tennis match, but lower. A guy was sitting, looking down on this young man, watching him copulating. He was smiling contemptuously. The fellow on the couch had his pants down and his fanny was wagging in the air and he was very passionate. The guy in the chair looked like a bastard-of-an-uncle of mine."

He said he woke up and immediately thought what a "cynical, contemptuous bastard" his uncle was. "He was completely the opposite of you." The patient expressed disdain for the man in the raised chair, and pity for the fellow who was so exposed on the couch.

His voluntary interpretation was a simple re-enforcement of his attempt to impress me with the fact that we shared the same values. He—as he imagined I would—condemned the contemptuous, uncompassionate attitude of the uncle-person.

The interpretive hypothesis I offered to him was in quite a different vein. I suggested that dreams almost always reflect some attitude of which we are unaware and which we are reluctant to acknowledge while awake. I proposed that this dream, coming just before his first session in analysis, threw some doubt upon his expressed admiration of me, and might be a reflection of a disdainful and cynical rather than an admiring view of me. Perhaps he feared that despite the impression I gave I was in reality like his uncle, and would secretly look with contempt upon him as he exposed himself, especially if he should openly express his deepest feelings. I assured him that his respect and admiration were accepted as genuine, but that he probably harbored also a contrary attitude of which he was unaware. If he had profound doubts about me, it was important to examine them and also to explore for evidences of cynicism in his relationships with others. Doubts about the genuineness of the qualities he admired in others could make him feel insecure in many of his positive feelings.

Thus this man entering analysis "protesting too much" his subscription to warmth and decent human values, was introduced to the possibility of a contradictory, fundamental, and utterly unrecognized aspect of his personality, namely, disbelief in the existence of genuine sympathy and concern. The analysis was begun on a sound basis—"getting right down to work"—by dealing at once with the crucial pathology revealed by the initial dream.

Had the therapist disregarded the exposure of it in this vivid dream, the patient's cynicism would have been re-enforced through a false sense that he had conveyed exclusively his admiration for the analyst, who would then be regarded as subject to flattery. The cynicism would likewise have been re-enforced if the positive aspects of the patient's behavior—his genuine respect for the analyst—had been rejected. Accepting his respect, while dealing at the same time with his contempt, fostered a forthright, realistic, and searching therapeutic atmosphere. (This is furthermore an excellent example of the pursuit of insight by exploration of the interpersonal relationship between the therapist and the patient.)

At the very outset it was possible to suggest to this patient the connection in himself between his attitudes and his behavior. Because of his hidden doubts about the character of the analyst, he had felt compelled to "protest too much" his admiration. This exaggeration distorted an initially genuine feeling to the point where it lost its authenticity and became flattery. The pursuit of the connection between attitudes and behavior is an essential and continuing activity in analysis, and cannot be incepted too early in treatment. Dealing with this initial dream made the connection demonstrable in the first hour.

Woman on Barren Beach

An unmarried social worker, thirty years old, came for analysis because she felt she was "getting old," had no close relationships, and went "around feeling angry all the time." She said she had only a year for therapy because she had job plans away from New York.

She brought with her a dream she had had recently, and which she regarded as expressing "perfectly" her whole present life and feeling.

"A young woman is lying face down on the beach. There is no

one else there. There is one barren tree. The water is still; everything
is still and quiet. There is just one thing that moves in the picture, the
clouds in the sky. They keep on moving constantly. The young woman
is hopeless and depressed. I couldn't stand the clouds keeping on moving. I wanted them to stop. I was angry that they kept moving. I
wanted them to stop."

She stated again that the dream was a "perfect" depiction of her
life and her feeling about her life. It was all hopeless and barren. The
young woman, she knew, meant herself. The patient was puzzled, however, about feeling angry about the continuous movement of the
clouds.

This patient came not only with an introductory dream but also
with an interpretive hypothesis. In the discussion of the general pano-
rama of her existence it was agreed that the patient's interpretation
of her dream was clear, that the dream appeared to represent her life
as being barren of rewarding emotional experience. The analyst's interpretive hypothesis, however, involved relating the barrenness and
hopelessness in a consequential way to her other feelings and to her
behavior.

It was suggested that some of the barrenness and hopelessness in
the dream was the consequence of the young woman's lying there
doing nothing. It was suggested furthermore that her anger related not
to any inability to get up and do something about her life, but to the
fact that while she lay there inert, motion and life were continuing to
go on about her. Remaining inactive herself, she sullenly desired all
movement on the part of others also to stop. The interpretive hypothesis was directed toward illuminating the connection between her general condition—depressed, hopeless, barren—and her role in bringing
this about.

In time (the analysis lasted several years) she overcame a great
deal of her obstinate inertness. Her introductory dream had made it
possible to "get right down to work" in the first session on a major problem and to deal on an affective level with her refusal to engage in the
activities necessary to free her from the barrenness of her existence.

Recurrent Dreams of Lionesses

A divorced woman of forty-two, a public relations executive, came
to analysis because, although she was successful in her career, her relationships with men were not meaningful and she dreaded the prospect of continuing to live alone. She had emotionally, and for the most
part financially, supported a weakling husband for over fifteen years

before acknowledging to herself the emptiness of the relationship and divorcing him.

Her manner during the first session was friendly, direct, femininely soft, alert and composed. Her story was that she had broken away in her late teens from a midwestern home where she had grown up masking her ambitions for a career and independence behind a compliant manner. In the east she had succeeded relatively quickly in the advertising business, and had settled into a childless marriage in which she had gently but utterly dominated a weak, petulant man by a skillful, self-deceiving maternalism. During the initial interview she was asked if she could recall any dreams. She replied at once that for twenty years she had had "recurring dreams of lionesses."

"In those dreams, though I sometimes feared the lioness, I generally tried to manipulate the lioness, tried to outsmart her. The lioness was always very strong and beautiful. I always managed to keep her under control, but it took some very careful maneuvering at times."

She added spontaneously that she never could understand what the dream meant or why it recurred. An interpretive hypothesis was suggested, based upon the dream in conjunction with the reported nature of her marriage, her fluency, and her conspicuous composure as she described strained life situations. This muted affect was apparent in the descriptions she gave of breaking away from her parents, of difficulties in her marriage and profession, and of frustrated relationships with men after her divorce. The interpretive hypothesis was that the lioness might symbolize an unperceived angry, destructive feeling in her that she feared would get out of control.

The idea "rang a bell" and she added that she had always felt proud of being able to control her feelings, to keep calm under provoking circumstances. With this hypothetical concept of strong, unperceived anger perpetually needing control—a theme which had been repeatedly experienced in dream form for twenty years—her therapy, centered around feelings, got under way in the first session.

Analyst-Chauffeur

A young man about thirty years of age, a social worker, married and a father, came to analysis to improve his marriage and to enhance his professional qualifications. He and his wife lived together without open friction but also without real intimacy. He was superficially amiable. Beneath this surface, a basic tyranny began to come to light in the first interview.

It was not possible to start him in therapy until time became available two months later. At the second interview, occurring after this lapse, he reported a dream he had had a few weeks after the initial hour. The dream had been very vivid.

"You had voluntarily been coming to my house for our sessions. After one session you were chauffeuring me about the city with your car." He spontaneously appended his interpretation. "I have dependency feelings. I want things done for me."

His translation of the dream seemed apt enough, but what did it tell about his personality? After a fuller pursuit of the patient's ideas and associations, an interpretive hypothesis that occurred to the analyst on the basis of the present and the preceding initial interview was introduced. The patient was asked what he meant by "dependency." His prompt reply was, "Wanting somebody to do things for you." As an example, his first association was his insistence upon having his mother "push me into doing homework. I never got started by myself. It was absolutely necessary to have my mother get concerned about it, and to push me before I would get started." It was suggested to him that what he called "dependency" was actually (as is so often true) the very tyranny we had talked about in the first session. His "wanting somebody to do things for him" was not merely a yearning for help but a powerful insistence. He had *compelled* his mother to take the responsibility for his doing his homework. The soft, quiet manner was largely tactical, to make him appear undemanding, noninterfering, and unselfish, while he was maneuvering to force others to do things his way.

At this point the interpretive hypothesis was offered to him that the dream of the Analyst-Chauffeur represented his demand that I take the initiative and the responsibility for his getting well.

In the succeeding hours, the tyranny of the patient in all his significant relationships—with his wife, children, supervisor, parents, and friends—began to show clearly, along with a variety of operational techniques, including that of the "tyranny of dependency" that had emerged from working with the introductory dream.

The dream material brought immediately into focus the patient's neurotic distortion of his working relationship with the analyst. The patient's new, more realistic apprehension of the collaborative nature of therapy inaugurated activity tending to be corrective to the pathology of dependency which he had sought to maintain in the therapeutic relationship. Finally, the extension of dream exploration into correlation of past and present behavior (the patient's parallel emotional orientation toward mother and analyst) served to demonstrate to him the contrast between interpretive activity and the making of a merely apt interpretation.

Skating Rink, Wading in Deeper, Shark in Swimming Pool

An intellectual businessman of thirty-seven, married, a father, busy in such community work as PTA, and an avid reader of serious literature, came for sporadic consultations every few months over a period of two years. He was an exaggeratedly kind and considerate man, a "do-gooder." His chief difficulties were in his marriage, which was characterized by a coolness and strain that did not seem at all to reflect the qualities with which he sought to invest this and all other relationships. Among his friends were many who had been or were being psychoanalyzed. He felt, however, that he had derived so much insight from his occasional visits (more, in his view, than a number of his friends had achieved over extended periods of a continuous analytic process), that he had never seriously contemplated intensive therapy for himself. Finally, however, because of the increasing emotional distance between himself and his wife, he came to seek treatment on a regular basis.

He brought to the first session a dream that he had had the preceding night. "I was at an ice-skating rink. All the skaters were going around in a circle. I was skating in a circle, too, but I was going in the opposite direction. I was having a good time."

The interpretive hypothesis was suggested to him that he had finally entered into analysis like many of his friends, but that he was still trying to maintain his special status, as represented by his skating in a different direction from the rest of the crowd. The session was devoted to exploring his secret sense of uniqueness. The discovery of this trait was extremely surprising to him, because he had always felt himself to be notably modest.

The importance of discerning his real feelings was emphasized. He was amazed at the course the session had taken.

He came to the next hour with the following dream: "I was at a beach and in the water, bathing. The waves were small, and I waded in deeper and was enjoying myself. Then the waves began to get bigger and bigger and I kept bathing, but I was worried. I wasn't sure I'd be able to keep from being overwhelmed."

He was puzzled because he loved swimming and had no fear of the water. He was asked how he felt about coming to the second session. He said he was a little afraid of what might come up. The interpretive hypothesis was suggested that the prospect of "wading in deeper" to look at his true feelings was very frightening to him. He was afraid of the emotions he might find welling up in himself, afraid that he might be overwhelmed by his feelings. The hour was occupied with exploring his attitude toward emotions. He despised those who were carried away by emotions, particularly such feelings as anger and self-importance. When there was a conflict, he always tried to be understanding and reasonable. He tried always to do more than his share, and he never looked for credit. In the course of examining these attitudes, it began to appear that he secretly felt that his humility itself, as well as his maintaining calm when others became angry, placed him in a category above other men. His supposed humility, in fact, concealed a marked grandiosity. (This theme had been suggested by the work with the Skating Rink dream.)

He had complained also that in his marriage he wished merely to have credit where credit was due, that he was very helpful around the house and felt he was deserving of more affection from his wife. It was then suggested that his disdain for people might include some disdain also for his wife, and that perhaps this tended to stifle his wife's affection.

He left feeling somewhat shaken, but expressed gratitude that he was being helped to see himself more realistically.

He came to the third hour with another dream: "I was in a large tank like a swimming pool. There was also a shark in the water. I was swimming frantically to get away from him."

He could offer no explanation of the dream, and had no awareness of waking fear. His association with the swimming pool was that it was about "the shape of this office." The interpretive hypothesis was suggested that he frantically wished to elude the analyst, that he was extremely fearful that the analyst, who could navigate more skillfully in the therapeutic medium, would destroy him by destroying the illusions about himself. His illusion that he was a humble man had been shaken after the first dream. After the second dream he began to see more deeply into his disdainfulness and to embrace the concept that he had significant feelings of which he was unaware. His self-concept of humility, of self-effacing solicitude, of an unqualified, fearless desire to examine himself, were seriously challenged.

For this man who was so proud of his calm, brave rationality, it was most important to recognize the force of his fear and the degree of his elusiveness. Unheeded, these could operate effectively against his healthy attempts to explore his problems and to change.

The three introductory dreams, coming successively in the first three sessions, successively gave impetus to therapy. The grandiose disdain revealed in the Skating Rink dream was an unhealthy aspect of the patient's personality that might have become a serious impediment to therapeutic progress. The anxiety and elusiveness revealed in the Wading in Deeper and the Shark in Swimming Pool dreams offered immediate therapeutic access to the problem of resistance, and provided the opportunity, always so valuable for a "hyperrational" individual, to focus attention upon unsuspected, irrational, and disturbing emotions.

All of the patients whose introductory dreams were discussed, with the exception of the woman of the Empty Suit dream, became engaged at once in the therapeutic attack upon important personality problems. Some of these problems were manifested in the therapeutic interpersonal relationship. The young homosexual of the Hot Dog dream began to see his seductiveness. The male social worker of the Analyst-Chauffeur dream was introduced to his dependent tyranny. The young psychiatrist of the Contemptible Passion dream began to recognize his own cynicism and contempt. The young woman who was Scared Shitless became involved, through her introductory dream, in viewing her fear of analysis itself and of exposing her emotions both in general and to the therapist specifically. The businessman found grandiosity behind his humble facade (Skating Rink dream), and in response to the rapid inception of therapeutic activity, soon comprehended, through the dream of the Shark in the Swimming Pool, his intense fear of the analyst.

In the examples of the patients who dreamed of the Lionesses, the Bird of Prey, Annoyed with Mother, and Woman on Barren Beach, all were brought into immediate contact with pathology that did not initially involve the relationship to the therapist.

In the first part of this chapter, the dreams of the man during the first few weeks of analysis revealed a number of personality problems and also indicated that behind his readiness for therapy there was also a desire instead to go it alone (Straight and Narrow). He found his fraudulent conscientiousness in the therapeutic interpersonal relationship as revealed in the dream Faking It, and a tricky competitiveness exposed in the dream of the Fight with an Antelope. Soon, however, he showed his capacity for change, and revealed the beginnings of genuine respect for the analyst and the analytic process in the Toaster dream.

Work with introductory dreams as here described does not, however, insure immediate inception of intensive, productive therapy. Sometimes excellent results do occur; at other times gains are partial; in still other situations nothing avails for a long while to induct the patient into a productive therapeutic process. What has been discussed is a potentially productive approach.

4. Sexuality in Dreams

Wᴀᴋɪɴɢ ᴏʀ ᴅʀᴇᴀᴍɪɴɢ, the total personality is expressed in the individual's sexuality. In the conditions that stimulate or inhibit his sexual appetite, and in his mode of seeking or curbing its satisfaction, there are reflected all of his feelings and conceptualizations about himself, about the nature of men and women, and about the nature of his relationships to them.

According to the classical view, the evolution and functioning of the personality are predominantly determined by sexual energy and motivation. This view was developed in the course of astute observation of clinical phenomena. To explain these, Freud devised constructs which were brilliant, original, courageous, and immensely useful in the time and the culture in which they originated. Support for them accumulated through what Freud described as overcoming the patient's resistance *"by firmly insisting on what has been inferred, and by emphasizing the unshakable nature of one's convictions."* [1]

[1] Italics mine. The full quotation reads as follows: "Having accurately diagnosed a case of neurasthenic neurosis under observation, and correctly classified its symptoms, one may proceed to transpose into aetiology the symptomatological knowledge so gained and may fearlessly require the patient's confirmation of one's surmises. Denial at the beginning should not mislead the physician; every resistance is finally overcome by firmly insisting on what has been inferred, and by emphasiz-

It is possible to continue in the present to explain phenomena psychodynamically within this historically well-established framework. Many clinicians, however, observe and deal therapeutically with the identical phenomena, but understand them differently. In the present chapter, problems which in the classical approach would be dealt with as fundamentally sexual, will be treated as aspects of the total personality. In the instances given, they have their expression sometimes in sexual and sometimes in nonsexual form.

Sexuality is neither prior nor governing, but is interrelated with all other aspects of the personality as this evolves out of interpersonal experience. When we study an individual's sexual behavior, we are continually interested in two questions: (1) What is the nature of this human being, what are the attributes and attitudes that cause him to respond or fail to respond sexually under certain circumstances? (2) What can we find in his forms of sexual activity, feeling, and thinking to illuminate our understanding of his personality in its nonsexual as well as its sexual aspects?

A patient once said, "I was thinking that my feeling about analysis was like my feeling about love-making—it was like my husband having to force my legs apart." Was she experiencing psychoanalysis sexually? Did her husband's approach represent to her something other than sex? Under what interpersonal conditions, common to her sexuality and her working relationship with the analyst, did she frigidify responsiveness? Did she angrily reject every type of penetration in all situations? When she dreamed about an obstetrician with his hand painfully tugging within her and making only a "bloody mess" (Induced Labor), was she having a sexual dream?

When another patient dreamed of standing, his body enlarged to heroic proportions, while a beautiful woman stroked his enormous erect penis, was his dream reflecting sexuality alone (Statuesque Masturbation)? Did the dream present, symbolized in sexual form, a wish of the same patient for the analyst's acknowledgment of his superior intellectual and social prowess? Was the dream image a symbolic reflection of a grandiose concept of himself upon which he based demands for worshipful indulgence by all, by women and men, in many contexts, some sexual, some nonsexual?

In the discussion of symbolism in dreams it was stated that it is only from the life history of each individual that we can derive the

ing the unshakable nature of one's convictions. In this manner one learns all kinds of things about the sexual life of men and women which might well fill a useful and instructive volume; . . ." From "Sexuality in the Aetiology of the Neuroses" (1898), in *Collected Papers,* Volume I. New York: Basic Books, 1959, p. 228.

meaning of his dream symbols. We seek the meaning of the sexual symbols and of the sexual activity of any human being within that context. A great deal of valuable biographical data may be discarded or overlooked, and a great deal of insight sacrificed, if the pursuit of symbolic meaning is restricted within the framework of sexuality. This psychoanalytic loss is threatened even in cases where sexuality is unequivocally indicated by the dream. Whether sexuality is explicitly manifested or is associatively derived from the nonexplicit symbols, if the interpretation is not extended into the multiple social evidences of whatever traits his sexuality reveals, and if, instead, it is confined exclusively to the framework of sexual behavior, the growth of insight is stunted.

The importance of the implications beyond sexuality may usefully be illustrated by a hypothetical dream: a man dreams of firing a gun and wounding someone. Let us assume that *by asssociation*—not by referring to any dictionary of symbols—he relates the gun in the dream to his penis. A great many interpretive possibilities immediately arise. The particular meaning or meanings could be determined by such specific elements of his life history as the following: He may, as a boy, have been forbidden the use of firearms; the use of the gun in the dream (or of his penis in waking life) might then indicate rebelliousness. On the other hand, he may have been given freedom to use firearms, and then been ridiculed as a poor marksman, and so have become diffident about his handling of guns. His firing of the gun in the dream might then reflect evolving health, the emergence of new self-confidence, represented either incidentally or importantly in sexual activity. The dream might, on the other hand, expose vindictiveness toward those who restrict him in sexual or other activities. Rebelliousness, self-confidence, or vindictiveness—only the affective associations and experiences of the dreamer can tell us which of these, or what other emotion, is the meaning of the dream for this dreamer.

The inherent factor of injury to another by his firing of the gun could have a variety of implications. It could mean that he associated sexuality with injury to others. The dream could represent a dawning recognition that those who derided him and tried to keep him diffident would be frustrated, hurt by his developing self-assertion and self-confidence. It could symbolize his desire to injure women or, on the other hand, represent his *fear* of hurting women. It might also stand for his fear of hurting people coupled with his desire to hurt them or his recognition of hurting them—men or women, or specific individuals such as his mother, wife, or father—not by sexuality alone but by any act of self-assertion. His firing of the gun might represent a technique

THE CLINICAL USE OF DREAMS

of protecting himself by means of sexual seduction from the real or fancied aggressiveness or hostility of women—elimination of his enemy by amorous conquest. The dream might also reflect his efforts, by seductive techniques, to eliminate *anyone* who threatened him. Seductive techniques as weapons of conquest could then be represented symbolically by the metaphoric action of aggressive sexual seduction, in his dream the shooting of a gun.

Moreover, these interpretive speculations need not be mutually exclusive, and the dream symbolism could then reflect many complex, multifaceted aspects of the dreamer's personality. All of these possibilities have as a common denominator an instrument of combat—the gun—and thus tend to indicate the consciousness of an individual who conceptualizes the relationships between himself and other human beings as entailing a combative problem in which some aspect of himself functions as a weapon.

Many of the same interpersonal problems could have emerged from this dream even if neither patient nor analyst had made an associative connection between the firing of the gun in the dream and the idea of activity with a penis. Extensive examination of such an individual's dream in the context of his whole existence might lead us to a deeper understanding of his behavior in many varied areas, including his sexuality. The translation of the dream gun to a penis tells us nothing significant about his problems and personality, whether in sexual or in any other situations, unless we intensively examine the context of the individual's life.[2]

It is clear that the further discussion in this chapter of sexuality and symbolism in dreams must diverge from Freud's basic belief in the universality of sexual symbolism. Freud expressed himself on this point most emphatically. "When we have become familiar with the abundant use made of symbolism for representing sexual material in dreams, the question is bound to arise of whether many of these symbols do not occur with a permanently fixed meaning, like the 'grammalogues' in shorthand; and we shall feel tempted to draw up a new 'dream-book' on the decoding principle."[3]

It is helpful to bear in mind that much of the sexuality popularly found in dream symbolism is based upon these psychosexual theoretical concepts, which are uncritically accepted by many as the basis for understanding human psychodynamics. But when such constructs as infantile sexuality, the universal Oedipus conflict, castration fear, penis

2 For a related discussion of the snake symbol, see pp. 36–37.

3 S. Freud, *Interpretation of Dreams*, J. Strachey, translator and editor. New York: Basic Books, 1960, p. 351.

envy, universal masturbatory conflict, and other orthodox theories of psychosexual development are not insisted upon as scientifically unchallengeable facts, then there is much in dreams that will be seen not as dream reflections of sexuality but as dream reflections of noninstinctual interpersonal and intrapersonal human emotions, conceptualizations, and behavior.

In the complex totality of human consciousness, there are many areas in which there is confluence of the innumerable components of the personality. Such areas as sensory experience, love in its nonsexual aspects, other emotions, memory, perception, conceptualization, and creativity all involve a dynamic interlacement of personality components. Sexuality is one of these crucial areas; an individual is likely in his sexuality to manifest many and perhaps all of the components of his personality.

In dreams, these behavioral, conceptual, or emotional elements of personality may be sexually represented without being sexually (instinctually) determined; likewise, aspects of sexuality may be symbolized in nonsexual forms. Any of these nonsexual dream representations of the patient's sexual experience, however, will never refer to functioning which is exclusively determined by or restricted to his sexuality.

In the following pages of this chapter these general concepts will emerge from the consideration of a number of clinically observed dreams. Some portray manifest sexuality—seduction, copulation, masturbation, fellatio, incest, rape, homosexuality. Some of the dreams focus in their form upon frank genitality; others, although they contain common "universal sexual symbols," are not dealt with as reflections of the patient's sexuality.

Basically all these dreams are concerned with the patient's feelings, attitudes, ideas, and practices across the total range of his interpersonal relationships. They reflect, for example, anger, contempt, respect, affection, stubbornness, remoteness, happiness, fear, grandiosity, gratitude, trust. They reflect such practices as exploitation, seduction, cooperation, evasion. Aspects of the therapeutic relationship appear in sexual form without the sexuality of the patient being even remotely involved. In general, while most of the examples below will show a form or a coloring that is sexual, the orientation of the chapter, as of the book, is the total personality.

Son Sucking Me Off

The patient, a man starting his third year of psychoanalysis, was making efforts to overcome his inability to express emotion. He had been examining himself conscientiously but had made little significant progress. Some fantasies of forcing intercourse at gunpoint had raised the question of his desire to put others in a helpless position. Considerable documentation of this perverted satisfaction came from the realms of both reality experience and fantasies. The fantasy material included his enjoyment of torture situations described in literature. This line of exploration of himself brought up many memories of feelings of helplessness which he had experienced at the hands of both his father and his mother. With a great deal of reluctance and pain, he verbally expressed intense rage, particularly toward his father, in recalling some of the situations of helplessness he had suffered. He recalled having to sacrifice his whole play space in the cellar for his father's hobby, while his father at the same time tried to persuade the patient that the hobby was equally for the patient's enjoyment. He also remembered, with a brief subjective wave of rage, how a brother much older than himself used to tantalize him by holding him at arm's length and teasing him while the patient screamed and kicked, completely out of range, unable to retaliate. These memories were accompanied by headache and tightness in the gut. Despite the intensity of the feeling, the memories were reported during the session in a manner scarcely more emotional than the characteristically modulated style of all his analytic communications. He was several times reminded by the analyst of the importance of facing and communicating his emotions fully. Such reminders were introduced during the recall of these incidents of childhood impotence and then during the exploration of his seeking to render others helpless and of his enjoyment of their helplessness. His response to these reminders was extreme hostility toward me. This hostility was reported to me in the same relatively even, subdued fashion in which he had reported the rages against his mother, his father, and his older brother, and was accompanied by the same headaches and intestinal tension. Finally, after similar developments for two succeeding weeks, toward the end of one hour he decisively took the responsibility for accepting and expressing his feelings, and immediately started to speak with considerable, although still not fully expressed, anger toward me. He voiced a desire to smash up the office, to smash the furniture, to smash me. It was the most overt expression of his feeling toward the therapist that he had yet achieved.

That evening by chance he met me with my wife in a theater lobby, and the same night had a dream. He started the following session by reporting many contemptuous thoughts about me and my wife after seeing us in public. He then went on to report his dream. He said that he could remember only three brief but nevertheless vivid fragments. He stated that he was very ashamed of the dream and was under great constraint in telling it. The three fragments were as follows:

"My little boy (a two year old) was 'sucking me off.' He didn't know that there was anything wrong in this, but I did. Then there was another part in which I had my penis between his buttocks, not in his rectum, but between his buttocks. My wife called. I did have the feeling that something wrong was going on, something that shouldn't be going on, but nevertheless we (my son and I) simply moved to another room. Then there was another part of the dream in which my little boy had semen on his face and I was wiping it off."

The patient went right on without any pause to say that lately he had been having many fantasies of women sucking him off. "In all these fantasies the women are blowing me either with a lot of enjoyment or by my forcing them to.

"When I was about nine years old a guy who worked in our house as a handyman would sometimes lean back against the wall when I was in there watching him and would hold my head against his genital region that I just reached up to, and while he held my head gently against his genitals, he would rock back and forth and sing. I felt uncomfortable but I was never frightened or aware in any way that anything sexual was going on."

"How did you feel during the dream?"

"Uncomfortable. Something was going on that shouldn't be, but when my wife called, when I had my penis between the little fellow's buttocks, we simply moved off to another room. I've been more affectionate to Henry (the two year old) than to anyone else in my life. I mean I've been more affectionate *lately*. I felt very uncomfortable the next morning thinking about the dream. I'm very uneasy now. I'm more uncomfortable than my tone conveys. I'm not uneasy in the sense of thinking that this could really take place, but in terms of what it means: it means *squashing my children*. I think the dream is about my having no respect for my children, no real feeling for them. My stomach gets bad as I say this. It's very seldom if ever that I blow up at the kids the way I used to when I first came into analysis. I never swat them, although I do chew them out verbally; but I do stop now when I realize that I'm pushing it too far the way I used to."

He remained silent for about half a minute, and then voluntarily explained his silence. "I've just been preoccupied with thinking about rendering others helpless and also about feeling helpless myself."

I asked him, "What's all this attack on Henry in the dream?"

"It's not really an attack on him. It's just his being *helpless*."

"It's more than his just being helpless," I said. "He was being *used*."

"Yes, but not by force."

He then went into a long description of the indomitable activities and spirit of his little boy, Henry. The child was described as constantly active, disappearing if he was given a moment outside the house without adult supervision. The child was vigorous and difficult to dress or undress. Then, comparing Henry with the older children, the patient spoke of his always "sitting on" one daughter and of how she had grown up subdued. He stated that he had tried the same with the next one, who never did accept being subdued, with the result that the patient and this second child were still fighting each other. Referring to the child of the dream, he said, "I can't sit on Henry hard enough. Nothing subdues him."

At this point I made an interpretive inquiry. "Perhaps your behavior toward Henry in the dream is related to your helpless feeling about dealing with his indomitability?"

"Maybe so," he said. "I just can't spend time figuring out how to deal with people—I just want them to respond the way I want them to." He was quiet for a few moments and then went into a discourse about free association, a topic that had suddenly come to mind, saying that he liked to have things under control and was afraid to just "let things come" and to say them without knowing what their implications might be.

I regarded this spontaneous discussion of his fear of free association as a tentative effort to return to the dream, and I said, "Take a stab at the dream—what does it mean?"

He responded immediately, "It has some relation to my anger toward you. I had those violent feelings about smashing up the office and smashing you in the face. That was just before the night of the dream. I was really feeling violent. I'd like to get you in the position where Henry was in the dream—where you're helpless, where I'm using you, degrading you, but with no struggle, not like my fantasies of smashing you."

In the course of two years of analysis the problem had frequently come up of his wanting to be taken care of, of using people for his own pleasure, and of his self-indulgence, as in eating and masturbating. He had been through frequent depressions when confronted with such responsible activities as buying a new house or bettering himself professionally, or when entering new situations in which anyone besides himself, his family in particular, would benefit from his activities. In this context we had discusssed his angry reluctance to afford the therapist any professional satisfaction from the patient's improvement. (His first dream in analysis, The Analyst-Chauffeur, showed the analyst going to give treatment in the patient's home and chauffeuring the patient about town, the dream expressing a preoccupation with satisfactions provided for the patient.) My long-term analytic background with this patient influenced my reply to his interpretation of the dream. I said: "In the dream you are using Henry, your little boy, exclusively for your own satisfaction—there is nothing in the dream for Henry's benefit."

He answered at once with manifest emotional agreement, "That's right!" Then he added, "I feel dizzy. I hate to think of anybody else. I hate to take my wife's needs into account. I loved it when she had to go away for a few days last month because of her father's sickness and we had a maid in our house. I didn't have to consider the maid's needs at all. I was really satisfied. Everything went along routinely. All the meals were on time. I had no worry about the children. I could come and go as I wanted to. I didn't have to discuss anything about myself. The maid had to take care of everything, and I didn't have to think about her. I really loved it."

The hour was nearly over, and I added my interpretation of the dream: "I think that your dream is related to your anger at me in two different ways. I think you are furious because you can't use me to get the satisfaction that you want from me (the way you use your little Henry in the dream). In the second place I think you feel a particular rage at me because you believe that I get a tremendous delight out of making you do what *I* want. You manage to agree with me, but if you go beyond that and actually change, then you feel that you are affording me an almost orgastic delight. This is the only way in which you can conceive of people relating to one another pleasurably—by dominating and exploiting. In the dream you find repeated orgastic pleasure in getting someone to submit to you completely. In your relationship with me you become enraged because you can't make me submit, and you imagine that I find my pleasure in subduing you."

In this dream there is an essentially nonsexual content in spite of its patently sexual symbolism. Homoerotic practices are portrayed, yet the question of homosexuality does not arise. The spirit and form of erotic practice are a vivid expression of the patient's interpersonal goals.

Homoerotic behavior is particularly manipulative and exploitative. However, all pathological sexuality, whether heterosexual or homosexual, is characterized by manipulation and exploitation. In waking life or in dreams, our concern as therapists is not with the form of the sexual practice but with the personality problem expressed by it. Thus when this patient dreams about using his little boy homoerotically, we do not become preoccupied with whether or not the patient is a homosexual. We are concerned with the pattern and meaning of his interpersonal dealings. The self-indulgent exploitation of the child in the dream was a pattern of interpersonal behavior that was also reflected in innumerable situations with others, people of all ages and of both sexes, connected with the patient in a variety of ways. Consistently, the self-indulgent, exploitative pattern of interpersonal behavior characterized his sexual approaches to his wife.

This dream occurred during a period of significant change in the personality of the patient. He had evidenced resistance in persistently colorless, nonaffective reports during his analytic sessions; in his psychosomatic expressions of rage and hatred for the analyst (intestinal tensions and severe headaches); in depressions; and in his derogation and contempt for the analyst following the public encounter. On the other hand, he had also given much evidence of significant constructive change. He had achieved a fuller (although brief) expression of feeling than he had yet experienced in two years of treatment when he stated angrily that he felt like smashing up the office. At home he had developed greater tenderness toward his little Henry than he had yet experienced toward any of his children. In spite of depressive reluctance, he had made recent important changes in a forward direction occupationally and domestically. In the session here described, he had engaged in a more cooperative, productive fashion, spontaneously and successfully overcoming his intense angry resistance.

The essence of this man's personality was: wanting to be taken care of, to use, to exploit, to have complete power over others, while no one was to get any satisfaction from him. This kind of role in life was utterly threatened by his becoming a more responsible father and husband and a more independent professional man. His life was changing. He was changing. God damn the analyst! Back to the joys of having people helpless in your hands, controlling them, using them. Back to being "sucked off"!

Tiny Cobras

The patient who experienced this anxiety dream was a young married woman who enjoyed frequent satisfying intercourse with her husband. She had a single, healthy, welcome child. In analysis she had been working during the previous three months on her problem of using timidity and helplessness, coupled with a general manner of excessive sweetness, for domination of her husband and others. The sweetness served also to disguise the fury she often felt toward those she could not dominate, toward any who were in a position to exert pressure upon her, and toward those who were superior to her in some way that had significance for her.

She had begun to face the existence in herself of rage and jealousy, and at the same time to develop a greater self-respect. She had been gradually achieving more directness in her dealings with people, and greater self-sufficiency and decisiveness both in her marriage and in her broader social life. This progressive success had been punctuated by frequent anxiety as well as pleasure and pride. Three months after the initiation of her determined attack on these problems, the following nightmare was presented.

"There were many tiny cobras. They were about a foot long and sandy colored. This was all in a room, and there were bookshelves. . . . The cobras were concealed everywhere. They came up everywhere I went. They could come out of a book. There were other people around and I was pleading with them not to do it. They had something to do with having these snakes come out. I pleaded with them not to do it because I was so scared of snakes. I didn't kill the snakes. I was too scared to touch them. I was pleading with the people. They were doing it on purpose. They were hiding the snakes. I was tense and scared. I woke up petrified.

"I kept waking up and I was too frightened to go to sleep again. I kept waking myself up lest I dream about the snakes again, but finally did get to sleep. I'd rather kill myself than a snake, because the snake would get me before I got him.

"The next night I began to feel frightened lest I get that dream again, so I lay in bed and started to analyze the dream so that I wouldn't get it again. I think it has to do with something in someone else that's in me. The other night Frank [husband] and I and another couple were at a large party together. I detest Isabelle. She spoiled our evening completely. I tried so hard not to let her disturb me. I was wearing a Spanish dress that Frank had brought me from Spain. Isabelle said, 'You'll be *so* upset. There's another Spanish dress here.' I said, 'I couldn't care less.' Isabelle was stunned. Saying 'I couldn't care less' was competitive. The whole evening was competitive among the four of us. The helplessness in the dream—I was pleading with the other people to kill the snakes. The snakes were like a challenge to my helplessness."

Here I interjected, "You were sorry that you said 'I couldn't care less.' You felt bad that you said it, is that it?"

She replied, "It's not a nice thing to say."

Then I said, "Your remark was quite appropriate under the circumstances, but your saying it did show that you are not at all helpless."

She elaborated the thought, saying, "I couldn't stand the success of what I said."

At this point I reminded her of a dream which she had had the night before going to visit the repertory company of which she had once been a member. The patient was quite proud of having left theater life and established herself in a good marriage and borne a child. She felt superior to the other people in the company who were still struggling to succeed on the stage. She had hoped they would look jealously at her while she would appear elated, sweet, still the ingénue. Before going to visit this group she had had a nightmare in which she was trying to sweep out a room in which there were many little vicious crocodiles (her own malice) running around on the floor. In the dream it was her job to sweep them out, and she was upset because she wasn't quite succeeding.

Her response to my reference to that crocodile nightmare was, "This girl Isabelle who made that remark at the dance is just like that bitch Jill in the repertory company." After a pause, she added, "I'm afraid of lashing out at Frank when he's unfair to me."

I then said, "You're really quite capable of handling Frank's unfairness and also the poisonous things from Isabelle and Jill and others."

She replied, "I'm afraid of real snakes. They are one thing I can do nothing about."

"But," I said, "if you had your child with you and you met a snake, you'd back away from such a situation."

"Yes," she replied, "but that's not handling the situation."

"Nevertheless," I said, "it would be appropriate to back away if there were a real snake. You don't have to become a snake-killer nor do you have to stand and shriek for someone to come and take care of you."

She replied, "I think there's a snakelike quality in me. It's sneakiness. I manipulate Frank by my helplessness."

Here I said, "You're really quite capable of taking care of yourself. You slapped down Isabelle quite effectively. What frightens you is that you can't expect to handle yourself capably in front of your husband and at the same time cry for his help because you're so helpless. When you strike back in front of him you're really destroying the effectiveness of your sweet, helpless manipulative role." Her response was to recall a relationship with a woman friend in which she had been quite docile and intimidated. That relationship had improved when she had begun to assert herself in a healthy fashion. When her husband was present, however, she would change her manner. She would hide her effective, self-assured behavior with this woman so that her husband could not detect the change in her. After a visit with this woman she would come to her analytic session and report the interpersonal progress she was making, but when she recounted to her husband the identical visit, she would describe it as a trying situation, conjuring up a sense of her helplessness in the relationship. She replied, "I'm like a snake with my husband. When a snake strikes, it's suddenly. It's right out of the blue. That's the way I pick on him. I suddenly criticize something he's doing in the midst of an otherwise peaceful situation."

The hour was ending at this point. I suggested that the fright from the tiny cobras came from two sources. First, she was recognizing her own snakelike qualities, her own destructiveness, her sneakiness, her darting attacks. Secondly, by the exposure in herself of this destructiveness toward others, she was destroying the manipulative effectiveness of her innocent, sweet, helpless role. In the dream she was pleading with people not to do things which would "bring out" her venomous (her cobra) characteristics. (In the dream others were responsible for putting snakes into the picture: "I kept pleading with them; they were doing it on purpose.") If only Isabelle had not made that bitchy remark at the party, the patient's venomously inflected "I couldn't care less" would not have suddenly, uncontrollably, popped out. The snakes represented her aggressive retaliation, and if she were revealed as self-sufficient in her own defense, capable of attacking, this public revelation would in itself destroy her. It would render impotent (kill, as snakes kill) the personality which operated effectively in a role of sweet helplessness.

While she and her husband often enough enjoyed well-functioning intercourse, she recognized that her destructive, viperous quality was from time to time expressed in a perverse yearning for sex when her husband was physically exhausted. The meaning of the tiny-cobras symbolism extended thus to her sexual life, not in terms of a classical phallic concept, fear of the penile serpent, but as an expression of the interpersonal pathology set forth in the interpretive discussion of the dream.

Long Corridor

The following dream, coming at a crucial period, had failed to be of use to the patient in her previous analysis (curative in many ways) because interpretation had been imposed which was based upon a belief in universal sexual symbolism. Thirty-eight years old at the time, she had already spent twenty years in a miserable marriage which she still hoped to reconstruct.

"I was starting to walk down a long corridor. It was the corridor of a hotel where we had spent the Christmas holidays in Palm Beach. It was a very long corridor, with many doors on each side. As I walked toward the far end, where our room was, I could hear voices behind the doors as I passed them. Behind the doors people were talking and laughing, children were singing and playing games. People were quarreling and gossiping, or just telling ordinary things to each other. In the dream I thought, 'So much is going on behind the doors, but here in the corridor I'm alone.' The light was very dim and bleak. The carpet was old and faded."

She recalled, "The dream came up at the end of the session and very little was said about it. My analyst made an immediate interpretation. He said the long corridor was my vagina, and that I felt neglected in my sex life. His interpretation was a shock to me. It didn't seem to ring a bell. There was nothing in it that I recognized, and I didn't feel excited in the painful but rewarding way that I used to feel excited when an interpretation was recognizable and gave me something to work on in my home life. Instead I was shocked and saddened, and I felt that something was missing in the interpretation, that there was more in the dream, and that I was losing the value of the dream somehow."

The dream remained vivid in her mind for years afterward. "I can still [nine years later] see the corridor with the many closed doors. I am certain now that the dream represented the way I felt about my entire life at that time. I felt that all doors were closed to me, that the rest of my life was going to be a long, bleak, empty journey. I had already unconsciously given up on my marriage, and I had no hope of getting out of it at that time. Other people were living together, having meaningful relationships. Things were happening to them. I was sealed off in an empty corridor. If I had understood the dream and consciously recognized how hopeless I felt about my marriage, I would have taken steps to get out of it at that time, instead of waiting five more long, miserable years."

The dream which had, meaninglessly for her, been interpreted in sexual terms, was, I believe, not at all a sexual dream. The patient might have obtained from it the insight that would have helped her out of the marriage before she was released from analysis, instead of five unhappy years later.

Three Bedraggled Cats

There are many words in the vernacular which support the interpretation of cats in dreams as symbols of female genitality. Nevertheless, when we seek to derive specific meanings from the life context of the individual dreamer, we find cats appearing in dreams without reference to sexuality.

The following dream came from a forty-year-old man who had begun to experience emergent healthy interpersonal feelings. "There were three cats and somewhere in this dream the three cats were lost. [He associated the cats with his wife and two children. The older child was a boy.] They strayed away or something. A couple of days later they came in through the window, one after the other, bedraggled, hungry, tired. It was very odd to me that a cat could find its way back. The minute they came in, two of them were somewhat vague, but one of them was very clear and came and snuggled up to me like a human being in its happiness at being back."

The dream occurred at a time when the patient, who had grown somewhat more aware of his wife as a person, and warmer toward her, had nevertheless established a subtle competitive struggle to keep her from extending the independent community activities which she enjoyed. He had, earlier, as an outgrowth of analysis, encouraged this and other activities, but then had begun sulkily and self-righteously to withdraw his support. He marveled in the dream at the cat's capacity to find her way back (his wife's ability to reach out to him with tenderness, despite his "leaving her out in the cold"). He marveled at the cat's looking for human warmth and attention from him, above everything else it needed.

"I thought that cats could get along by themselves" [that women needed only material provisions and sex, not human responsiveness]. He also said, referring to the cat in the dream, "I petted her, which is the last thing I'd do to a cat. This makes me think of all the affection and warmth that I have been withholding all this time."

To treat this material as a reflection of problems of sexuality would tend to deprive the patient of insight into both the evidences of and the obstacles (such as his emotional parsimony) in the way of his increasing humanity and maturity.

Statuesque Masturbation

A brilliant research engineer in his early thirties expected endless attention and admiration from his wife, who resented these demands.

When the first baby came he begrudged it the priority of solicitude it required, even to the extent of raging one morning because the formula was started before his breakfast eggs. At that period, in order to rectify his outraged sense of general deprivation, he entered into a clandestine extramarital affair. His mistress adequately worshipped the neglected scientific hero. She was a completely submissive young woman, adoring, sexually acquiescent, available, someone who he felt really loved him. That affair had ended before he came into analysis. At the time of the dream about to be reported, he was trying to understand the role of his excessive demands in bringing about the unhappy state of his marriage. In the atmosphere of this incipient insight, he returned home one evening with an optimistic outlook and flushed with a sense of being a good husband. He and his wife had planned to hire a baby-sitter and to go together to a movie that both wished very much to see. As they were finishing coffee the sitter's mother called to say her daughter had become ill and would not be able to sit for them. After a few hurried calls they found no available substitute. With a genial, expansive, equalitarian gesture, the patient turned to his wife and said, "That's all right, darling—let's toss a coin for it. The loser will stay home and be the sitter." So they tossed, and *she* won. But then she did not say, as he had confidently expected, "Oh that's all right, dear—you go." She accepted her victory and went off alone to the movies. Outwardly a good sport, he was nevertheless inwardly furious. Shortly after his wife left, he sat down in the living room and masturbated. That night he dreamed.

"I was standing like a tremendous statue, a colossus. My arms were akimbo and my legs sort of astride. I was huge, and I had a gigantic erection, nearly six feet long and a diameter that was proportionate. At the end of my penis, on top, there was a little safety valve, like the kind on top of a furnace. As I stood there with this tremendous erection, beneath it there stood a beautiful naked woman reaching up with her arms and stroking it back and forth. She just stood under it and stroked it back and forth like a slave. At a certain point the safety valve went off and there was a great big spurt upwards. That was the end of the dream."

His chief associations were the incidents of the coin toss and the masturbation when he had been "steaming mad," and memories of his erstwhile mistress.

Certainly this man's grandiosity was strikingly symbolized in the dream. A great deal more, however, than sexual potency was represented. He not only saw women as diminutive, but in his aloof, statuesque posture and proportions he towered above all other men as well.

The ingredient of aloofness in his grandiosity was emphasized as he presented himself for the satisfaction of his needs in a manner that precluded intimacy or reciprocation. (Likewise, on the evening of the dream he had been puffed up with a sense of generous equalitarianism, but had offered his wife only a counterfeit of affectionate respect.) The penile safety valve in the dream reflected the way he had of "blowing off steam" by going to his slavish mistress, an act which he reproduced through masturbation on the evening before the dream. Acquiescence and adulation were responses he demanded, not only from his wife, but also from his parents, siblings, and colleagues. When frustrated by any of these, he became angered and sought emotional harmony through the compensatory satisfaction of his pathological requirements elsewhere. Sometimes this was accomplished in academic or social surroundings, by the evocation of admiration, the commandeering of services, or the elicitation of special favors. The dream of the glorious statue being masturbated by a female slave presented in vivid sexual symbols his basically nonsexual personality pathology.

Contemptible Passion

Another patently sexual dream was that of the young psychiatrist entering "training analysis," who stated that he had chosen me because he liked my personality and my views. During the night before his first analytic hour he dreamed of a young man passionately engaged in intercourse on a couch under the derisive, contemptuous gaze of an older man. The dream suggested much about the patient that had no specific or primary relation to sexual pathology. He was exposing cynicism, a secret belief that the analyst whom he lauded for compassionate qualities was actually profoundly contemptuous. The dream also reflected the patient's fear of the analytic process, specifically a fear of appearing ridiculous if he freely expressed any passionately felt emotions.

Sexual passion in this dream was a symbol for deeply felt emotions of all kinds, while intercourse represented the expression of such feelings. It was essential to recognize and to deal with this patient's distorted attitude toward expressing all intense emotions rather than to restrict the therapeutic exploration to his feeling about sex. It was similarly vital to investigate with him his cynicism, manifested by doubts about the very qualities he had praised in the analyst, rather than to concentrate upon his attitude regarding the analyst's responses specifically to his sexual behavior.

The relationship of the patient with his analyst is often expressed sexually by the patient in his dreams.[4] The young research engineer of the Statuesque Masturbation dream provided repeated examples. It was painful for this intellectual colossus to engage in the intimate exposure of himself that is necessary in analysis without the consolation of some sense of worshipful solicitude from the analyst, something akin to the awe-struck dedication of a mistress. The analyst's clinical objectivity, combined with an appropriately sympathetic and friendly but unimpassioned regard (recognized as no different from the response toward any other analytic patient), was for this patient insupportable. In addition to a number of dreams reflecting these problems—some despondent, others homicidal toward the analyst (see Sledgehammer Attack, p. 163)—he had several sexual dreams. In one, he visited a most beautiful woman who was quite ready to receive him as a lover, but who made him feel humiliated and frustrated because of her independence (Independent Mistress). She was attractive and she was available, but her independence and unconquerability were unbearable. The dream was an expression of the patient's desire to make a conquest, to subordinate, and was clearly not a symbol of a homosexual approach to the analyst. The patient could accept me as his analyst, admire me, seek me out, look to me for help and comfort, if I could only be overwhelmed by his caliber, be to him in a subordinate relationship analogous to that of an adoring mistress. For him, a mistress who had her own integrity, her self-asserted equality, her independence, was no solace whatever, no matter how attractive and available in other ways. Similarly, the analyst's friendly and competent collaboration was for this patient no substitute for the pathologically demanded adoration. It was so hard for him to need an analyst simply the way anyone else needs an analyst!

Grandiosity and the desire to dominate, here specifically focused in the analyst-patient relationship, were the aspects of pathology reflected in the patient's dream in the form of sexual metaphor.

The same patient had another dream, in which he was in bed with a woman, impotently and clumsily trying to make sexual ingress through her side (Sideways Approach). This dream reflected his seductive tactics carried to a stubborn, persistent extreme. It referred immediately to the relationship with the analyst, representing his intense desire somehow to penetrate the analyst, but was associated broadly with many tough interpersonal situations involving both men and women. The problem of the dream, expressed only incidentally

[4] Examples of this are more extensively presented in Chapter 7.

in sexual terms, was his continuing attempts at conquest, with, however, the use of indirection—a "sideways approach."

At one productive point in his analysis I became more energetic in seeking to engage him in exploring a problem. This led to a dream in which he found himself in bed with an old Negro prostitute, who was pleading with him to make love to her (Old Negro Prostitute). In the dream he was revolted by her eagerness for him. Work with this dream revealed that the very sight of another person wanting an honest exchange was repellent to him. Others were expected to reach out worshipfully to indulge him, like the slave under the statuesque penis. By revealing a genuine eagerness for him to go further in the pursuit of an insight, I had engendered only his contempt for me. Subjectively he recoiled as from a hungry old whore.

The patient revealed through the sexual pictorialization in the dream another facet of his pathology. The dream did not indicate fear of what he might have misconstrued as homosexual overtures by his analyst, nor a general recoil from heterosexual contact. In this dream the analyst's overt concern and recognizably felt desire to make contact with the patient was represented as a sluttish approach that invoked his disgust and recoil. More broadly, there was implied the contempt of this superior and remote scientist for any human emotional needs.

This patient's pathology was deep and damaging. It would be bound to isolate him from, among other experiences, any significant sexual love. More than this, it would insulate him also against responsiveness to the need of his children for him, and to the need of his wife for him; it would insulate him against friendship, against being responsive to the need for him of others outside the family. The more he insulated himself from the need of others for him, the more he rendered himself incapable of developing the capacity or the freedom to experience or to express meaningful need for others.

An approach to the whole problem of the need of human beings to make meaningful contact with each other, and his distorted attitude about this, was first made through the analytic relationship. It was explored in terms of the patient's genuine need for the analyst and the analyst's healthy need to function spontaneously and productively in response.

A clear view of his emotionally distorting, emotionally isolating, and emotionally retarding pathology developed for the patient in the course of his therapy. It began to evolve through its expression in a dream, and was initially symbolized in sexual images.

Old Woman Masturbating Him

A picture with some similarity to the last dream was presented by a young man in his early twenties. In the dream an old woman was paying him for the privilege of "jerking him off." "She was working her hardest to make me come. I just laughed and lay calmly aloof."

Like the patient of the Negro Prostitute dream, this patient manifested grandiosity in his contempt for any display of emotion and in the pride he had in his capacity to "play it cool." An additional problem, his sadism, was expressed most characteristically in his enjoyment of *withholding of expected responses*, especially emotional responses. He took pleasure in *not* being upset when scolded or deprived by his parents, *not* responding sexually to girls after he had succeeded in attracting them, or, in the reverse situations, in *not* restraining himself sexually when a girl wanted him to do so. He loved to keep a straight face when someone told a funny story. He enjoyed remaining indifferent when someone else was enthusiastic. In the dream he enjoyed *not* having an orgasm as the concerned old woman masturbated him. Consequently, it was of considerable importance that we should not become lost in speculations regarding possible homosexual transference to the analyst. Pursuit of the explicit problems set forth in his dream—his cultivated anesthesia and his cruel enjoyment of frustrating—did, however, prove extremely fruitful. This pathology characterized his interpersonal relations with both sexes and functioned in the analysis itself, where his enjoyment of frustrating the analyst's efforts was a barrier to the patient's productive participation. The dream presented, in blatantly sexual terms, his pride in his impassiveness and his sadistic pathology which, while it permeated his sexual activities, was not fundamentally a sexual problem.

Just Friends

A genuine affectional feeling for the analyst may be an entirely healthy outgrowth of productive therapy. It is important not to relegate such an emotion to the area of pathology.[5] In the dream that follows, the patient revealed both a healthy, friendly feeling and a pathological sexual urge in relation to the analyst. It was necessary to recognize both feelings and to distinguish the one from the other.

[5] Affection for the analyst: See Chapter 6, pp. 226–228 and Chapter 10, p. 290; see also You Hold Me Close, pp. 275–278.

In the session three days before this dream occurred the patient attained the fullest degree of immediacy and the most honest communication of feeling that she had thus far achieved. In the analytic session that immediately preceded the dream, there was an upsurge of craving for intimacy with the analyst. Her emotions were a mixture of genuine affection and a strong sexual urge. In the discussion of these feelings I suggested to her, and she tentatively accepted as valid, that this emotional upheaval was associated with two principal factors. One was her gratitude for the assistance she was getting in orienting herself emotionally, in learning to feel both honest with herself and safe in intimacy with another. On the other hand, I speculated, her acceptance of feelings that she had so long fought against acknowledging, either to herself or to me, had had the emotional implications for her of submission to me, conquest by me. She had always feared the influence of others—parents, men, friends, husband, her analyst, and even her children. In her view, to be influenced by others was to be enslaved by them. One of her ways of conquering enslavement by men was through sexual conquest of them. In competitive response to her "submission" to my therapeutic guidance, she had therefore developed a great desire to make a sexual conquest of me.

The night following that analytic discussion—a discussion that relieved her of the agony of sexual desire with which she had come in— she had a dream.

"You were a homo or in some way inaccessible. It was a silly dream. It was not you. It was a man—almost asexual. There was no detail. I wanted him sexually, but he was inaccessible so we decided to be just friends."

Then she quickly added, "It makes me angry to think of him being inaccessible—nobody is going to tell me what to do! Oh, now I remember what we were talking about yesterday—my fear of enslavement."

The achievement of trust in another seemed like being conquered. In spite of the patient's inordinate competitiveness and the resulting emotional confusion, she was able to represent in a dream what she was reluctant to acknowledge when awake—the realistic situation of being *friends* with her helpful analyst. At the same time, in a sort of counterattack, she symbolized her desire to conquer him; this was the upsurge of sexual desire (a common psychosomatic preparation for interpersonal conquest in our culture). Her healthy attempt to abandon this approach to an interpersonal dilemma was only partially successful. Somewhat reluctantly she resigned herself to the impossibility of the pathological solution. She expressed the emotional compromise in her dream through the desexualization of the analyst. Through this dream therapeutic gains were made by the delineation and separate consideration of its definitely sexual aspects, in this case pathological, and its definitely affectional aspects, which were clearly healthy.

Homosexual Incest

A young woman of twenty-five who had been brought up never to show emotion had begun, after some time in analysis, to achieve a measure of courage and the capacity to accept and reciprocate warmth and friendliness. Her distrust of the genuine interest of others was both an excuse for keeping them at a distance by hostile or superficial behavior and a technique for squelching her own spontaneous friendliness. The distance she maintained deprived her of friendship, and this deprivation in turn made her feel worthless. Convinced that she was worthless, she then felt re-enforced in her certainty that all friendly overtures toward her were insincere.

"Grace is willing to satisfy my need for people, but it is not because she likes me. She has no feeling for me, therefore there must be something manipulative going on. If people have no feeling for me, their friendliness must be manipulative. So their friendliness must be seduction." This was the way she speculated about Grace, her only durable friend, after an especially friendly visit to the apartment of Grace and her husband. The night of that congenial visit she had the dream that follows. She said it was a "horrible dream," very hard for her to report, "because it has two horrible things" in it—homosexuality and incest, and these, furthermore, with a sister whom she neither liked nor trusted.

"My sister and I were sleeping in the same room. I woke up—Oh God!—and as I wake up in the dream I find her about to start petting me. Her hand is creeping toward my vagina, up my thigh. I had two strong emotions. I felt terrible revulsion from it and also a great temptation to enjoy it. I woke up from the dream with both feelings."

With no hesitation she went right on to associations. "It's the same feeling I have with her whenever I'm with her. It's the same feeling I get from her behavior, which is in a way very warm and friendly and admiring—she's always full of admiration—and I always have that feeling that she wants to seduce me, though not in a sexual sense. I always have this uncomfortable feeling she is trying to suck me in and at the same time I'm tempted to enjoy her attention to me. Yet I know so firmly it's all an act: one, because of the way she's treated me, never with any consideration or love; and two, because she tears down other people behind their backs; and in the third place, when she's talking to other people I can see very clearly that she's acting. Yet, when she's talking the same way to me, I'm deluded it's real."

I reminded her of a nightmare (see Crazy Woman, pp. 73–77) she had had a year and half earlier, when she had begun her first timid efforts in the realm of the emotions, had first permitted herself to acknowledge their existence, and had dared to express some feeling in analysis. In that nightmare the analyst was represented as an insane woman making wild demands on her. The patient responded to this recall by saying, "I was afraid of feelings in the Crazy Woman dream, and I saw expressing feelings to you as a nightmarish thing—now I'm afraid of having feelings in social exchanges, of having feelings socially, with other people."

The patient came in to the next hour and remarked at once, "It was wonderful that you thought of the Crazy Woman dream. That woman [an emotionally unstable actual acquaintance who represented the analyst in the dream] is someone who *is* nearly crazy. She was a symbol of something I *was* afraid of, and my sister is, too. That woman was sick, and I saw emotions as something sick and to be afraid of. I see everybody as having just under the surface what she showed openly. I don't trust the reliability of emotions.

"My sister is a sick person, and I see her as being insincere, which I'm sure she is. She is a symbol of the insincerity of all people. Just like the incest dream, she could seduce me coldly, calculatingly, without any real feeling for me at all. If I succumb, what I'm afraid of is giving her the pleasure of seducing me without her giving me something genuine. Then she'd have me under her thumb and it would be a terrible humiliation.

"In real life I want friendliness and warmth; that's what's symbolized by desire for sexual satisfaction in the dream."

Then she expanded on these nonsexual feelings about being seduced, enslaved, humiliated, and also on her yearning for genuine closeness. She made the connection between these feelings and the interpersonal situation in her actual sexual relationships, too. "I just started thinking of feelings I've had during intercourse with men. They're the same feelings as in the dream. He has no interest in me as a person. I know it. I have a great desire for sex and a great desire to satisfy it, even if the guy is not what I want and it's all dirty. I just can't visualize a healthy situation between me and another person. It's all a matter of people using me and me using people. The real thing doesn't exist. That's why it's dirty to me. Because it's not *real intimacy.*"

This seemed to be a complete return to and restatement of her feelings at the beginning of analysis. She could no longer, however, accept so barren a state of living. She thought some more. The dream had, after all, followed an evening of more than usual friendliness at Grace's. She associated the analyst (as in the Crazy Woman dream of a year and a half earlier) with the sister-woman in this dream. "Maybe I've got things all twisted up, and it's healthy things I'm resisting. If the dream is my cynicism toward people generally, and it's you in the dream, the temptation would be a healthy thing. It would be reversed. The temptation to open up, to give, to want, and to take would be healthy. That's what I would like for it to be. That seems so much to the point of what we are trying to get at. I fear being used and manipulated . . . the truth is I do feel less isolated, more of a human being than I did. I care more . . . I want more."

This dream of homosexuality and incest was a sexual metaphor for the patient's feelings concerning the whole range of intimate human relationships. During the course of her changing through psychoanalysis, she began to strive for warmth, for the enjoyment of the friendship available, and for the establishment of more friendships with both sexes. She had been worried that the enjoyment of others, for which she yearned, was a dirty, nonmeaningful use of them, or else an exposure of herself to a dirty nonmeaningful enjoyment by them. The response to friendly overtures, or the intensification of an established relationship with a female friend or a male analyst, was for her like lending oneself to the seductive blandishment of an insincere, destructive older sister in real everyday life, and like engagement in homosexual incest in dream life. To this patient, sexual relationships and intimate nonsexual relationships had a common foundation—both were dirty, like homosexuality and incest, like seduction, getting people under your thumb, exploitation. She had equal doubts about the possibility of healthy friendship and healthy sex.

The dream had been precipitated by the doubts and fears engendered in a completely nonsexual friendship context—the evening with Grace—and augmented by her increasing trust of the analyst. She was saying in this dream, in overt sexual symbols, that friendly and affectionate overtures frightened her, and that she was more threatened and revolted because what might turn out to be false and humiliating was, if genuine, so attractive to her and so yearned for. Although the metaphoric language of the dream was sexual, the problem was clearly not limited to nor determined by sexuality; her pathology was that of interpersonal disturbances involving profound cynicism toward and fear of the emotions of intimacy. These disturbances applied in precisely the same manner to nonsexual and to sexual activity, and to the areas of her relationships with both men and women.

Three Condoms

A final clinical illustration of a nonsexual aspect of personality expressed in clear sexual form is the dream of the Three Condoms. This was reported by a thirty-year-old bachelor, experiencing, as he approached marriage, a mixture of anxiety and depression because of the crescendo of emotional demands upon him. He had been raised as an only child by a superficial, falsely gracious, middle-class mother who considered most people beneath her family in quality. Both parents had hovered over the patient throughout his childhood. His mother had been opportunistic about her son's every cramp or sniffle, having sought to use all such minor physical signs to cordon him off from his peers while she ministered to his every need except that for independence. After college, medical school, and Army service, even after he had become a successfully developing ophthalmologist, she would still call him on snowy mornings to advise his wearing galoshes. After he was already comfortably self-supporting, it had once been a momentous and anxiety-ridden step, as he took leave of his parents at the end of a routine visit, for him finally to use his own money for the subway.

By the time of the dream reported below, he had made much progress in becoming independent of his parents, had concluded several relatively long-term affairs with women, was well established professionally, and was on the verge of marriage to a sound and affectionate woman. The occasional dutiful visits to his parents were, as in the past, unrewarding.

After visiting them alone one Sunday afternoon when his fiancée was out of town, he had the dream: "Three people were sleeping, wearing three condoms. They were all in one very big bed. They were supposed to be using the condoms for some active sexual activity, not necessarily with a prostitute, but certainly someone with whom there was no attachment. Instead they each had a nocturnal emission with the condoms on, and the thought crossed my mind in the dream that it would be messy and wet and a waste of the condom. The three condoms cost forty-five cents.

"It was weird. I had a feeling that the three people were vaguely *me*, my *father*, and my *mother*, and that my mother had given out the condoms, but her having a condom doesn't seem right—a female doesn't need a condom."

His first association was, "Yesterday afternoon I went with my parents to a neighborhood movie. I got up and bought chocolate bonbons for the three of us. They cost forty-five cents. In one scene of the movie a girl who reminded me of my girl said something about the difference between genuineness and superficial trappings." He then went on to discuss a relationship with a woman in which he had sought to avoid superficiality and to have a meaningful contact.

I asked him what his *feeling* was in the dream and he answered, "*Death warmed over* is the feeling I had in the dream—that phrase comes when I think of feeling in the dream."

When I asked what he thought was the meaning of the dream, he replied slowly, "I don't know—something about sterileness, our family's sterileness—I'm included." He was silent for a few moments and then added, "I think it's a concern about my ability to bear fruit in a relationship."

"So you really see yourself with the same kind of sterility as your mother and father?"

"Yes," he said, "I've had no relationships that have really borne fruit. What was the forty-five cents for condoms? Oh, that was the forty-five cents I paid for the bonbons. That was the extent of my participation with my parents."

Again I carried his thought along, saying, "That's as much as you have to offer them, or they you? The relationship among you is about as fruitful as the three of you lying there having wet dreams into condoms."

His thought shifted to his future wife. "I suppose I'm concerned about not having much to offer the girl I'm marrying."

Often he had spoken with contempt of his mother's emotional stinginess and falseness, of the inhospitable atmosphere in his home as he grew up, of the lack of family friends, of the lack of affection between his parents, and of his mother's having "worn the pants." He had often spoken of his mother's quick smile but complete lack of warmth. The patient in his own life had, in spite of many contacts, experienced little intimacy or friendship. His fiancée's abundant, genuine warmth had been to him, nevertheless, the most attractive aspect of her, a determining factor in his marital decision. With his decision to marry, however, a characteristic reserve had tended to become re-enforced in him and he had tended to withdraw from socializing rather than to continue his trend toward expansion of more meaningful friendships.

After his expression of concern about not having much to offer his fiancée, I said, "You felt in the dream that your mother had given out the condoms. At the movies it was actually you who had given out the bonbons. It's as though you feel that what you offer is the same as what your mother offers, that you are like your mother. That is the sterility in your relationships with your parents and others. What could be emptier, more sterile, than a wet dream into a condom?"

He concluded the hour with the remark, "But I've been feeling warm toward my girl. It goes in cycles."

My own final comment was to the effect that he did feel his greatest warmth toward the woman he was going to marry—that the problem of the dream was not his warmth, which he did show at times, but his concern about the lack of it. This was the basic problem which he had to explore, the sense that his engagement in human relationships was like "death warmed over."

This lack of warmth was a generally consistent deficiency that had again to be pursued. It had been repeatedly investigated in the past with, however, less urgency and less awareness. The similarity between his personality and that of his mother's was shocking to him. A few weeks later, after an interval during which he had grown closer to his fiancée, both in activity and feeling, he said at one session when suddenly and obviously affected by recall of the dream, "The stark sterileness of it makes me shudder now." Thinking about it further, he added, "I remember going to that movie—the three of us sitting there. There was no intercourse—the only intercourse was my getting them the bonbons. The movie was the ejaculation—a pleasant sensation, no more. My mother being masculine that way and distributing the condoms—she's been the initiator of that kind of sterile activity." It was this kind of sterile human intercourse that became illuminated by the dream as an important aspect of the patient's feeling and behavior.

In this final clinical example it is again abundantly clear that sexual symbolism can be understood as reflecting basic interpersonal pathology. In this instance, the problem can be characterized as an emotional sterility, a withholding of warmth, an avoidance of affectional intimacy. The problem was exacerbated by the imminence of marriage.

Naturally the presence in the dream of the adult patient in bed with both of his parents in a sexual context, and at a time in his life when he is disturbed by the prospect of marriage, offers rich speculative possibilities for Oedipal interpretation. Such an interpretation would, however, be arbitrary. It would be the application of a construct from outside of this patient's biography, and would result merely in substituting one set of symbols for another. There was a real and immediate problem to tackle—the problem of his unwillingness to fructify a relationship, to give himself to the enhancement of another.

The sterility manifested in dramatic, passive sexual symbols in the dream was present also in the patient's sexual life. There his emotional sterility was manifested in an *active*, although unconscious, form, in the practice of premature ejaculation, which was his refusal of full engagement in intimacy, a refusal to give himself to another person. The patient completely overcame premature ejaculation. On one occasion, however, later in the same night on which he had achieved his most intimate experience of intercourse, he masturbated. During this masturbation he had a fantasy which could be regarded as compensatory: masturbatory orgasm was achieved with a spontaneous visual flash of premature ejaculation! This dramatically expressed his resistance to his growing capacity for affection and intimacy.

In the tradition of orthodox psychoanalysis, the human being has been regarded and dealt with clinically as a *predominantly instinctual, primarily sexual* individual in both the emergence and the functioning of his personality; dreams have been correspondingly dealt with as the reflection of such an individual.

It is the orientation of this book that basic functional aspects of the total personality—conceptualizing, communicating, responding affectively, creating, engaging in all types of human behavior including sexual activity—are never limited to nor determined primarily by the individual's sexual constitution or experience.

Most of the dreams in this chapter have shown manifest sexual symbolism. These and numerous others throughout the book abundantly demonstrate the possibilities of sound clinical use of dream material without recourse to classical psychosexual concepts and their derivative symbolism. All dreams, all feelings in dreams, all dream symbols, sexual or otherwise, ultimately refer to aspects of the total personality of the patient as it operates through the broad range of interpersonal and intrapersonal function.

5. *Anxiety in Dreams*

THE BASIC CAUSE of pathological anxiety, in dreams or in waking life, is a feeling of bankruptcy or of the impending failure of an important way of functioning. Personality evolves from interpersonal processes; its functioning produces a subjective experience, the sense of self. Personality functioning, furthermore, to be effective, requires (as in a game of tennis) the consummating response of others. The human being, even in isolation, *even while dreaming*, functions always in terms of interpersonal referents. When the functioning (including the consummating response) is threatened, the derivative sense of self is also threatened.

The interpersonal processes in our culture are pervasively competitive in nature. There is a constant contest to prevail over others, to use them to fulfill one's own functional effectiveness, and to avoid being used—as indicated in Chapter 2, "Feeling in Dreams." This competitive struggle is a constant and prevailing source of anxiety, accentuating the anxiety stemming from all of the processes to be discussed in this chapter.

Human functioning is infinitely complex, and during anxiety, as during any other experience, the behavioral, conceptual, and affective processes are going on simultaneously. Elements of the totality may, however, be delineated to facilitate examination. The "sense of self" refers to the basically nonconceptual, subjective *affective* sense of being that derives directly from the functioning of one's personality, from functional effectiveness. There is, in addition, the *conceptual* aspect of the functioning personality, the "self-concept" which is an interpretation—often a misinterpretation—of the meaning and consequences of one's functioning and of the kind of person it denotes.

In Chapter 2 it was pointed out that there is often a discrepancy between the individual's emotions and his concept of his emotions. In the area of interpersonal activity a parallel discrepancy may exist between the individual's behavior and his concept of his behavior. The discrepancies involving emotions and those involving behavior are in fact more than parallel—they are inseparably interwoven.

This was illustrated in the case of the young bachelor who thought he was *feeling* "compassionate" and *acting* "protectively" toward the badgered husband, when in fact he was feeling contemptuous and sadistic, and acting in such a way as to augment the husband's misery (see pp. 62–63).

A man like the benevolent and domineering patient of the Shark in Swimming Pool dream (see pp. 126–127), who manipulates people into doing what he wishes, gets a sense of self from this characteristic form of functioning. (I use functioning here to mean both the man's activities and the consummating responses of others.) By misinterpreting the nature of his influence on people and of their response to him, the man continues to elaborate and support his self-concept of benignity, generosity, and uprightness. One important source of his sense of self is his effective control of others; his self-concept enables him to maintain his gentle demeanor during his disguised tyrannical practices; and, reciprocally, the subtly controlling practices produce in others the docile responses which confirm his mistaken self-estimate as a gentle, generous, family man. His functioning, with its derivative affective sense of self, and his ideational self-concept are thus mutually supportive.

Likewise, the absence of consummating responses of others (ineffective functioning), or their outright attack upon his self-concept, are disrupting. If people do not respond, the individual may, nevertheless, in an effort to maintain his familiar sense of self, continue for a time in the same kind of functioning. But when the essential interactive responses from others persistently elude him, leaving his activity unconsummated, then the sense of self wavers, and the self-concept supported by this familiar functioning is also threatened. The patient's established activities may become anxiously intensified in his effort to stave off a sense of interpersonal bankruptcy. Other types of people, such as the depressive, shrink into inactivity, which is often a hostile and desperate emergency measure to activate responses no longer available through the old techniques. Both types of response—the anxious intensification and the depressive behavior—are bulwarks thrown up against reality's intolerable disruption of the patient's ways of living.[1]

Sometimes cumulative failure, or a single deeply shocking experience, may cast a significant doubt upon the individual's self-concept, and motivate him to recoil from the interpersonal functioning which supports it. (For example, an ingratiating magnanimity might lead to the end of a courtship, accompanied by angry but penetrating accusations that the seeming generosity was insincere and enslaving.) The more realistic appraisal, then, while it inhibits the pathological functioning, undermines the sense of self and is accompanied by anxiety.

The nightmare of the Tiny Cobras (see pp. 138–141) reflected the threat of functional bankruptcy. The patient, it will be recalled, was a young married woman, formerly an actress. She conceptualized and comported herself in the manner of an unfailingly sweet, genteel, dependent, and defenseless person. In covert and unaware ways she was also sharply and effectively competitive. By maintaining the facade of a shy, small-town girl in the big city, she was usually able to keep herself out of open contention and to maintain intact both her operative style and her self-concept.

At the dance which she and her husband attended with another couple, she successfully and caustically handled the "bitchy" assaults made upon her by the other wife. Her behavior challenged the authenticity and perpetuation of her sweet, vulnerable demeanor. Her venomousness, not a new development, but now exposed—particularly to her husband—represented a lethal threat which resulted in the terrifying dream of tiny cobras coming after her in a domestic setting.

Here then was the frightening, anxiety-raising threat; as a competitive and secretly superior person she could not bear to seem too stupid to comprehend and answer the subtle public assaults upon her of the other woman; her competent and venomous retaliation, however, threatened to annihilate her primary ingenuous weak style of interpersonal functioning, and the related sense of self and self-concept.

Another patient, threatened with the failure of a similar type of functioning, reflected her resultant anxiety in a nightmare of a murder trial (Murder Trial; see below). She was a married woman in her late thirties, a highly successful executive in the publishing field. Her behavior was nevertheless frequently timid and diffident, and she con-

[1] Elaboration of this concept of the depressive appears in the author's chapter, "Dynamics and Psychotherapy of Depression," in J. Masserman, ed., *Current Psychiatric Therapies*. New York: Grune and Stratton, 1962. (These dynamics have, in addition, important implications for psychotic processes.)

ceived of herself in those terms. She was the patient of the "another olive" incident described in the discussion of waking symbolism (pp. 42–43), and it may be recalled how she sweetly and unconscionably, and in a manner of helpless desperation, maneuvered to alter all of the vacation plans she and her husband had made with another couple. Then at their first meal in the shared cottage, she had asked in a mousey voice, "Does anybody mind if I take another olive?" The appropriate explosion, triggered by her pretense of being undemanding, frightened and angered her, and led to the analytic exploration of tyrannizing-by-dependency. When others recognized her helplessness as a demand, the effectiveness of this style of functioning would be lost, and a disintegration of the associated sense of self became imminent. With this, extreme anxiety as well as anger at the attacker was engendered.

The olive incident led to a further penetration of the problem, with particular reference to her marriage. One night about three months after the olive episode she lay in bed "thinking some more about how I use weakness to dominate." She fell asleep and had the following dream, and then "woke up so scared that I couldn't bring myself to get up and go to the bathroom, though I needed to."

"There was a murder trial going on. There was a horrible, gruff, uncouth, trampish man on trial and it looked as though a conviction would come. *A little boy, who had really committed the murder,* was darting in and out through the trial. I felt it was awful that the man should have to take the rap. *There was a shyness, a patheticness about the little boy and I hoped he wouldn't be found out.* In the dream I felt the little boy was I. I had terror for the kid—that he was going to be found out. *I felt I knew, and should inform.*"

The patient's first association was the feeling she had had that very morning, Election Day, in the voting booth. "I had fear in the voting booth—yet I have a *right* to vote." She unquestionably had a right to her one vote, just as she had a right to an olive. She had not, however, the right or power to force everyone else to vote her way, nor the right endlessly to push her friends around. The conscious exercise of her one-person franchise was, it appeared, subjectively very close to a violent wish to force her will on the electorate (as she had forced it upon her friends, and as she frequently tried to impose it upon her husband and her analyst). In the context of her nightmare and of the pursuit of this pathological functioning, even the modest but overt act of casting one vote was a dangerous occupation, and was therefore her first association with her anxiety dream of the deceptively innocent, murderous child.

In the course of the same session she said, "I was thinking the other night how I hated to have to talk to you about my dominating through weakness." She stopped. "Just as I said that, I had the fantasy of going at you with that brass letter-opener you have." The fantasy was reminiscent of the nightmare's pathetic little boy who "really committed the murder."

She had spent much effort in analysis painting her husband as the one who was murdering the marriage—the "horrible, gruff, uncouth, trampish man on trial." She had also, however, begun to recognize her own culpability. In the dream this was represented by her feeling that the horrible man (her husband) should not "take the rap" for her. But her strongest feeling was "terror" for "the kid," that he would be "found out." Exposure of the murderousness lying behind her innocence meant death to her (having to take the rap for murder), just as the exposure of the tiny cobras, the previous patient's venomousness, meant the threat of death. Here again was a situation which threatened to bankrupt an important way in which the personality functioned, experienced by the patient as imminent dissolution of the derivative sense of self.

Entrance into therapy generally has as its premise some failure of personality function, and is, for all the sense of relief that may accompany the final arrangements to get expert assistance, a threat to the only familiar criteria of self that exist. In the enforced intimacy of the analytic relationship, most of the patient's modes of interpersonal behavior will be activated and intensified. The prospect of engaging in a penetrating reappraisal of his self-concept, the exposure of his often ill-defined ways of living, and the impending challenge to change them, to give them up, to *be* something else, are subjectively equivalent to engaging in the weakening and dissolution of whatever it is that the individual conceives and feels as self.

The threatening quality that inheres in the failure of any form of functioning has led the patient to cultivate and operate within relatively (or distinctly) narrow ranges of interpersonal activity. Influences tending to move him into unfamiliar territory cause fear, since he lacks confidence in his ability to develop adequate new ways of functioning. The individual is thus often caught between the unsatisfactory, inflexible activity and the fear of moving outside the accustomed range.

Analysis in particular, among extraordinary life situations, is a constant force tending to drive the patient outside the familiar patterns of his pathology. His established pathological forms fail in the therapeutic relationship. He anxiously and often angrily intensifies his efforts to make his pathological functioning succeed with the analyst, and offers intense resistance to interpersonal exchanges tending to move him beyond the narrow range of his sick, familiar, and sometimes successful functioning.

A strict and inordinate control of the emotions is fundamental to the interpersonal functioning of many people in our culture (see p. 53). A number of the dreams already given have reflected both a sense of self and a self-concept based upon this control (see pp. 53–60). For such an individual, the anxiety-potential in everyday living is very high, especially through the vicissitudes, surprises, and frustrations of intimate relationships, but also through the infinite range of possible stimuli to the emotions in either chance or routine activities. This anxiety-potential becomes still greater through the influence of analysis, which tends to remove the cultivated barriers to detection and recognition of feeling, and fosters in the anesthetically isolated individual his human capacity for the emotions of intimacy.

The young patient of the Crazy Woman nightmare (see pp. 73–77), whose subjective sense of self had always rested upon maintaining and acting in accordance with cynical distrust, was terrified at the demand to expose her feelings. Her anxiety reached the intensity of terror because her progress toward trusting the analyst had made such exposure a realistic prospect. This new way of feeling and relating threatened her with emotional and operational disorientation, with a destruction of her familiar sense of self.

Affective control may be applied by any patient differentially to a variety of emotions, or it may be focused in one specific emotion. Hostility is frequently the specific emotion that must be subdued or concealed to preserve the integrity of the personality. It is often disguised—deceiving even the individual in whom it occurs—as depression, as a charade of benignity, as psychosomatic manifestations, or as a combination of these.

Hostility threatening to get out of control is widely recognized as a major source of anxiety. The eruption of anger not only shakes the self-concept of emotional control but also disrupts the familiar course of behavior that subjectively characterizes the individual. We hear him "apologizing" for the smallest manifestation of anger: "I forgot myself [meaning "Anger is not part of me"]; please forgive me." "I don't know what happened—it's not like me." The phrases represent not so much an apology as a plea for others to erase from mind the anger that was exposed. The compassionate reply, "I understand perfectly," is an insult, not a consolation.

For this kind of person, frustration of any sort is exceptionally threatening. If he accepts a refusal and withdraws, outwardly calm, the frustration inwardly angers him, and this is subjectively dangerous. If he presses harder to overcome the refusal, and also to avoid the anger at the refusal, his commitment and therefore his stake in prevailing increases. With that, the anger and the threat of explosion grow. He becomes furious toward the agent of his frustration. If the fury cannot be contained, and the individual does explode, the anger that is revealed is then much greater than the immediate frustration might warrant: by this time the fury has been greatly intensified by his resentment at the fact that he has been made angry. He furthermore feels terror because he has lost control of himself. This kind of patient fears that he is "going to pieces," because of the loss of control and because of the obvious discrepancy between the scale of the frustration and the intensity of the ensuing rage. Not only is he frightened when he actually becomes enraged, but he also has anxieties in situations in which he may possibly become enraged.

The patients just described are characteristically depressive and psychosomatic reactors. In frustrating situations they undergo painful physical "disguises" of the anger they suffer, have exacerbations of migraine or lesser headaches, asthma, colitis, ulcer, and the somatic components of depression. The threat of existing or impending rage and consequent disruption of their personalities is reflected in the great anxiety, often of panic proportions, found in their dreams. These dreams are frequently the initial or the strongest clues to both their fury and their fear of disintegration, as illustrated by the following three patients (see also White-Hot Car, pp. 59–60).

The outwardly calm, composed researcher of the Statuesque Masturbation dream [2] (who incidentally expressed some of his rage psychosomatically in depressions, bladder urgency, and migraine attacks) was so frightened of feeling and manifesting his anger that he thought he was becoming psychotic after an episode of swearing out loud to himself while having angry thoughts. In one nightmare he mashed to a pulp the head of a man who would not die (the analyst), after which he woke up in terror (Sledgehammer Attack). Many factors entered into his anxiety, including his sense of impotence against the analyst, his incapacity to function effectively by compelling the analyst to respond "appropriately," i.e., with admiration and deference. An essential factor, however, was the open expression of rage, which violently disrupted his concept of himself as a man capable of *consistently maintaining magnificent composure.*

[2] See Chapter 4, pp. 143–145.

Another man, in some measure depressive, characteristically gentle, empathic, generous, and also seductive, was in a relationship of mutual enslavement with a subtly demanding woman. He could not conquer her by functioning with "kindness," an important source of his sense of self and a prominent element of his self-concept; nor could he openly object to her annoying activities lest this appear ungenerous; nor could he express the fury that developed out of all the frustrations he felt from pursuing his passive and nobly considerate course. He had a vivid, brief dream in which he was a "whirling dervish, a tornadolike, flame-colored, spinning spiral about to go off like an explosive." He woke up in heart-pounding terror. For him the expression of rage in this pyrotechnical symbol of himself was so utterly incompatible with what he conceived himself to be that it meant imminent disintegration.

Another man, whose subjective image of himself was compounded of fairness, conscientiousness, and composure, a man who withdrew and sulked but "never got mad," was reluctant, late in his analysis, to probe still more deeply into his hostility. In the course of reapproaching the problem in connection with his marital relationship, he had the following dream (Atomic Reactor).

"I am entering an atomic energy plant. The guide and I board a steel car which will carry us into the heart of the reactor. Before entering, I touch the steel over the car and find it very hot. *I enter the plant with trepidation,* and wish I were far away. When we are deep inside the reactor, the guide tells me that the Geiger counters have been registering at high speed and that the staff has been *trying very hard to keep the plant from becoming overactive and turning into a bomb.* The guide also suggests that rather than going into the reactor chamber, we go downstairs where we could visit some of the theoretical exhibits."

He had worked on the dream, and added some interpretive comments. "I feel that I am referring to myself as an atomic reactor. *I feel that the dangerous energy refers to my emotions. These were particularly explosive* over the weekend, especially toward Vivian and Ralph [wife and son]. I wanted to avoid entering the reactor—my emotions—and would rather go downstairs where I could engage in a theoretical discussion."

The dream depicted the patient's reluctance to go to the "heart" of the matter of his hostility. This would involve his looking directly at his anger and openly, feelingly expressing it. In the dream he has anxiety ("trepidation") as he approaches the problem of his "dangerous" emotions. His sense of the peril of *disintegration of the self from anger* is suggested by his dream metaphor: ". . . trying very hard to keep the plant from becoming overactive and turning into a bomb."

In contrast with the previous patients, the young woman of the Crazy Woman dream was terrified of the emergence of tender and trusting feelings. Many women in our present-day western culture fear disintegration if they express or even acknowledge to themselves the tender feelings that earlier generations conceived of as properly feminine. In its simplest juvenile form this phenomenon appears in the "tomboy," whose criterion of self depends upon combative toughness. The Elevator Nightmare discussed in detail in the next chapter (pp. 218–226), was dreamed by a mother who unawaredly feared that maternalism would undermine her stoicism, in which her sense of self was rooted. Many men of our culture are also frightened by emotions within them which have popular connotations of softness and femininity.

Spontaneous sexual arousal may also be a threatening feeling. One young, unmarried woman who had had years of experience with intercourse and its numerous variations, and who considered herself a sexual virtuoso, was impelled into psychoanalysis in a panic after her first and totally unexpected experience of intense sexual desire. During her analysis she married. When she began to evolve toward healthy sexual enjoyment, she had a nightmare in which she battled desperately against being dragged (by the analyst) to a large chamber where great numbers of people were engaged in orgiastic sexual activities. An important subjective criterion of her individuality was that of being above sexual need. To use man's sexual need to control him, to minister to it with tender condescension, was one thing; to burn with desire was quite another thing, a frightening assault upon her self-concept. Her experiencing sexual desire was a substantial disruption of her smooth, enslaving activities with men and, subjectively, rendered her helpless and threatened her with personality disintegration.

One individual can thus feel the anxiety of weakening and imminent collapse, while another experiences the anxiety of possible explosive disintegration. In either case the anxiety, whether in dreaming or waking consciousness, comes from the eruption into his functioning and into his self-concept of an emotion which seems to the patient to threaten an important way of living and its derivative feeling of self.

The ability to control or conceal feelings is not, of course, the only subjective criterion of self which produces anxiety when threatened. Grandiose self-concepts, supported by appropriate functioning, are common and occur in a great variety of forms; they are always potential sources of anxiety because, through shifting circumstances, unpredictable and uncontrollable, they are so vulnerable to repudiation. Actually, the individuals cited above whose subjective sense of personality resided in their ability to inhibit or conceal emotions can also be included among the grandiose; control of the emotions sets them, in their own inner view, above ordinary human beings. The unhappy, scholarly intellectual of the Pissing Dream (see Chapter 2, "Feeling in Dreams," p. 87) expressed this attitude quite explicitly, using the symbolic language of his dream: "I was embarrassed that *I* have to urinate, *too*." At this point he remembered an author who wrote that he "hated to see his women piss, hated to see they were human." These patients develop anxiety when unwanted emotions arise, because in addition to the disruption of functioning there is threat of destruction of the self-concept of superiority to those who, in the patients' view, are contemptibly and helplessly buffeted by emotions.

A dream of a physician-analysand is another example of anxiety resulting from the threat to a grandiose self-concept. The patient, because he was a psychiatrist, felt the need to be immune, not to emotions, but to emotional pathology. Yet, as an honest observer, he could not altogether deny experiencing an inappropriate anxiety; judged by ordinary clinical standards, his anxiety (he dimly recognized) was pathological. He felt nevertheless that his ability to control himself and to behave with outward calm, and above all, to understand what was going on, removed from his inner tension the stigma of "neurosis."

He had already achieved psychiatric status with hospital and research connections and had been in practice for several years. His manner was affable but professional, and his whole bearing was designed to evoke friendly deference from the laity and respect from colleagues. He entered treatment as part of psychoanalytic training, and at once felt threatened by his "patient" status. By coincidence, therapy began very shortly before he was scheduled to present a research report at a large departmental meeting. In anticipation of this event he suffered excessive anxiety, which he attempted to minimize by referring to it casually as a reaction he could "completely understand" and "handle." I said it was a "sick" reaction requiring psychoanalytic investigation.

The interchange was followed soon afterward by a brief anxiety dream (Positive Throat Culture), which he reported at the next session.

"My throat culture showed positive organisms. They were an *epidemic* strain. About two hundred and fifty colonies. I wouldn't be able to be on the research project. I was frightened. I had anxiety when I realized I couldn't be on the project. I was anxious and disappointed."

His association was the discussion at the previous hour regarding his intense anxiety in anticipating the presentation of his research report. He recalled my statement that his was a "sick" reaction. Three symbols pointed toward the analytic situation as the source of the anxiety in the dream. The throat culture was positive, indicating that he was "sick"; the organisms in his throat culture were of an epidemic variety (he was sick *like any other patient*—the most threatening aspect of the sickness question); the specific number of colonies, two hundred and fifty, was a multiple of the twenty-five-dollar fee. This was an analytic sickness.

The feeling of uniqueness is a very common pathological criterion of self, and the challenge to it is a common cause of anxiety during therapy. That this patient's illness was of "an epidemic variety" was so serious a finding that he "wouldn't be able to be on the research project." If he could not maintain a self-concept of being above the laity, he would not be able to function professionally.

I said to him, "It seems that you have anxiety lest the existence in you of an authentic emotional disturbance should disqualify you for professional activities [research project in the dream]. Your sense of your professional ability is threatened by the existence of emotional pathology [the positive throat culture]. In actuality, learning that you have some emotional disturbance could not conceivably disqualify you from any activity in which you are already successfully functioning. Your professional status is not in the least threatened. As you explore and come to understand better both your irrational and rational feelings, you will be in a position, like any patient, to deal with your problems in a healthier fashion. Your actual functioning and enjoyment of your professional activity will be considerably enhanced."[3]

The investigation, to his surprise, revealed also a highly exaggerated sense of the importance of his report and, to his credit, he began to see that his earlier anxiety derived, at least in part, from the grandiosity and unreality of this estimate.

The chief source of the patient's dream anxiety was the challenge to his grandiose style of functioning and the related self-concept, that of being, in a psychiatric sense, above illness.[4]

Besides the feeling of self-aggrandizement associated with affective control, there are other forms of grandiose criteria by which people may subjectively judge their personalities. A grandiose self-image may be based on a sense of exceptional goodness. The man who dreamed of the Shark in Swimming Pool (pp. 126–127) was quiet, soft-spoken, very active and effective in business and in social enterprises, a "good" neigh-

---

[3] The connection between the maintenance of the self-concept (being immune to real emotional pathology) and the ability to function (as a psychiatrist) is unusually explicit in this dream.

[4] Many individuals remain in analysis for long periods without regarding themselves as patients.

bor, a "good" friend, and trying hard to be a "good" husband and a "good" father. This was, however, a misinterpretation in many instances. He would, for example, most reliably put out the garbage every night. In handling that problem he set an exemplary standard of neatness, diligence, and efficiency. But he had polluted many mornings of the first two years of marriage by trying, at first patiently and later petulantly, to train his wife to roll up the toothpaste tube from the bottom. By handling the garbage with neatness and efficiency, he had established the right to demand that she handle the toothpaste tube with neatness and efficiency.

Throughout their marriage he had not been able to understand how he had failed to elicit real affection and sexual responsiveness from his wife, because his own affectional style seemed to him a manifestation of his superior humanity. He had failed to recognize the extent to which he had made demands for, rather than offerings of, real affection, when he used an affectional style palpably deficient in substance to manipulate his wife into fulfilling his sexual and other desires. Much of this material, of course, came out during the later course of therapy, but it nevertheless made up the life context of the early anxiety dream about the shark. His way of functioning and the related grandiose concept of his "good" personality were inseparable, and together were threatened by initiation of therapy.

In his second session, the dream Wading in Deeper indicated the beginning of anxiety over "getting in too deep." Some searching questions about the nature of his interpersonal behavior had been raised. Was he accurate in conceptualizing his activities as kindly? Were his notions about his role as a husband false? The formulation of these questions began to shake the conviction of superior goodness which was the mainstay of his self-concept. The problem which arose was his having to change the very type of functioning which was a central source of his sense of self. Superficially he was intrigued at the first hour, eager to examine himself more intensively and to change his ways; at the end of the second session he again expressed a conscientious interest in the new insights. But to the third hour he brought the anxiety dream in which he was frantic, caught in a tank (the analyst's office) pursued by a destructive shark (the analyst).

In reality there was some genuine kindness, honesty, and cooperativeness in this man. With these assets he would be able to enjoy a sense of self, arising in the course of healthier interpersonal functioning, and would be able to achieve a more rational and substantial self-respect. The shark dream revealed, however, that to uncover the fact that he was not a *superlatively good* person was to threaten him with destruction. The sense of impending failure of the important techniques of living, and dissolution of the derivative self-concept, constituted the essence of his anxiety.

The man whose dream of the Analyst-Chauffeur was reported earlier (pp. 123–124) had achieved a sense of almost magical control over people. Smooth manipulative functioning was much of the time the source of his sense of self and the basis of a highly inflated self-concept. He said early in analysis: "I thought my case would be so interesting . . . you'd treat me without a fee," and, "if I can't manage people, I'm nothing." After a few sessions in analysis he recalled a repetitive anxiety dream (The Wand and the Apes) from his twelfth year, a period in which he had also begun to read avidly on hypnosis.

"I was a magician with a magic wand with which I could perform miracles. The dream would end by my being in a huge, long, high room in a castle. The room would be besieged by giant apes who would crash through the windows and overwhelm me. I would wave my wand but it would be useless to stop them. Then I'd have anxiety."

He added, "When I thought of this dream in connection with analysis, I felt all my power would be neutralized and I'd be helpless. I was fearful lest my techniques of dealing with people wouldn't work in keeping off insights here."

One of his techniques was the use of intellectual agility, another was his seductiveness. He referred to a social worker who had been his supervisor: "The more authority a person has over me, the more passive and seductive I become—and the more anxious, because with some the technique won't work, the wand isn't potent." Then, associating to his intellectual maneuvers, he said, "This connects with the treatment situation. After leaving last time I thought, 'Dr. B. is too clever for me'— every time I have something figured out, he says, 'Yes, but there's also this.' "

In his childhood dream, the apes crashed in uncontrollably; and when he became an adult he could not control the independent working and influence of his analyst's mind. The patient's intellectual ability and his seductiveness often made it possible for him "magically" to immunize himself from influence, to mold the minds and responses of other people. The carefully elicited responses—wonderment at a well-timed casual introduction of crucial information, or trepidation because of his inscrutable countenance—responses that made him appear unique, were unconsciously divorced from the manipulations that produced them, and so gave him a sense of mystical power. When he came up against a situation in which his manipulative techniques failed, then in spite of his real intellectual endowment and genuinely attractive personal qualities, he felt, both in dreams and waking consciousness, impotent, worthless, and filled with anxiety. The only criteria by which he felt aware of himself as a personality were threatened with paralysis and dissolution—as in the dream the magic wand became impotent against the overwhelming apes.

The healthy individual develops consciousness and a sense of self through response to and response from other human beings. He lives with a basic confidence in his ability to comprehend and respond adequately and appropriately to others, and to engender appropriate responsiveness in them. His concept of himself is close to the reality about himself, and no major efforts are required to muster support for this concept. His interpersonal functioning feels neither precarious or strained. Limitation in his own responsiveness to an interpersonal situation does not signify an incapacity to function at all adequately, a functional bankruptcy. A limited response *to* him does not make of him a person insufficient to be responded to. If there is an interpersonal failure in either direction, it is emotionally and conceptually absorbed as only a limitation, one which may be either his own or the other person's.

The individual with personality pathology, in contrast, must constantly exercise his techniques of living, constantly test his effectiveness in *making* others respond.[5] Irrationally, furthermore, he senses the adequacy of his total functioning and the whole integrity of his self-concept according to the success or failure of *each instance* in which an interpersonal technique is involved.

The threat to manipulative techniques is a major source of anxiety in analysis, and it compounds the anxiety that is already activated by other impending changes. Frustration or attenuation of influence upon the attitudes and activities of others (which includes failure to counter their influences) is a factor in the anxieties of all the cases in this chapter. The young woman of the Crazy Woman nightmare (see pp. 73–77), already terrified by the threat of exposure of her feelings and of placing trust in another, suffered still greater anxiety from loss of her fending-off and other operational techniques.

[5] The cynicism of our western culture, discussed in Chapter 2, is largely derived from the fact that people, while practicing the outward forms of love and friendship, are using each other to bolster their self-concepts and to maintain a subjective feeling of functional effectiveness. In so many people, the vital importance of manipulative techniques is the basis of a great deal of resistance in psychoanalysis and of a great deal of anxiety in the course of evolving health.

Effective functioning has for a surprising number of people a particularly strong subjective requirement of control over the lives of those intimately involved with them. This is a major source of marital and child-parent pathology. Genuine cooperativeness is never tolerable to these people, because a margin of power must be maintained.[6]

The following dreams are examples of anxiety engendered by interference with an excessive control over another person. The first is an introductory dream already presented, Empty Suit (pp. 117–119). It will be recalled that in the dream the patient was climbing with her husband through the rafters of a huge indoor stadium. She was guiding him. "It was my responsibility to get us to safety—he fell and I looked down and it was an empty suit lying in the form of a man. . . ." Later she was walking with him, again a man, outside. "I'm helping the man who was an empty suit." She is leading him away from a villain [analyst] who is trying to get them to enter a coach which was "nothing but a hearse. . . . I was scared, too. The villain was going to get us. I was mostly worried about my husband because I was in command of my faculties and he was dazed."

For this patient there was something lethal about analysis, and her husband was more susceptible to its influence than she. The analyst would undermine her own dominant role in the marriage. ". . . I felt he should have some kind of treatment less intensive than psychoanalysis, *so he could be weak and need me.* . . ." Her desire to retain the dominant position is expressed in a common euphemism of solicitude—*to take care of*: "Not needing me *to take care of* him will make me weak." Because her primary subjective criterion of being a person was her effectiveness in dominating her husband, there was basis here for her extreme anxiety in his movement toward health and independence.

Another woman, although much healthier than the wife of the Empty Suit dream, revealed a similar source of anxiety. She, too, was concerned lest control of the marriage relationship slip from her in the course of her husband's analytic progress. She felt inadequate as a wife and as a mother, although she was competent in both roles. As much as she wanted her husband, who tended to be preoccupied and cold, to become warmer and more responsive, she nevertheless paradoxically, whenever he was at his best, tended to be critical, petty, and contentious. Then he would react to her attrition with his worst.

[6] The man of the Statuesque Masturbation dream, in the very context of offering his wife equality, had been enraged when she won the coin toss. In the Independent Mistress, Sideways Approach, and Sledgehammer Attack, he reflected, in symbols of sex or violence, attempts at conquest of the analyst.

The problem was delineated through a three-episode dream of a single night (Disturbingly Adequate Husband). In the first dream she was sitting behind him in a plane while "he was at the controls." She felt willing for him to be at the controls and confident of his ability, and at the same time she suffered anxiety. In the next episode she was pregnant, and all her friends were concerned over her being alone, unmarried, and pregnant. They were trying to find her a man to be her husband and to be father to her child. That episode ended with her realization that, "of course I have a husband, all the search is ridiculous." In the final episode she was playing cards and bid a grand slam, followed by immediate anxiety lest her partner not play his cards correctly. She was then "surprised and happy" to find her partner playing his cards capably. One of her associations to this dream episode was her concern a year earlier, when her first baby was born, that there were many things that she would not be able to do to insure the baby's developing properly in physical and emotional health. She had had a "feeling of inadequacy." Her infant nevertheless enjoyed a robust, successful first year.

The dream led to an important recognition. She had achieved enough solid health to welcome, in all three of the dream episodes, her husband's increasing adequacy. She nevertheless experienced some anxiety within the framework of his adequacy. By following up her anxiety feelings she saw that she was more competitive than she had thought, that she sought to maintain a competitive advantage, to be the stronger, the controlling one in the marriage. She saw her unwillingness to accept her husband's independent and contributory role. When in the dream he was at the controls, she experienced this as dangerous, even though he was entirely adequate. When pregnant, she anticipated being inadequate *alone* to supply all that would be necessary for a baby, and she had to accept the necessity and existence of a husband. If she had a good hand at cards (in playing her cards throughout life) she needed a partner with whom to fulfill her bid. In her waking life, if she gave up the maneuvers that kept her husband cold, petulant, and in need of her "handling," she would be giving up her dominion.

On the other hand, if she could accept and healthily relate to the independent role of others, especially such significant individuals as her husband and her baby, she would have a reality basis for feelings of adequacy. For example, the patient discovered that her husband was adequate, *not* because of her wise handling of his shortcomings, *not* because she somehow evoked what otherwise would not exist, but because of his independent personal assets and his independent spontaneous strivings. Similarly, her baby had in a year evolved into a happy, stable, healthy child, not only in response to her efforts, but also because her husband had been a good father, and because of the spontaneous independent role of the baby in his participation with both of his parents. It was unnecessary for her vigilantly and anxiously to plan, elicit, and guide all their behavior. By recognizing and engaging with their healthy, independent capacities, she became a more relaxed, spontaneous, healthy individual.

Basically there were two foci for this woman's anxiety. First, as her husband progressed in his analysis, there was a threat to her functional effectiveness as the dominant partner in the marriage. Secondly, there was anxiety connected with the undermining of her self-concept, because of her real inadequacy to fulfill the double or triple responsibility she construed as her own—a responsibility greater than one person could conceivably encompass. The direct exposure of these two interrelated sources of anxiety, subtly camouflaged beneath a degree of healthy personality integration, was achieved through exploring together the conditions for the anxiety that were brought into focus by the episodic anxiety dream.

Just as there are individuals whose sense of self is rooted excessively in control of others, there are also people whose sense of self is rooted excessively in functioning designed to nullify interpersonal influences upon them. The patient who dreamed of the Three Condoms (pp. 153–154) was a product of excessively manipulative parents. He resented the merest attempt to influence him, but sometimes enjoyed playing contemptuously with those who tried. It may be recalled that one of the psychosomatic symptoms of his problem was premature ejaculation, through which he in effect made use of the woman while making certain that she did not "use" him. Later on, this patient made considerable progress; his marriage was basically sound and sexually was characterized by reciprocally fulfilling intercourse. He suffered, nevertheless, occasional anxieties associated with the idea that he was being handled by his wife. One evening she prevailed upon him to put up some kitchen gadget over which he had successfully procrastinated for several days. He started his next session by reporting the dream that followed this incident (Rat Eyes).

"I was in a place that was immaculate during the day, but it was full of rats at night. The rats' eyes lit up. Then they started to come at me, and I had anxiety and then woke up."

He then recounted the circumstances of his wife's asking him to install the appliance. "I remember how she looked at me when we were sitting on the couch and she asked me to do the chore. She said, 'My lazy husband doesn't want to work and I'm finally going to get him to put this up.' As she said it, her face lit up. I couldn't get out of it."

I interrupted him to say, "That's the phrase you used to describe the rats in the dream . . . their eyes 'lit up.'"

He responded at once, "Oh yes—the rats' teeth lit up, too, like her smile." And he added, "Sometimes I feel she's at me, like my mother."

This patient had been compelled to develop techniques to avoid being consumed by his mother. In that process his whole personality had been molded. He was so sensitive to "being used" that he would be enraged whenever, after a pleasant conversation with him, anyone parted with the remark, "It was nice talking to you." That simple amenity made him feel he had been "taken." When he succeeded in maneuvering others, especially when he made it awkward or unpleasant for them, or when he frustrated the attempts of others to maneuver him, he would report these incidents with a great belly laugh—a belly laugh that was his most intense, spontaneous expression of feeling. The laugh expressed exultation in his manipulative and antimanipulative effectiveness and in the resultant strong subjective sense of being a somebody. If, however, he failed in these maneuvers, if the exultation was the other person's, if another's face "lit up," then he felt threatened and angry. The dream delineated the basic conditions for anxiety in this patient. Was his self-concept of being too smart for people becoming threatened? Could the marriage relationship, which appeared so "immaculate," perhaps be infested with manipulative, ratty, gloating elements that he might not be able to control? Such a question, so easily stirred in him, must in such a personality inevitably engender anxiety.

In this patient, as in many of the others whose dreams have been presented, competitiveness was an active motivational force compounding the sources of anxiety (see p. 86). It is common for all the techniques of pressure, evasion, and seduction to become aspects of a general sparring for position in which the whole self is the tactical instrument for winning. If the tactic fails, it is a failure of the total self. (This is, I believe, a basis for the anxiety of some psychotherapists in their therapeutic interpersonal relationships.)

Guilt

Guilt, referred to in Chapter 2, on feeling, as one of the fuzziest words in psychiatry (see p. 97), in a vast majority of cases is not any sort of self-condemnation but is rather anxiety, based upon anticipated failure of some pathological interpersonal operation. It frequently relates to the fear of failure to evoke the desired response or produce the proper attitude in another person—an attitude requisite to successful functioning. The woman of the Tiny Cobras nightmare might have expressed herself as feeling "guilty" about her venomous remark at the dance, instead of saying, more perceptively and accurately, "I couldn't stand the success of my remark." The success, which exposed her competence in combat, threatened to undermine her effectiveness in manipulating her husband by timidity and helplessness.

Similarly, the woman of the "olive incident" woke up in terror because the little boy (her ingenuously functioning self) was recognizable to her as guilty of murder (as she was guilty of murdering her marriage). The guilty terror in this dream came, not from high-minded self-recrimination, but from fear of being exposed at the trial (analysis) —something which would curb her tyrannizing-by-dependency, and begin to extinguish the sense of self derived from this kind of functioning.

The subject of guilt should and has filled volumes; a few statements of opinion are in order in the context of this discussion of anxiety. A sound and rational *recognition of and sense of guilt need have in it no element of anxiety whatever*. It would healthily contain awareness of injury to another, remorse, sadness, and desire to undo or compensate for the injury for the sake of the *other* person and to restore one's self-respect. When voluntary compensatory or corrective action is possible, guilt is the emotion expressed in such *action*. When a patient speaks of feeling guilty, he may be referring to feelings of embarrassment, sadness, inadequacy, very often competitive hostility, and almost invariably some measure of anxiety closely related to fear of being found out and having some important functioning of the personality rendered thereby ineffectual. Under any circumstances, in therapy it is essential to reject the term "guilty" whenever it is offered, and to direct the patient's efforts toward delineating the precise nature of the uncomfortable and anxious feeling designated by the term (see p. 97).

Rejection as a Source of Anxiety

It is not in the patient's best interests for the analyst to approach all his feelings of "rejection" with compassionate concern. The unhappiness that appears to be experienced from lack of love may instead be a sullen sense of frustration due to the failure of a manipulative demand. Often the individual who feels rejected has already experienced anticipatory anxiety because he has pitted himself against the other person, seeking to force acceptance or love. The man who dreamed Kept Calling Up, for example (see pp. 89–90), originally came to analysis because of anxiety attacks in which his knees literally buckled under him. In analysis *all* these attacks were correlated with competitive defeat in relationships with parents, cronies, business associates, and later with wife and children. Referring to the woman with whom he was involved in the dream, he said spontaneously that what he couldn't stand was her dropping him "before I dropped her." Unless a relationship could be worked out on his terms, he felt rejected, and when there was a threat of this kind of "rejection" he was tormented by anxiety.

In general, feelings of "rejection" are a mask for rage, are frequently associated with anxiety, and in great numbers of cases are related to the pathology of control, manipulativeness, and competitiveness.[7]

Security and Needs

Security and needs, like guilt and rejection, are vague concepts clinically associated with anxiety. Insecurity and unsatisfied needs have pathetic aspects which tend to obscure their pathological nature. In the common phrase "neurotic needs," for example, the word "needs" has a commanding force that tends to determine our response to the complete phrase along lines that are not therapeutically constructive. In the mind of the patient, and often in the mind of the analyst, social worker, and family, "needs" implies a claim for indulgence.

The establishment of freedom from fear and the right to security are unimpeachable goals in every avenue of life. The therapeutic goal is emotional security based upon rational, cooperative functional effectiveness, relatively free of anxiety. Clinically, however, *it is essential to examine the individual's criteria of needs and of security,* and to confront him with his demand for freedom from anxiety based upon the fulfillment by the environment of the conditions for his pathological forms of functional effectiveness. The man whose wife is always available for intercourse on demand, regardless of her own feelings, may feel secure, and may be expansively generous. He is, however, not likely to be a secure man any time she hesitates.

In our culture a great deal of energy is devoted to establishing particular conditions for the fulfillment of special "needs." The special conditions involve activities which re-enforce the individual's sense of self through competitive victory in manipulating others. The victory may be in eliciting sexual submission, where the "need" is satisfied by little

[7] Rejection as a form of depression: see the author's chapter, "Dynamics and Psychotherapy of Depression," in J. Masserman, ed., *Current Psychiatric Therapies.* New York: Grune & Stratton, 1962.

more than the sensation of conquest. Or the need may be satisfied by victory in eliciting some service or some attitude such as special attention, admiration, deference or general subservience. Sometimes the pathological need (e.g., a vindictive or sadistic one) is fulfilled through success in evoking negative reactions, such as frustration, embarrassment, or fear.

Our culture is full of people "on the make," out to make others do what they want, whether by bullying, helplessness, desperation, bribery, or seduction. The anxiety-laden maneuvers include a great deal of affectionless sexual activity (during recent decades an increasing proportion of this is homosexual activity, which is characteristically affectionless). Such people spend much of their lives in activities directed toward allaying the anxiety that arises from their constantly frustrated competitive interpersonal efforts. Relief is sought in alcoholism and other addictions, and in all kinds of social, hobby, speed, and power distractions.

These patients come into treatment feeling anxious, frustrated, insecure, depressed, withdrawn, worthless, or hopeless, and functionally ineffectual. They seek in analysis new aids to the establishing of pathological security through the successful fulfillment of their pathological interpersonal needs. In this context we face our vulnerable, unhappy, anxiety-prone patients. It is essential that we not be diverted by a misplaced compassion, if we are to help them fulfill their real needs and achieve healthy security.

Anxiety and Sex

Most of the anxiety associated with sexuality, including that called guilt, arises, not on the basis of specific psychosexual ontogenesis and its disturbances, but as a manifestation of primarily interpersonal pathology reflected secondarily in the sexual area. Sexual satisfaction requires the participation of another human being, and thus all the interpersonal techniques come into operation, all the elements of intimacy, and all of the most deeply competitive functioning. One exposes oneself to being seduced, enslaved, used—and reciprocally one becomes involved in seducing, enslaving, and using. Much terminology related to sexual experience expresses competitive interpersonal strivings. People are "on the make," they are "making a conquest." The competitive vocabulary of nonsexual activities makes use of such sexual terms as "Screw you!" and its variations. A striking expression of exploitative competitive feeling, that of taking without letting the other person receive, is the designation of intercourse as "tearing off a piece."

The research scientist of the Statuesque Masturbation dream sought to correct the intolerable independence of his wife by the sexual enslavement of other women. This patient often experienced anxiety as he approached his analytic sessions, and in the dreams of the Independent Mistress and the Sideways Approach he sought in the symbolism of sex to correct the competitive imbalance of the therapeutic relationship.

The controlling and anxious woman of the "olive incident" and the Murder Trial nightmare sought, in the competitively unequal activities of analysis, to restore her threatened sense of self by sexual conquest of the analyst: she openly proposed that the analyst should spend a weekend with her, so that she could show him that she was a "real woman." (She would be in a more favorable position to make the analyst admire and respond to her.)

Because so much of the neurotic sense of self is laced through with the competitiveness of our culture, and because this competitiveness is almost inevitably present in sexual activity, there is a consequent high anxiety potential in the sexuality of our culture. Examples are readily found of anxiety associated with competitive disadvantage in the sexual relationship. One man, referred to earlier (Son Sucking Me Off, pp. 133–138), maintained his feeling of functional effectiveness by masturbating with fantasies of raping women tied to the stake, or at the point of a knife or gun. He later developed anxiety, highly correlated with new behavior, as he began to achieve tenderness and affection toward his wife; this was a surrender of his dominant role.

An extremely controlling woman, with strong sexual appetite, used to masturbate regularly as she awaited her lover and then, quite in the ascendancy, would tenderly commiserate with his fruitless efforts to give her orgasm.

Culture, Sex, and Anxiety
(A Re-evaluation of Some Freudian Concepts) [8]

The techniques of manipulation, influence, seduction, withholding, all aspects of competitive pathology, permeate interpersonal sexual relationships just as they permeate all other forms of interpersonal activity in our culture. It is the genetic influence of this broad constellation of life experience upon sexual pathology, rather than the reverse influence, which, I believe, accounts for much of the pathology that Freud observed, creatively distilled and structuralized in his sexual psycho-

[8] See also Chapter 4, "Sexuality in Dreams."

dynamic concepts, and then applied universally. The concepts of Oedipus complex, castration fears, and penis envy, for example, may readily be viewed as arising from Freud's observations of intra-familial competitive strivings. In the Viennese culture of Freud's time, it is likely that the hostility of the domineering father toward the infant boy arose because the child had invaded the life of the mother and made an influential demand upon her solicitude, which weakened the total control of the father over his wife. Freud saw this as the child being a *sexual* rival for the mother. The child felt the hostility of his competitive father, whose functional effectiveness and sense of self were subversively threatened by any reduction of his control. The little boy's clinging still closer to his mother for protection, comfort, and affection was a response to the anxious hostility of the father, and had only a speculative, not a verifiable, connection with sexual desire for his mother or with fear of genital castration at the hands of the father. Even in the cases where genital castration was explicitly threatened, it was at least presumptively in an atmosphere in which that threat was but a re-enforcement of a more diffusely destructive or "castrative" threat.

In those cases where the child became witness to a "primal scene," the child's anxiety was postulated to have come from his own copulative desire for his mother, and fear of castration as punishment. He is more likely to have been terrified by misinterpreting the act as violence consistent with his sense of his father's hostility. The act could symbolize his father's potential for overpowering him, and for overcoming the mother who was the child's source of affection and protection.

The concept of penis envy is consistent with the generally patronizing attitude toward women in Freud's time. It is a denigration that indicates a quite remarkable absence of any grasp of the ecstatic sense of fulfillment women achieve through the creative individual development of maternalism itself. Particularly in Freud's male-dominated Austro-Hungarian capital, the arrival of a child meant for its mother the possibility of a much higher degree of healthy functional effectiveness than was afforded her in other spheres. Some mothers, however, sought to compensate themselves for their subservient family role by their own subtle or overt methods of domination over the children. Under the guise of maternalism these women could be excessively controlling toward their sons. The son, as he developed into manhood, might then become active sexually in defiance of the hovering and perhaps infantilizing mother, throwing off the maternal influence by assuming a culturally determined, manly, domineering sexual role, and feeling with each act of intercourse that culture's equivalent of a defiant

THE CLINICAL USE OF DREAMS

"Screw you!" For another man, intercourse might be too dangerously close to an overt expression of an otherwise unaware competitive hostility toward his mother. For such a covertly hostile man, the prospect of full engagement in a symbolic "screw you" activity could engender enough anxiety to incapacitate him in heterosexual activity, or could lead to his avoidance of sexual contact with women. This would not be Oedipal fear, but more likely a fear of bankrupting a personality which evolved in interpersonal experiences with a dominating mother and functioned in a style of sweet, passive submission to any strong female. Such a development in a man could be comparable to the anxieties of the women of the Tiny Cobras and the Murder Trial dreams, who affected weakness in order to control, and who developed terror over the exposure of their competitive hostility.

It would be impossible here to attempt a fuller critique of Freud's psychodynamic concepts. Some suggestive observations have however been necessary, because reifications and popularizations of his constructs are used to explain so much of the anxiety that exists. My own belief is that little if any anxiety or so-called "guilt" derives specifically from the sexuality of human beings. The anxiety associated with sexuality is only incidentally expressed in the area of sex, and is basically the fear of bankruptcy of major ways of interpersonal functioning.

It is in the anxiety areas that the individual is least ready and least equipped to explore alone. Anxiety, whether reflected in dreams or in waking circumstances, is therefore always to be taken as a signal for more determined therapeutic pursuit, rather than for withdrawal, which would be an abandonment of the patient. Contrary to the more usual view, I feel this applies particularly to the schizoid individual,[9] because his resources, due to his insularity, cynicism, and anxious caution in living, are the least available for his independent use. He is the least likely to take the initiative anywhere for developing his potential in the indispensable milieu of interpersonal exchange.

These considerations apply from the onset of treatment. A number of the previous clinical presentations of introductory dreams, for example, indicate the application of this general psychotherapeutic principle during the initial phases of analysis.[10] Whether early or late in therapy, however, it is the therapeutic context itself, the constructive, intimate, cooperative activity of fully operative psychotherapy, which

[9] See the author's "The Pursuit of Anxiety-Laden Areas in Therapy of the Schizoid Patient," *Psychiatry*, 22: 239–244, 1959.

[10] See The Eliminator and associated early dreams of the same patient; see also, Wading in Deeper, Shark in Swimming Pool, and others in Chapter 3.

provides experiential and emotional evidence to the patient that he will not become functionally paralyzed nor experience dissolution if he changes his established ways, that he can function effectively in different ways. The analyst knows that successful new experiences will bring with them a new and more realistic security and a new healthy sense of functional effectiveness, and so he presses ahead against the patient's fear until the patient, by many anxious risks, learns experientially an expanded way of functioning that is free from anxiety.

6. *Resistance in Dreams*

 THE TERM "RESISTANCE IN DREAMS" refers to the reflection in sleeping consciousness of all the forces operating within the patient to avoid alteration of the personality, to maintain functional effectiveness in forms the individual feels to be the only possible basis for the survival of his personality. It involves fighting against the impingement of the analyst on his way of living.[1]

The patient comes into analysis with some sense of interpersonal functional bankruptcy, yet he seeks to make all that has failed in other relationships nonetheless operate successfully in the therapeutic situation. He manifests the same pathology in all areas of his life; the term "resistance," however, applies specifically to his interpersonal struggle in the therapeutic situation. Through his resistance maneuvers, the patient tries to hide the sources of anxiety, to have the neurotic structure supported rather than revealed, to have the pathological goals fulfilled rather than challenged. In this context the overcoming of resistance is identical with the process of cure.

The prevailing competitiveness of our culture not only appears regularly as pathology, but also operates to prevent the recognition of all pathological functioning, including the competitiveness itself; it is

[1] For a discussion of *transference,* see introductory portion of Chapter 9 (pp. 268–270).

a major difficulty that must be dealt with during the therapeutic endeavor, for it intensifies all resistance. In Chapter 2, on feeling, there is a discussion of the reciprocal relationship between competitiveness and cynicism in the genesis and characteristics of much of the personality in our western culture. Briefly, it was suggested that the trend, beginning with the parent-child interaction, is for the individual to use people, to relate to them primarily for his own benefit, and to do so under the guise of love, friendship, solicitude; and at the same time to fend off all influences upon himself, the genuinely solicitous as well as those patently calculated for the profferer's own aggrandizement. The continuum of experience in fending off influence and in influencing others, not only expresses, but tends also to foster, amplify, and validate the patient's competitiveness and cynicism.

In therapy the patient's disbelief in the analyst's genuine concern, the patient's efforts and techniques to fend off his influence and even actively to defeat, frustrate, and incapacitate the analyst, are the cynical and competitive factors in resistance behavior. The anxiety factor in the patient's motivations, discussed in the previous chapter, will be further elaborated below. All of these factors are reflected in resistance dreams.

The patient's resistance involves all his efforts to preserve the competitive, manipulative, cynically rooted, lonely, and miserable yet familiar and reassuring forms of interpersonal functioning, against the efforts of the analyst to involve him in detecting, understanding, and changing these painful ways of living. The overcoming of resistance is achieved in a process in which the patient engages with the analyst; with increasing trust, increasing commitment to exposure of distortions in himself, he undertakes to alter the very behavior and conceptualizations which have been his subjective criteria of self. He becomes involved in a new, friendly, unfamiliar, and frightening experience—the cooperative activity of psychoanalysis.

Throughout analysis, whether progress is nonexistent, slow, or excellent, some resistance is always present. One common problem that generates or intensifies resistance is the patient's endlessly, often unawaredly, often indignantly, stubbornly, and vindictively pursued *demand for an unrealized childhood.*[2] Many patients have never received what was appropriate and necessary in the course of early development—the affection they appropriately craved, the genuine tenderness and anticipation of their needs when they were children. As adults, they continue to experience a gnawing sense of deprivation. They

---

[2] Much that has been traditionally categorized as "infantile" and "dependent" may be alternatively considered in the ensuing framework.

often continue in their efforts to elicit the desired responses from their parents; and the parents continue to frustrate them, while making their *own* demands for filial devotion. This gives rise to reciprocal tension, criticism, complaints, hostility, mutual manipulation, retaliation, and attempts at seduction. But there is no parental love. These patients look for it from husband or wife, friends, sales clerks, neighbors, and analyst. They do not recognize that the situation of childhood has passed, its necessities and yearnings never to be fulfilled, that the unreceived parental concern has to be written off as "uncollectable," that there can never be a loving-protective-responsible parent or parent-surrogate, because there is no longer a child. These people often hold on to their demands, becoming increasingly punitive to those who will not respond, stubbornly unwilling to participate in life on an adult level. And, of course, they then miss most of the satisfactions of adult life. As this occurs, their bitterness increases; the deprivations of adulthood have been added to the deprivations of childhood, swelling the total of life's indebtedness to them. It becomes increasingly difficult for them to benefit from the ordinary, often abundant sources of satisfaction, for against the background of life's enormous and growing debt to them, almost any available gratification is too small a payment to be accepted. Analysis is the very antithesis of their demand for the golden childhood privilege of having others bear the responsibility for their happiness. In childhood, the sense of their own worth appropriately depended upon being loved by parents. In the adult state a sense of being accepted is prevented by their tenacious clinging to the same unachievable, anachronistic criterion of lovability. Their clamoring, unappeasable, disgruntled, and often spiteful behavior tends to guarantee a continuing lack of loving response, and in a viciously circular way this increases their bitter vindictiveness and with it their sense of worthlessness.

For these patients, the therapeutic orientation toward their taking the responsibility for their own happiness carries with it the imagined risk of disqualifying themselves as capable of being loved.[3] What is more, it deprives them of a consoling pathological sense of power experienced in vindictive retaliation. Therefore, they hold stubbornly, with a false sense of integrity, to their demands, refuse to make efforts to achieve their own happiness, and, in retaliatory fashion, frustrate the efforts of those who would help them to engage in gratifying adult activity.

These have been general considerations of psychodynamic factors

[3] ". . . to be strong is to be unlovable"; see Captain-Woman dream, p. 257.

in resistance. There now follows a more detailed and categorized examination of resistance—its clinical setting and its reflection in dreams.

Outwitting and Eluding the Analyst

The woman of the Induced Labor dream (pp. 31–32) revealed during much of her time in analysis amazing intuition and remarkable intellect in the grasping and correlating of dreams and other data. Nevertheless, she rarely moved forward therapeutically. She was skillful at ranging close but not looking directly into her problem areas. This behavior was, in the therapeutic relationship, an expression of her major interpersonal problem, provocativeness. Such activity was frequently accompanied by anxiety, particularly if to any degree she glimpsed the nature of her behavior. She had a genius for preparing, in and out of the sphere of therapy, for harmonious joint activity and then disrupting it. In the course of exploring this problem, she brought in the following dream (Escaping the Photographer).

"I was in some kind of an enclosed place, a building that gave me asylum. Each time I came out from shelter I risked my life being exposed to a photographer who wanted to take a picture of me. So each time I encountered him, I retreated."

She briefly alluded to the photographer as the analyst, and to her retreating as her usual withdrawal from problems after "dancing close."

This dream of resistance (characteristically brought forward at the very end of the session) was never fruitfully pursued. It had preceded, by a month, a summer vacation during which she made no significant effort to work on her problems independently. The following year was her most unproductive single year of analysis, and an unhappy year in family and other phases of interpersonal existence. In analysis she continued her practice of briefly exposing herself and then running back to shelter before it was possible to get a clear picture.

The same patient, in a more productive period of her analysis, had another resistance dream reflecting an aspect of her personality related to the provocativeness, her sadism (Enjoying Her Frustration).

"I was climbing over some repetitive obstacle like repeated hurdles. I was trying to reach some goal, but didn't know where I was trying to get. When I finally did make it there was a great feeling of satisfaction at frustrating my sister, the feeling that I had the key and she couldn't get it—I had a *terrible* hatred for my sister. As I woke I had a terrible feeling of hatred, a great feeling of triumph over her." She interrupted with the association—*"like my feeling here,"* and continued reporting her dream. "I had the key, and she didn't. I could open my own door or jewelry. She can't get it, and I have it. I'm frustrating her. I *enjoy* frustrating her."

She was silent for a few moments and then I suggested that she associate with this enjoyment of frustrating her sister. She snapped a denial that she had reported frustrating her sister in the dream, and insisted that *I* had introduced the theme of frustrating her sister. Then, with an immediate healthy reversal, she said that my question had sounded like past remarks of mine implying that she enjoyed frustrating others, ". . . and so I wanted to steer away."

I said to her, "Your competition against me comes out clearly right now. You wanted so strongly to avoid acknowledging something merely because it came from me, that you denied a remark you had made only a few seconds before. You actually said it was *my* statement, not yours, when I was quoting your own report of your dream."

She continued to deal constructively with her own resistance. "When I had the dream, I hoped I'd come up with associations of childhood competition with my sister. Not until I came in here did I have associations with you, and here."

"What associations do you have with enjoyment of frustrating?"

"I thought, 'gloating over my sister's defeat.' *Gloating*—that's the word I thought and didn't say."

"Because you have been so miserable getting this gloating kind of satisfaction," I reminded her, and then asked, "What is the key in the dream?"

"The key is the truth. In the dream I was glad to show *you* the key, and *you* can't have it. A large part of my analysis has been my walking out with the key. If I have it, you can't have it. I *enjoy* frustrating you!" A characteristic analytic maneuver of hers had been to indicate awareness without developing it, and in this statement, made during a predominantly constructive and self-searching session, she faced her enjoyment of her own typically resistance behavior.

A dream somewhat comparable to "Escaping the Photographer" was reported by a young husband (Battle Tactics). He had started analysis because of marital friction, and had shown rapid therapeutic movement during the first weeks. He was enthusiastic about the therapeutic process until he began to feel the burden of the accumulating insight and of its growing imperative to change his behavior in the marriage relationship. Then, in contrast with his previous willingness to examine a single incident collaboratively and intensively, he launched upon a period of digressive, cluttered, session-cramming recounting of great numbers of incidents. This went on for several sessions, and then the patient had the following dream.

"It was war. A bunch of us were hiding alongside a rough kind of wall—like this one. [He touched the wall alongside the couch.] Every once in a while one person would run out from cover and get shot— killed. I said, 'If we go out one by one they'll get us each time. Let's run out in a bunch—then we'll have a better chance of some not getting hit.'"

The elusive, competitive, tactical orientation toward interpersonal relationships, which characterized the marriage from which he came for assistance, and which was developing (as resistance) in the therapeutic relationship, was graphically reflected in his dream.

Slowing the Pace

The previous dreams fall into a loose category of resistance characterized by outwitting, eluding, somehow triumphing over the analyst. There are other types of resistance behavior reflected in dreams. During productive phases of therapy, there are often periods in which patients express resistance in the form of slowing the pace, seeking to maintain part of their stake in pathology.

One patient, having gained considerable insight and having started to try new and more rewarding interpersonal behavior, was smitten with occasional fright and uncertainty. He dreamed that with happy anticipation he was about to go through a doorway into a new kind of country, where he would live permanently. All one had to do was empty one's pockets of all the old currency (the pathological currency with which he was used to making his way). He pleaded with a little old man at the gate for permission to keep "just one coin!" He would have liked to keep just one little bit of his old pathological integrity (Keeping One Coin).

A somewhat similar attitude was expressed in the dream of a young medical student who had been making slow but definite therapeutic gains for several months. He entered the office one morning feeling depressed, saying that he wasn't doing well enough in his courses, that he wanted to learn more without studying more. (His wish to achieve result without effort had been a problem already productively tackled. There was nothing new or surprising about the remark, and it did not explain his depression.) He spontaneously launched into his previous night's dream (Growth Pills) and into interpretive activity.

"I dreamed this morning about getting some kind of growth pill, a pill that makes you grow—but I was a little anxious. I was *worried that the growth couldn't be stopped,* and that's like cancer.

"My first association was 'growth without effort,' and I laughed. I know I want to learn without having to study. My fear, though, seems to come from my definite feeling that I've *been* growing, definitely maturing in the past few months." He suddenly interpolated, "The depression has gone already."

"What is threatened by your growing?" I asked.

"That's what I'm wondering," he said. "Why should I fear health? Something just popped into my mind—a line from Shakespeare: 'I am myself alone.' I think my uniqueness is *me,* and so I'm clinging to it. I'm feeling schizy—kidding myself, sometimes, like not brushing my teeth before going to bed, or reading and not absorbing, or listening intently without hearing. It's schizy because it's making believe for myself, trying to twist reality. I don't actually say, 'I won't brush my teeth.' What I do is say to myself, 'I'm mature, realistic.' Then I brush my teeth superficially, without really cleaning them. What do I get out of brushing my teeth superficially? It bolsters my uniqueness—the laws of decay don't apply to me."

He would like to maintain a small toe-hold in his illusion of immunity to reality (to tooth decay) and thus delay the assumption of manly, adult, realistic responsibility for himself. His anxiety was sharply reflected in his association that too-rapid growth was "like cancer." In spite of his reluctance, however, this patient was not fighting, outwitting, or eluding the analyst, but only slowing down the process.

The imminence of the analyst's summer vacation will cause an exacerbation of resistance in some patients. The patient of the following dream had recently started in a new job with great increase in responsibility, and had moved into a new home. During his year and a half of analysis he had been slowly but successfully struggling with his unwillingness to accept responsibility as a professional and a family man, and throughout his maturing had experienced considerable resentment and hostility toward the analyst. (This was the patient who had dreamed of the analyst as his chauffeur.)

One of his techniques for avoiding influence from the therapist had been the preparation of an agenda for his analytic session. He would characteristically "cooperate" by spending time during the therapeutic session on the problems which had been focused upon by the analyst—but his productions were usually a careful reconstruction of thinking already accomplished outside the analytic hour. Analytic "exploration" had often appeared fluent, copious, and conscientious, and yet it often served to defeat immediate and spontaneous exploration of himself on the couch. An example of this is the spirit in which he brought in the dream to be reported.

The prospect of the summer break of two months found the patient with his hard-earned maturity and independence, his new acceptance of responsibility, all of which he must now carry forward alone. He came in for his last session before the vacation, complaining of a headache of nearly migrainous proportions which had begun as he left home to come to my office. After stating that his headache was growing worse by the minute, he said conscientiously that he wanted to report a dream (Wheelbarrows) he had failed to speak of at the previous session. He could not remember all of it, but the setting was the analyst's office.

"Your office was a huge place. I was talking with another patient of yours whom I know, and while we talked somebody brought in a wheelbarrow. He was returning it. You had a whole pile of them behind your desk. I was there to return my wheelbarrow, too. I was talking with my friend about keeping it for a longer time, instead of returning it right then."

The patient made no attempt to work on the dream, but instead went into a long discussion of how brilliantly he was doing in his new professional position. After this had gone on for some time I interrupted and said, "Let's get back to the dream. What are your associations with the wheelbarrows?" He said, with some surprise at having been interrupted, "You mean my association right now?" I said, "Yes." He replied at once, "A load of shit." (This was his first spontaneous remark of the hour.)

I said, "So you feel that my other patients are turning in their wheelbarrows, while you want to hold on to yours a while longer."

He laughed aloud, and blushed. After a few moments he said, "I'm glad this is my last session." He paused for a few moments, and added, "I'm left to handle things myself this summer. Things are going better than I anticipated, but yet I'm apprehensive."

In the dream he was asking symbolically for permission to stop the difficult process of growing up and to continue bringing in "loads of shit" to fill the hour instead. The prospect of carrying on alone during the summer had stimulated his resistance in the form of repudiation of already recognized therapeutic advance.

The resistive slowing up, as contrasted with eluding and strongly contravening therapeutic influence, is related to an ongoing process of change. This type of resistance is sometimes complicated by the patient's competitive struggles against others. He may be unwilling to permit a resented spouse to benefit from the change in his personality—the partner doesn't *deserve* a good marriage, and particularly not as the fruit of the efforts of the long-suffering patient. Furthermore, change would be a competitive defeat in the home battle, a humiliating acknowledgment of having been at least partially wrong in the past. In this framework, a spouse in analysis often paradoxically contemplates divorce just as his therapeutic efforts begin to create a happier marriage.[4] On the other hand, he or she may prefer to stay in the marriage and *not* change, in order to "get even."

In the competition of marital partners, resistance thwarts the therapeutic search for reasonable equality. There is a great desire to maintain a strategic "edge" over the other, a great fear that without an operational margin of safety the balance of power might shift adversely.[5] There also may be the unexpressed, even unrecognized, concept that pathology is a privilege. "If *he* doesn't [if *they* don't] change, why should *I* have to? They got away with it, why shouldn't *I*?" A negative therapeutic reaction, a depression, a backsliding, frequently will follow contact with other neurotic members of a closely related group, particularly the patient's family. The witnessing of the open franchise for the rest of the world to be sick without having to struggle to change often intensifies the battle against the analyst, lending to resistance the added force of righteous indignation.

For some patients, the retrospective recognition that during a holiday period away from analysis they have made some independent progress (with the logical inference that they are ready on returning for accentuation of the collaborative therapeutic effort) will bring forth a fresh denial of change. Although the therapeutic influence had been put to rewarding service *at a distance* during vacation, there may be the added factor of recoil from the *direct* influence of the analyst.

The following dream (Screwed Up) was experienced just after a constructive long summer by the man who dreamed of the wheelbarrows just prior to the vacation. He returned for his first session of the new analytic year and filled the hour by talking about several

---

[4] Maintenance of pathology in order to be punitive, or to continue to deny having been wrong, is also a strong resistance factor in young adults whose parents are the ultimate target of resistance. (This is dramatically expressed by the patient of the Rabbis' Curse dream; see p. 293.)

[5] See Empty Suit, Disturbingly Adequate Husband, Death of Husband, Statuesque Masturbation, and Very Contented, But . . . .

crucial problems, which he illustrated with pertinent accounts of various interpersonal events. At the end of the session it was pointed out to him that while he had, as was his custom, dealt with the crucial data about himself, he had done so in a very detached, affectless fashion. It was emphasized to him that no real change could take place unless we could thoroughly explore his feelings, both those that he experienced while discussing his problems and those that had accompanied the reported experiences.

He started his second session by saying that he had been shaken by my parting remarks. "I realized that there was a great reluctance, actually a refusal, on my part to talk about my feelings."

He then reported a dream. "I was teaching some students. I was reading from a book. It was a book you had written. I was reading incorrectly and after several tries it continued to come out wrong. I was aware of your being there, and I was embarrassed. Then I made some remarks to the students making it clear that the whole difficulty was in my reading and not in your writing. I could read the ideas in the book clearly enough. I could read what was there, and understand it. But in reading aloud, I somehow made it come out screwed up."

He went on directly to associate. "I think of your interpretations. I may understand them, but I can't put them into practice. I recall the time that we talked about my obesity. I decided then to go on a diet. That day, instead of having my usual sandwich for lunch, I had a piece of pie, a tall glass of orange juice, and then a large dish of ice cream for dessert. Only after I got back to work that afternoon did I realize that that was the day I was going to start on a diet."

His association to the resistance dream was the comparable waking resistance to dieting. In the dream he comprehended and endorsed what he read, but when he tried to give the ideas audible articulation they came out "screwed up." In his waking life he understood his overeating, but his plans to diet got "screwed up"; he accepted the responsibility to resume analysis intensively, and tackled crucial problems at the first session, but that too came out distorted, because he refused to include emotions.

The patient's resistance was even more strongly expressed when he left this second post-vacation hour, which ended just before his supper hour. He had bought a candy bar in case the restaurant where he usually took a quick bite should be closed. He found the restaurant open, and decided to eliminate dessert and substitute the candy. As it turned out, however, he ate his dessert and then absent-mindedly started to eat the candy, too. Catching himself, he had the impulse to throw the candy away. Instead, he consumed all of it, thus again validating our joint interpretation of his compulsive "screwing up" in activities involving insights to which I had contributed.

There are patients whose pathology may be deprived of the fullest therapeutic efforts of the analyst because resistance is neither flagrant nor intense. These are people who have developed a fair degree of poise, sensitivity, and adaptability. They have considerable resources of health, tend to be direct, friendly, and conscientious. Their ready engagement in the analytic process, the willing, intelligent examination of problems, the relatively steady, realistically slow modification of behavior becomes deceptively rewarding to the therapist, and at first encouraging to the patient. Cooperation appears to be on a high level and thus therapeutic pressure seems unnecessary. For the analyst, the patients are welcome; the sessions tend to be a relief from more exacting clinical encounters. There is some change, some progresss, but the patient feels an unidentified anxiety, and the analyst becomes aware of an almost imperceptible slowing of the pace. The patient has been apparently straightforward in some areas, but has nevertheless acquired a mainly superficial grasp of the problems.

The analyst begins to detect that what has appeared to be insight has often been largely sophistication, that what has appeared to be courageous self-confrontation has sometimes been only bold generalization. In reality these patients have a great potential for commitment to the analytic process, but what looks like commitment is largely a skillful adaptation to analytic activity. It is important to detect their lack of adequate penetration and to press them to deeper search. They are more afraid and more capable than they know, and they will overcome their anxious resistance if given adequately particularized and persistent prompting.

One young wife [6] came to analysis primarily to help her husband who, like a number of their friends, was finding his own analysis an emotionally painful experience. Partly because of his preoccupation and detachment, she felt some inadequacy as a wife. Once started in her own analysis she worked hard, but her productions, even when she welcomed help in the direction of insight, often tended (particularly as seen in retrospect!) toward vagueness, generalization, and superficiality. Partly out of conscientious involvement, partly because of psychological sophistication, she followed new leads without challenging their potential fruitfulness, but for a long time she did not probe

[6] This is the patient of the Disturbingly Adequate Husband dream, pp. 172–173.

long enough or deeply enough into any one area. After a while, with much prompting, she began to realize that her inadequacy to deal with her husband's problems was not her only trouble—that she had some authentic pathology of her own, and that she had been holding back from exploring it fully.

Basically she was grateful for the therapeutic pressure. She was *not* a hostile, strongly fending-off, seductively evasive patient. Her recognition of her own anxious resistance enabled her to take more deliberate initiative in spite of it. When she began to probe more deeply into her personal pathology, the frightened resistance engendered by this intensification of self-exploration was revealed in a dream (Execution).

"I was in a room—like a cocktail lounge or a hotel lobby. (It reminds me of the lobby of this building.) It was dark, with weird lighting glimmering on dark woodwork, lots of shadows in dark corners. The atmosphere was eery and rather frightening. There were six or eight people there sitting about the room—all, I knew, were waiting to be executed. I was sitting with one of them, I think a man, and I seemed to be very much concerned about this person. My role was that of a *visitor* to these people—particularly to this one. They had all received some sort of injection under the arm; the injection seemed to be a necessary preparation for the execution by gas that was to follow. At one point a guard came over to me. I was very much afraid he would think I was one of the prisoners. I showed him that I had had no injection as proof that I was only a visitor. They began leading the prisoners out, one by one. I was talking with this one person—I seemed to be trying to soothe, reassure, and support him through the ordeal. Then I was alone in the room and one of the guards came and told me that the execution hadn't 'taken' on this person I was interested in, and that therefore he would be pardoned. I felt a tremendous feeling of relief and pleasure."

She went right on with associations and interpretations. "The dream seems to reflect my feeling about analysis being something that involves suffering and eventual execution. I see myself as a visitor to analysis—not really a patient. In fact, when a guard [the analyst?] begins to treat me like the rest, I become anxious and have to prove that I am only a visitor—I show him that I have had no injection, that is, no suffering.

"I have had this feeling about analysis. I felt that since I did not seem to have the same amount of torture that I had been led to expect from it, I am not really in analysis. Actually, *I am afraid of being involved in such a terrifying experience.* The one prisoner I am most

interested in is my husband. Since he has been in analysis I have usually felt that it was my role to soothe and help him through his ordeal.
He always pictured it to me as an ordeal."

The fears of paralysis (in the dream, imprisonment) and the fears
of disintegration of the personality upon entering more deeply and
directly into the arena of analysis (in the dream, annihilation) are
clearly indicated. The patient had not suspected how much of herself
she would have to commit to analysis once she was in: "I was very
much afraid he would think I was one of the prisoners . . . [whereas
actually] I was only a visitor." She was above the therapeutic needs of
her husband and other friends in analysis, and the analyst was not supposed to "treat me like the rest."

In another dream of the same night, this wife revealed her resistance to penetrating beneath the surface view of herself and accepting the affective impact of achieved insight. She had begun to discover
her feelings over a broad area, broader than her marriage and her
analysis. She was only beginning to feel the quality of her girlhood
relationships with her mother and brother. The patient had talked of
her mother often and with impatience, but had tended to formulate her
reactions in sophisticated psychological fashion, with some honesty but
essentially little feeling. She was often in the neighborhood of the
problem, but only after a year and a half did she become willing to
go to the heart of it. In the dream that follows she experienced shame
rather than anxiety over the persistent penetration into her emotions
(Crude and Ugly Things).

"I am driving with someone; he was vague, but it was a man.
I drive past some shops with ugly old furniture and bric-a-brac in the
windows. I tell my companion that my mother has that kind of junk
in her house, and that I don't like it. Then driving on I point to a spot
and say that my mother's house is there—but it is not there, and I feel
quite dismayed not to see it. The place where it used to be is surrounded by modern new apartment houses. We do some further driving around the area, and then I see that the house is there after all,
though it had not been visible from the road, as it used to be. I want
to show my companion the inside of the house. When we go inside
I am very much ashamed to see that the house is dark and very old-
fashioned, and filled with old and crude and ugly things. The feeling
is surprise and dismay, even though I had said that this was the kind
of thing that was in the house. It is not as I remember it, though I
know as I look at it that it was always this way."

The patient went on with spontaneous associative and interpretive
activity. She said, "My first association with the man next to me in the

car is you. I know that it is you. I seem to be showing him my past. In a *casual, generally vague* kind of way, I can accept and let him see that there are things I don't like in my past—like the ugly furniture and things like that *in the shop windows.* The modern houses surrounding my mother's house are, I think, *the newer ideas and attitudes I have acquired in order to avoid looking directly at my real feelings and at my past—but they are there when I look hard enough.* My feelings about the inside of the house are feelings I have had in talking in the analysis about my experiences and relationships of the past. Even though I had said *in general* that there was ugliness there, *I am surprised and ashamed when I really find specific examples of it*—and I know that it was this way. For instance, facing the fact that my mother never really loved me the way I wanted her to, and not just because she was busy or worried about other things; or looking at the really intense rivalry I had, and still have, with my brother—*not just dismissing it casually* with the assumption that 'of course I had some sibling rivalry.' "

At the end of the session I asked her to tell me what she felt the two dreams of that night (Execution, and Crude and Ugly Things) meant, taken as a whole. She thought for a moment. "The two dreams seem to show my changing attitudes and confusion about the analysis, about myself as a patient, and about your [the analyst's] role. First I see 'real' analysis as something frightening. I see myself as an outsider, not really a patient and not wanting to be. Then I see you as a prison guard leading his prisoners to execution. At the end [Crude and Ugly Things] I seem to reach the point of trying to look at things with you, and I have some desire to show you things about myself. But I find it is not easy or pleasant. I don't like the idea of finding all these things in me that other patients have. Even though I have always said, and thought I believed, that of course I am just like anyone else and *I* have problems too—still, really looking at them is another story."

These dreams, and the pursuit of feeling in an intimate endeavor with the analyst, led soon to the intensification of the patient's positive feelings toward the analyst. This was disturbing to her; she sought to avoid the subject, and explored it only in response to constant prompting. In the dream that now follows there is an echo of the resistance theme of her being "only a visitor" at the execution. The focus here, however, is the reluctance to deeper penetration into her positive feeling toward the analyst (Driver Does Not Stop).

"I am on a bus and the only passenger left. I pull the cord to get off, but the driver does not stop there. He continues on many blocks further. I am angry at him and tell him what he did and that I don't like it. He says nothing, but keeps driving. I gradually stop feeling angry and just wait to see where we are going. He takes me home to his house. He has a big family. It was the kind of thing like when a boy takes a girl home to meet his family."

The patient summed up her feelings about the meaning of this dream as follows: "The bus driver is you. I feel that you are taking me in this analysis further than I had planned on going. Part of this is a reaction to your getting me into discussing my relationship with you in the last session. I still don't like to feel that I have all of these feelings about you—I still can't stand getting entangled in all this business just as I knew other patients do. The big family I think must be all the other patients. I'm not too sure of myself in all this but at least I'm going along and seeing what will develop."

In these dreams the prospect of increasing intimacy in the cooperative pursuit, while producing shame, anger, and some anxiety, did not generate the resistance and terror found in less healthy patients. There was here none of the overwhelming sense of annihilation that produces intense anxiety and hostility, and that often and for long periods utterly thwarts progress in therapy. This is a fundamentally cooperative patient (like the one in the Screwed Up dream, above), who demonstrates, rather, a slowing-up type of resistance.

Intense Resistance

The first dreams in this chapter focused chiefly upon the outwitting and eluding of the analyst. The next dreams indicated the slowing-up of productive work. Anxiety was present in these dreams of resistance. Until a good deal of health has been achieved, it often happens that the more rigidly the patient opposes the analyst, the less anxiety there is in the patient's dreams. By contrast, as the rigidity and the resistance are reduced, anxiety is more likely to appear in the patient's dreams during periods of effective therapeutic influence and productive analytic work (see Chapters 8 and 10).

The two dreams that now follow are examples from a single individual illustrating intense determination to preserve the pathological self against the inroads of cooperative, self-exposing behavior.

In the first dream (Japanese Battlefield) the patient feels that the competitive odds are strongly against him, and there is temporary panic. In the second (Bear Man) the same patient has "emergency resources" readily at hand, and there is no anxiety, because there is no forward movement in the analysis.

"I was on a kind of Japanese battlefield. A very tough-looking soldier came, and I was down on my back. I felt helpless, but had decided submission was the best course. I placatingly lifted up my leg toward him. He had a big sword, and with a swish he cut off my foot. I was somewhat shocked, for it was more than I had expected. Then my face was ripped open with a knife. I now felt some panic as I realized this was really serious, and was going farther than I had anticipated. I was scared, and a little belligerent. Then a steel rod was shoved up my spine, and I had a rather silly helpless grin as I realized I was really paralyzed. But I was still alive."

The patient followed with a few comments. "I offered up my foot as a kind of sacrifice. This didn't bother me too much. I was really upset when my face was cut. This was more than I had bargained for. When the rod was shoved up my spine I was resigned but also quite adamant, and felt proud, and wouldn't give in."

The dream reflects the patient's grim conceptualization of analysis as war between the analyst and analysand. Lying on the couch is being helpless on his back. The analyst is tough, alien, and out for conquest. Working together is, for the patient, either triumph or submission, and in this case he hoped that submission would prove to be a clever tactic: "I had decided submission was the best course." His foot was cut off, his face slashed, and his spine reamed: as though he were saying he didn't have a leg to stand on, had lost face, and was paralyzed through the cruel, ruthless analytic process. The resistance, in spite of the panic, is however somewhat glorious: "I was . . . also quite adamant and felt proud, and wouldn't give in."

That determined nurturing of the lingering spark of pathology— "I was still alive"—was examined in the interpretive exchanges. During the next month, the patient made some of the most effective progress of several analytic years. At the end of that time, however, he was due for increased status and occupational recognition. He responded to this with great self-inflation, and reassertion of his pathological strengths, a return to the "adamant, and felt proud, and wouldn't give in." Just before the occupational advance he had another striking dream of resistance, which this time he did not employ constructively. The dream heralded his therapeutic regression (Bear Man).

"I was in a room and there was a huge giant of a man with me, who seemed to smile a very knowing and self-assured smile—a bear of a man, with huge hands and a condescending look and smile. I felt he was going to just crack me with his big paw. I held a gun, but it was a sort of air pistol. I had great difficulty in getting it to work.

Finally I did, and shot him in the stomach. It stopped him, but only made a little hole. He came again, and I had trouble with the complex mechanism, but got another shot away. I prepared again, and this time it got easier. But he stopped before I shot, and went and lay down on a bed. It was now like a hospital. I called the doctors' dining room and said that it was an urgent emergency. Three doctors came. Someone said I should have seen how they jumped when I called. I was pleased. But they stood there looking at the two little holes oozing blood and I felt, 'Why don't they do something?' "

Immediately after telling the dream he went on with attempts at interpretation and association. "The giant was me. I recognized the belly as my own when I gained weight in the army—that was the time that I was most grandiose. I felt quite good that I was getting the hang of the gun and able to stop him; but I was disturbed that he was very hurt, and this meant a change in my feeling in the dream. Now I was very anxious that I shouldn't die and kept feeling that the doctors should do something instead of just looking at the little holes."

Occupational promotion brought with it an overwhelming resurgence of resistance, intuitively previsioned in the dream. The pathological personality was "transfused"—the grandiose, bullying "bear man" was revived, and the pathological integrity restored. The "doctors"—the real people who promoted and congratulated him just after this dream —performed, alas, a successful transfusion and plugged the holes in this "huge giant of a man . . . a bear of a man with . . . a condescending look and smile." The two shots, probably his two weekly sessions, "only made a little hole." The two conflicting trends, healthy effort to change and pathological restoring and preserving of the earlier self-concept, are here dramatically symbolized. The "change in my feelings in the dream" was reflected in waking life as a marked shift from the most productive period of analysis to a solid four months of resistance.

The Tactics of Resistance in Waking Life

All of the dreams in this chapter have reflected the patient's fight against personality change. They reflect the competitive struggle, often angry or anxious, to fend off the analyst's influence. The patient's resistance may utterly block his progress, may slow its pace, or may tend to nullify the progress already achieved.

Since the action of all dreams is a reflection in the patient's sleeping consciousness of his waking activity, resistance dreams have their counterpart, as already demonstrated, in the behavior of the patient's waking life—in his interpersonal life in general and in the analytic relationship in particular. This section of the chapter is concerned with the patient's devices, aware and unaware, for immunizing himself against the influence of the individual by whose influence, paradoxically, he has undertaken to gain help.

There are three reasons for considering the tactics of resistance in waking life in connection with resistance in dreams. First, these tactics pervade the behavior and feelings of the psychoanalytic experience [7] and thus form the substantive base of a great many dreams. Second, they operate against fruitful clinical use of the patient's dreams. Finally, these waking counterparts of resistance in dreams become foci for consensual validation. When this consensual validation is integrated with interpretive activity applied to resistance dreams, the resulting correlations serve to illuminate for the patient the relationship between his dreams and his personality.

The waking expressions of resistance are categorized below as follows: (1) Pseudo-conscientious forms of resistance; (2) resistance through direct and indirect challenges, antagonism, refusals to engage; (3) resistance through helplessness and diversionary self-pity; (4) resistance through seduction. The categories tend to overlap somewhat. All the activities, whether the patient is aware or unaware of the fact, represent anxious or angry competitive interpersonal operations, aimed at fending off the analyst's influence.

PSEUDO-CONSCIENTIOUS FORMS OF RESISTANCE

Every patient entering analysis is at least in some degree carrying out a voluntary decision. He is acknowledging his need for help, is ready to make considerable sacrifice to get it, and is presumptively committed, in his own best interest, to responding as fully as he can to the requirements of the therapeutic process. The conflict between this commitment and his desire to maintain the pathological integrity of the personality, results in many protective maneuvers. These maneuvers, while often appearing to be conscientious engagement in therapy, are in fact unawaredly designed to make the therapeutic process ineffectual.

One of the commonest of the pseudo-conscientious maneuvers is the *presentation of data in abundance*. The essence of the evasion lies in the patient's unwillingness to examine what he presents while at the same time he appears to be making his life an open book. He may occupy a whole session in presenting a dream, or two or three or five

---

[7] See Chapter 2, "Denial of Feeling," pp. 53–59.

dreams, in such detail that no component is ever correlated with life experience. The copious presentation allows no time for contemplation, for interpretive activity, for responsiveness between patient and analyst. The abundant data, dream or otherwise, may at times even represent a particularly careful gleaning of what the analyst seems to "want"—anamnestic, sexual, dream, childhood, occupation data, or even material indicating grasp of a certain insight. The tactical goal of such reporting is to prevent insight and change.[8]

Self-recrimination, good resolutions, and pious hopes are other common forms of resistance.[9] Often it becomes important not to be misled by a patient's earnestly expressed resolutions to change a mode of behavior. The resolution to change often substitutes for the process. It tends to lull the patient into a reduced rather than a heightened awareness of the need for therapeutic effort. Although the patient is usually self-deceived, he is, nevertheless, fundamentally employing a competitive maneuver to call off the efforts of the analyst. It is the readily recognizable present and active engagement in examining the distorted interpersonal practice that leads to future change.

Earnest hope for change or for maintenance of gains is also a frequent and transparent evasion of therapeutic effort. Sometimes after the patient has made genuine effort he devoutly sighs, "I hope this lasts!" Such a prayer is commonly the precursor of relaxed therapeutic activity on the part of the patient. It may reflect his resentment of the successful influence of the analyst, and a competitive compulsion to counter the analyst's effectiveness.

Self-recrimination, resolutions, and hopes do not modify personality, and are likely to be subtle manifestations of resistance.

Another manifestation of pseudo-conscientious resistance is the *"confirmation" of an insight with an inappropriate documentation.* One patient described to me the generous help she had given to a sick friend living alone. She stocked and prepared food, cleaned the apartment, furnished her with extra fluids and urged her to drink them, and then came to analysis acknowledging for the first time, by this inappropriate example, how she really did like to manipulate people!

Another patient, a mother who skillfully combined martyrdom with tyranny, was gradually coming to recognize her strong dominating tendencies. Her two boys, about ten and twelve, had grown highly

---

[8] The dream Battle Tactics, pp. 186–187 of this chapter, beautifully symbolizes this massive-data approach.

[9] The Elevator Nightmare, below (pp. 218–226), offers a good example of self-recrimination as resistance.

rebellious and abusive in response to her control. The day before her analytic hour she had picked up one of them and his playmate after school. On the drive home her son had become arrogant and contemptuous, was distracting her from her driving, vilifying her, and in general carrying on in an intolerable fashion. She reported to me that she had finally stopped the car a half-block before their house, and had (quite appropriately) ordered her son to get out and walk the rest of the way. Finishing the conscientious account, she burst into tears, saying, "I see, you're right, you're right, I'm really a tyrant. I was cruel and tyrannical toward my poor boy!"

If I had permitted this incident to become the ultimate basis for her conviction that she tyrannized, she could rest easily on a doubt of the validity of the insight, and thus, like the previous patient, effectively insulate herself from therapeutic influence and change.

Seeming therapeutic cooperation that is a common expression of resistance is the *escape into genesis,* or escape into dynamics. A patient who has rejected a formulation about his personality and who has shown consistent reluctance to consider relevant evidence, will suddenly begin to investigate the origin of the very pathology whose existence he has refused, even hypothetically, to acknowledge. He asks, "How does this sort of thing come to be?" or "How did I get this way?" One cannot meaningfully probe the dynamics or origins of something whose existence one has not genuinely recognized and acknowledged. Such "whys" are usually answered by the patient with a number of "supposes" ("I suppose it's because . . ."). When, instead of such academic speculation, associative activity is seriously undertaken, it may bring substantiation of a serious formulation, or a modification of it, or even a valuable repudiation of it, or the pursuit of a new and meaningful aspect of the individual's personality.

Avid acquiescence is another pseudo-conscientious resistance tactic. It may sound very much like a conscientious self-confrontation, but it is in effect what may be termed an *acceptance-out-of-existence.* Any therapeutic formulation is only the beginning of an exploration. A formulation offered to a patient is a recommendation to explore further, either by correlating previously reported data with new associations, or by searching for associations to a newly engendered concept or impression. When the patient says, "Yes, I agree, that's true, I *am* like that," the acceptance is too fast and too easy; he is going further than the situation warrants, unless the response is a bridge to further contemplation. The patient is justified only in acknowledging that what the analyst suggests "feels" right and, if he is genuinely conscientious, he then *begins to look.* With a hurried endorsement the formulation no longer exists as an analytic problem—it has been accepted out of existence.[10]

Resembling the deluge of data, the *analytic filibuster* is the unnecessarily confused presentation of material. This type of resistance is difficult to detect and usually difficult to deal with effectively. Any patient may be genuinely confused, and the analyst does not wish to discourage spontaneity or to encourage predigested, well-ordered reporting. A patient who is fully committed to searching and exposing himself may be halting, fragmentary, sometimes perhaps irrelevant and scattered, but if he is working honestly, the genuine commitment becomes apparent. Pseudo-conscientiousness, however, eventually reveals itself as a cluttered circumstantiality during which a focus of feeling or significance does not and cannot crystallize.

In the presentation of dreams, for example, the patient may make such constant shifts from dream element to association, often eliding almost undetectably from one to the other, that the result is a tangle of data in which individuals, surroundings, emotions and events, dream experience and waking experience, recall and interpretation are all present and unavailable for clinical use. When this kind of circumstantiality or confusion of dream with association is pointed out, the more committed patient learns to avoid it and to foster a more fruitful exchange. He will accept the suggestion that to overcome the tendency to confusion, a dream or waking event should be communicated in the session without interruptions, or with only the briefest footnote type of reference to the most significant associations. He will strive to fix in mind associations occurring during the report and return to them later. The evasive patient frequently responds to the criticism competitively by giving a very orderly presentation from which he withholds significant associative elements, thus substituting one form of resistance for another. The unnecessarily confused presentation of dream or other data, like any form of resistance, can be overcome to the extent that it is accepted by the patient as a problem with which to deal actively.

Another technique of resistance difficult to detect behind a facade of conscientious involvement is that of *repeatedly getting close to insight without going all the way.* It is a sort of analytic "brinkmanship." A patient will come to many sessions with incidents illustrative of the

[10] The value of detecting all of these evasive tactics is demonstrated below in the work with the Elevator Nightmare. After her "Why do I do it?" and numerous other maneuvers, the patient finally spoke with genuine dismay: "I guess I really am hurting her," and added with horror a substantiating association, "My God, I don't even feed the child!"

current problem, and describe in detail everything but the essential aspect. The woman of the Induced Labor dream for years pursued her pervasive problem of provocativeness, always emphasizing her justification, or her having known better, or her self-recrimination, or her sad acknowledgment that she knew "what you would say," but somehow always managing to leave out the essence of her provocativeness, her *desire* to produce a discomforting resentment in someone else, combined with her own deep *satisfaction* when the discomfort became evident (Enjoying Her Frustration, pp. 185–186). Another example is a sadistic homosexual man who for years brought in many examples of how he subtly hurt people. Always, with tears, tension, self-justification, or confusion, he disrupted the account short of clearly examining his hostile feelings and his role in the incident. Both of these patients brought in quantities of pertinent documentation of the problems, but never quite fully brought it all together to consummate the effort with insight.

The chapters on feeling and on introductory dreams included some discussion of resistance arising from the desire to control and conceal emotions.[11] A related phenomenon, the *synthetic exaggeration of feeling*, belongs in the present context of pseudo-conscientious forms of resistance. Some of the patients who are unwilling to expose their feelings resort nevertheless to dramatic displays of them as a sort of therapeutic opportunism. They cry with more distress than they feel, or ostentatiously swallow back their sobs, or speak their anger with forced intensity and clenched fists. Often there is an underlying genuine affect which makes the performance aspect difficult to evaluate. Still, detecting the false note is important for the avoidance of several possible therapeutic pitfalls. First, the exaggeration impedes treatment, because the patient's efforts are aimed at impressing the analyst rather than examining himself. The patient hopes that by proving his conscientiousness, he will gain the relaxation of the therapist's demands. In addition, if the pseudo-conscientious maneuver succeeds, the patient's respect for the analyst diminishes, and this permits a degree of disengagement from the therapeutic endeavor. The most serious danger, however, in the therapist's failure to detect this resistance technique lies in the fact that the patient's synthetic exaggeration obscures for himself his genuine emotion. In his pathological need to deny, control, and disguise his feelings, he leaves the session believing, aware or unaware, that whatever emotion he displayed was really just "put on." The therapist, too, needs all his astuteness, while detecting the synthetic quality of the display, to keep in sight the genuine underlying feeling that may also

[11] See Chapter 3, "Introductory Dreams," Scared Shitless dream, pp. 114–115, and Chapter 2, "Feeling in Dreams," Crazy Woman nightmare, pp. 73–77.

be present. A feeling cannot, after all, be exaggerated unless to some degree it exists.

Following is a brief account of three psychoanalytic sessions in which two dreams and the waking behavior of the patient within and apart from therapy reflect some of the forms of pseudo-conscientious behavior. The dreams are presented fully here, not only to illustrate the types of resistance behavior, but also to emphasize again the interrelatedness of personality, dream, and the patient's practice in the therapeutic relationship.

The patient was a married woman in her early thirties. These sessions occurred at an important nodal point in treatment, the first significant loosening of her resistance after one and a half years of analysis. At the immediately preceding session the patient had arrived in a mood of depression and open hostility, grimly withdrawn from the roles of wife and mother. She had, nevertheless, engaged thoroughly in the examination of her resentment of family life, had experienced a productive hour, and had left encouraged.

She returned for the next session manifesting in her spontaneous approach to her problems and in her total bearing some genuine improvement, which she proceeded to dwell on at length. She reported having been in excellent spirits since the previous hour, and expressed the feeling that the quality of life at home had had a salutary change: her husband and she were happier with each other and with their children. She described particularly what a good time she had been having with the children, whose burdensomeness had previously oppressed her.

Without her accustomed sense of harassment, she had taken the children to a movie. She had managed them in a pleasant, friendly, good-humored fashion, meanwhile noticing other mothers who were having difficulty with their children in the holiday crowd. During the outing she was pleasantly aware of her own superiority, thinking that others must be constantly noticing how loving and capable she was with her children.

I suggested that her self-conscious sense of superiority may have detracted from the realistic pleasure of being a good mother. The association occurred to me, and I reported it to her, of King Midas, who, through his hunger for gold (like the patient with her hunger for superiority) deprived himself of the simple enjoyment of his child. At this point she recalled a dream (Death of Husband). In it, the husband of a friend of hers had died in an automobile accident. "I was at the services. I felt a great compassion for the man who had died, because he had been about to go into a new venture which promised success.

His children were playing on the floor in the chapel. His wife entered dramatically with a gesture indicating, 'I'm here now, so you can start the services.'" With this the dream ended and she had awakened from it continuing to feel deep compassion for the "nice guy" whose enterprise had been unfulfilled because of death.

She went on associating spontaneously. "This woman has two children who are hypothyroid. The last time I was here and I was complaining about my children you said that if they were cretins I would not be able to have all the fun with them that I now do." She talked discursively and circumstantially about the woman in the dream, about the woman's sister and brother-in-law. There followed observations about her own sister and a discussion she had had with her mother about this sister. She glibly speculated that the widow in the dream was herself, and without pause went skipping along lightly, making other interpretive suggestions about who represented whom, but without any serious attempt to detect the problem in the dream.

I interrupted, "I think there's something in this dream you don't want to face." She paused for a moment, and then said emphatically, "I certainly don't want to lose *my* husband. If I had dreamed this a few nights before, it might have meant that." Then she talked animatedly about the family relationships of the woman whose husband had died in the dream, and again came up with a glib suggestion that perhaps the dead man represented her own father-in-law. "Maybe I hope my father-in-law would die?" Again I interrupted and reminded her that throughout her year and a half in analysis she had never hesitated to express her annihilative hostility toward her father-in-law; she would not, so to speak, have to waste time dreaming about *his* death. Besides, his death would hardly evoke the strong compassion she experienced during and following the dream. Her interpretive suggestion that the dead man might be her father-in-law had been offered cheerfully and with a questioning inflection which invited confirmation rather than consideration, as though the interpretation of dreams were a game.

At this point the patient's pseudo-conscientious resistance—already manifested by exaggerated emphasis upon her health, by filibustering, by playing a game with her dream—was now expressed in another form. In response to my fully expressed evaluation of her activity in the session, her comportment changed suddenly, and she said with concern, "You know, I'm scared now, and I can't think." I suggested again that there was a problem in the dream that she did not want to face, and pointed out that her thinking had been very fluid so long as she was not genuinely exploring for the problem; suddenly at the suggestion that she search for the real meaning of the dream material, she developed anxiety and an incapacity to think (psychosomatic confusion). She thought silently for a moment and then made the following offering: "I want to boss my children. I want to make them fit into a pattern." This was pathology that she had confronted frequently in the past.

By this time the therapeutic session was nearly over. I said, "I think that your raising the question of your wanting to boss your children and make them fit into a pattern is an evasion of the problem in the dream. It looks as though you are bargaining, offering to talk about being a tyrannical mother if you don't have to look for what is involved in the dream. You'll talk about this problem if you don't have to discover another problem." [12]

Something about herself in the dream remained for the patient to investigate. I offered an interpretive hypothesis. Perhaps the somewhat regal wife at the funeral was herself, and perhaps the husband who had died just as life became promising was her own husband. For some reason she wanted to eliminate her husband's participation at the start of what she considered a new career for herself, a new, happier, optimistic self-assertion. If she did seek to eliminate him, it would impede her own happiness. If she crushed her husband, she could not develop as a wife. She would instead be a lonely woman with a dramatic flair, her eye on glory. This attitude was reflected in her dramatic entry for the funeral in the dream, and in her reported self-consciousness in the public role of superior mother, and was associated with her previously acknowledged longing to be a prima donna in the theater.

I told her also that the dream, through her experiential strong compassion, indicated something very positive in her feeling toward her husband—a feeling that she did not want to lose him and did not want him to have his career (perhaps his career as a happier husband) stifled as it began. Because of this positive feeling and its potential for making her a happier wife, she had every incentive, I pointed out, to investigate, starting with associations to the dream, what forms her destructiveness toward her husband might be taking.

She left without expressing any acceptance or confirmation toward the interpretive hypothesis that had been offered.

In the immediately following session, she described in a sober mood some successful and happy times with her children and her husband, but did not refer to the dream.

At the second following session, a full week after the report of

[12] *Bargaining with insights* is a relatively common resistance tactic of the pseudo-conscientious type. The patient suddenly seeks evasion of an immediate problem by showing readiness to pursue a prior problem, sometimes one that has been eluded in its own relevant context.

the funeral dream, she began by stating that she hadn't felt like coming. She'd had a cold the day before, and had thought of calling up to cancel the session. Now, having overcome that resistance impulse to cancel, she wondered why she should have been so conscientious. Nothing was disturbing her, and there was nothing about which she especially wanted to talk. She began to recount a few matters in a rambling fashion. I interrupted, and reminded her that at the end of the session when she reported the funeral dream we had barely arrived at some concept of the problem in it, and that she had made no further reference to the dream. She immediately said, "I agree, but I can't do anything about it." When I inquired what she agreed about, she said, "About the problem in the dream,[13] but I can't do anything about it."

She was in no position, I pointed out, to agree about the interpretive hypothesis without exploring it; and she was in no position to decide whether there was anything she could do about the problem in the dream without first establishing the existence and the exact nature of the problem.

I then suggested that she examine her marriage, associating with my hypothesis that she was trying to extinguish her husband, to prevent him from growing into more of a person, more of a father, doctor, and husband.

After a moment she said, "With the children, *my* word is important. What I say goes. I justify that by saying they are with me more, and get used to asking *me*. I often correct my husband's English—it's a way of taking him down a peg, making his *thought* not count. I just pick on his words. When he explains to me something about his work, I don't let him have the pleasure of teaching me something. I just shrug my shoulders and say 'I don't understand—it's too complicated.' When I work with him at anything, I don't like to take orders. I like to do it *my* way. I've always resented authority. With my husband, I want everything my way. I like to make the decisions. Whenever he does anything wrong, I like to let him know it. I keep hacking away at his faults."

I asked, "For example?"

"Sometimes when he tells me about one of his consultations, I feel he didn't handle it well. I tell him he was hostile, smug, overbearing. Then when he clams up I get sore at him for that. When he offers to help me in the kitchen, I want things done exactly my way, or I get annoyed."

[13] An example of the pseudo-conscientious technique of accepting-out-of-existence; see p. 201.

I said, "To sum up, then, you try to make him feel inadequate in all these areas—as a doctor, a father, and a husband."

She immediately answered, "I left out sex, too. I want relations with him when *I* want it. If I'm tired, I just don't achieve orgasm."

At this point I said, "Let's get back to the dream. This guy in the dream was killed just at the beginning of his career. What does that mean?"

She replied, "He's going to take his boards in medicine . . . and he's made such tremendous strides as a father and a husband . . . he's beginning to be a *good* father, and a *good* husband. He's really been wonderful with the kids." Then she paused for a moment. "Last week we had a fight. I went to bed and felt, 'I'll fix him. I'll quit analysis. I'll write Walter and tell him I'm quitting. I won't try to be a loving wife and mother any more.'

"That raises another point. By coming here, I'm not just helping myself. I'm helping my family. I'm helping my husband and the children. When I was mad at him, I didn't want to help him." [14]

I said, "And that's why you come in here feeling you have nothing to talk about. If you talk and examine yourself honestly, you'll improve, and then your husband and the children will benefit. The feeling that you had at the beginning of this hour was unwillingness to pursue analysis."

Her reply was immediate. "Yet I get so much out of it. I have such a good time with the children, and I was so happy when my husband came home. The children have been so cute, I just felt like laughing, I was so happy watching them, and it was so good when he came home and I told him about it and we both went up and said goodnight to the children." She paused, and then continued, "There are times when I feel closer to him than I've ever felt to anyone in my whole life. Yet I'm always trying to cut him down. This is my problem with everybody, not just with my husband. How can I suddenly change?"

I said, "The problem with your husband is the most difficult for you, precisely because it is to him that you can give the most. You can enhance him more than you can enhance anyone else in the world. And it's a lifetime commitment, too. You pull back hardest from the marriage because it represents the greatest threat of change to your whole consciousness. You've been competitive, you've always cut people down, and you've fought against becoming the agent that benefits or enhances the life of anyone else. We've seen that this first developed in your family when you were a child. Except for your physical needs,

[14] This is an example of resistance complicated by a relationship outside analysis; see pp. 189–190.

your mother had no interest in your development. She always criticized you, always wanted you to act in a way that would enhance *her*. She exploited and frustrated and humiliated you. And you developed your personality in such a way as to insure that you would not be exploited any more. But how do you see 'exploitation'? To you, whenever you are enhancing others, being a nutrient to their lives, no matter how much *you* gain from the activity you still feel that you are being exploited. Now you've begun to get enjoyment out of doing things you used to fight against. You *enjoy* helping your husband and your children. But in this very activity with your husband in which you can develop yourself most fully, you feel the greatest assault upon your old personality."

She said, "Yes—all my life I've had my nose in the air. I must stay on top. If I make a mistake, it's an accident. If they do, or my husband does, it's characteristic."

I suggested, "You see that you've constantly worked to tear others down. It's not just a question of standing out above them. There is something more. When you predominate, you blot out any possibility of lending yourself to their growth, to their better functioning. Nevertheless, whenever you *have* enhanced the functioning of your husband or your children, you've been happy."

At this point she turned around with a big smile and a warm glow on her face: "You know, I had a very good dream the other night!" She went on to report the dream (Dancing Teacher).[15] "I was at a dancing studio and was trying to do something, and asked a famous dancer to help me, and she said yes. I was very surprised, because famous dancers are usually very snooty and have no interest in helping others. She started to show me a way of doing what I was trying to do, and I said, 'Ugh, not that horrible Humphrey-Weidman way,' so she said, 'Okay, let's try it another way,' and she asked me to show her what *I* had in mind. We tried it, and it didn't work very well, and I asked her to try the first way again, and that started to go very well, and I felt very good about it."

Without any hesitation she proceeded to the interpretation—which she had, in fact, worked out a couple of days before coming to the session. "This dancer might be you. At first I didn't want to do it your way, I wanted to do it my way. Then I found out that what you were trying to show me worked very well, and I wanted to work with you."

The second of these dreams reflects clearly the competitive nature of her resistance (do it *my* way) and symbolizes in addition the patient's

---

[15] Note the moment of association; see discussion in Chapter 7, pp. 234–235.

healthy efforts to overcome the resistance. "What I was trying to do . . ." she associated with her previous efforts to treat her dreams with pseudo-conscientious and evasive techniques. That approach was tried first, "but it didn't work very well."

The second dream illustrates well the concept that resistance in the therapeutic interpersonal relationship is an expression of the individual's general personality pathology. The patient had said, "When my husband tries to explain something to me, I don't try to understand and give him the pleasure of having taught me something. . . ." In the analysis she wondered aloud why she should be reluctant to cancel, implying that getting what the analyst offers isn't worth the effort, anyway, so why *not* cancel. And these influence-avoiding and derogating aspects of her personality were then reflected as well in her resistance dream—she recoiled from the willing assistance of the dancing teacher with an "Ugh, not that horrible . . . way." Nevertheless, the patient fought to overcome her resistance patterns of functioning at home, in the analytic session, and also in the dream.

RESISTANCE THROUGH DIRECT AND INDIRECT CHALLENGES, ANTAGONISM, REFUSALS TO ENGAGE

Hostility to the analyst characterizes much resistance, and is manifested in an infinite variety of behavior, according to the style or mood of the individual. The pseudo-conscientious forms of resistance discussed above may themselves be covert expressions of antagonism. The categories of resistance which are presented after this section on direct and indirect challenges, and which are formalistically referred to as "helplessness," "diversionary self-pity," and "seduction," may also be oblique expressions of inimical feelings toward the analyst.

Hostility may be manifested as open, noisy anger or as silent, grim, sulking, or depressed refusal to engage in the therapeutic process. It may be expressed in many active forms of elusiveness, or in direct challenges of many sorts regarding the analyst's methodology, concepts, motives, or competence. Hostility is often connected with anxiety, sometimes with contempt.

At times the open direct expression of anger at the analyst is an honest and welcome attempt on the part of the patient to express his feelings, but this is not always the case. A patient may also manifest anger openly as a diversionary action. The following is an unusually open statement from a patient who more characteristically practiced hostility covertly.[16] As a child, she used to torment and provoke her

---

[16] This is the patient who had the Induced Labor dream.

father, often getting him to scream at her in impotent rage while she listened with great contempt. One day she started an analytic session with the following declaration: "I'm beginning to feel toward you like I felt toward my father—I hate you, but what can I do about it? You're still my father—you're still my analyst. I have no way out. I feel I don't really have a choice. You can't change a father—you just go on living with him. I was going to say, 'You just go on *pissing* on him.' So I fight back tooth and nail." Her open statement, itself an overcoming of resistance, referred to hostile resistance usually expressed by her in covert forms.

Hostile resistance in most patients is predominantly covert and often unaware. While patients may block and have no associations for many reasons, including anxiety, there are times when the declaration, "I have no associations" is an angry, challenging statement. When a patient has, however, been in analysis for some time, and is familiar with the method of free association, the statement that there are "no associations" is a refusal to explore in the area of the problem. After all, the patient's statement is a prediction that no matter how long he waits or how hard he searches nothing will come into his mind. This is an impossibility. The prediction cannot be supported; it is therefore a determination not to communicate, and is frequently an angry, willful blotting out of imminent awareness. This was once expressed by a patient who came in stating, "I woke up this morning trying to forget a dream." Trying to forget a dream is, in a sense, intuitively seeking to blot out troublesome associations before they reach the context of waking consciousness. It is like trying to block off associations while awake, as a means of fending off illuminating data that would add to awareness in a crucial context. Fending-off of associations is frequently a reflection of hostile and competitive attitudes toward the analyst, based on the patient's belief that the analyst is seeking to manipulate him with standard therapeutic tricks at which he is an expert. As the patient sees it, the analyst's is a waiting game; the analyst opportunistically makes unwarranted inferences, assumes false correlations, and gives undue weight in dealing with all too fragmentary data.

Often the patient believes that the analyst's silences are stubborn or punitive. The patient may take up the apparently personal challenge in a battling frame of mind: "If he won't talk, I won't talk; I can out-silence him."

Sometimes when a patient who has previously been composed and affectively restrained has at last succeeded in expressing deep emotions, he will turn about and become angry, feeling somehow tricked. Retrospectively he will try to correct the situation, saying that the analyst has merely forced him, by some clever maneuver, to express himself in an emotional way. The patient thus repudiates the genuineness of his previous spontaneous reaction. This may be an anxious retreat from the recognition that there has been a significant change in his consciousness and behavior.

Quite apart from the general problems of cynical distrust, competitiveness, and hostility that have to be dealt with in therapeutic activity, it is necessary to examine the specific suspicion regarding "tricks" with all patients who are troubled by it. Needless to say, I am in total disagreement with analysts who manipulate the therapeutic situation in such a way as to produce anxiety or any other kind of reaction as a therapeutic tool. It is totally unnecessary to synthesize experiences in order to examine the nature of the patient's reactions. Every patient's life is replete with behavior and feeling available for mutual investigation by analyst and patient, and there is plenty in addition that occurs in the ordinary course of therapeutic exchange which can be examined. The artificial synthesis of circumstance not only insidiously re-enforces the patient's sense of being manipulated but also, for *both* analyst and patient, counteracts the essential cooperative spirit of psychoanalysis.

There is a great variety of indirect expressions of the patient's hostility to the analyst, such as starting out late to appointments, forgetting to get off the bus, train, or subway, forgetting to make the turn off the highway or, on other occasions, completely forgetting the appointment. The patient's hostility toward the analyst may determine whether or not an illness such as a cold or a difficult menstrual period is severe enough to justify a cancellation. When a patient observes that "I didn't want to come today," this is almost invariably a statement of antipathy to analysis and hostility to its agent, the analyst. It may also be communicated in a constructive spirit, the patient being aware of his resistance and already dealing with it. Much more often, however, the announcement of not wanting to come is a signal of unwillingness to be involved, and resistances may be anticipated during the ensuing session. The patient is likely to avoid independent, productive activity and may engage in argumentation, digression, or academic investigation, in lieu of exploration and interpretive activity.

More overtly, patients will angrily refuse to talk, will feel insulted, wrongly accused, will become contemptuous and challenging. One very distraught woman came for a first consultation because her marriage was breaking up. She nevertheless maintained at the outset a ladylike and composed facade. She had not talked very long before she began to cry, and then expressed resentment at having to expose herself in this humiliating fashion. As I sat listening to her, I had moved my fingers in my lap. She quickly said, "What are you twiddling your thumbs for? Are you nervous? Do you want a tissue? Maybe you have to blow your nose, too." She was angry at having to show her own instability and distress, and resented the greater stability of the physician whose help she needed. In thus revealing her hostility and competitiveness, she had exposed some of the source of her marital difficulty. It was then possible to focus on an important area of her relationship with her husband by calling attention to what had happened right there during the consultation.

Anger may be voluntarily generated as a self-protection against other, more painful feelings. An extremely ingratiating young patient came in one day after about three months of analysis, and, with a great deal of tension, lay down and began to talk under considerable pressure. "Either I'm anxious from trying to manipulate you to like me, or I can say 'Fuck you—you're the son of a bitch that makes me anxious.' You're not helping me. My anxiety is worse. Why should I try to please you? It hasn't made me great in your eyes. Maybe after a while a patient gets sick and tired of those techniques that make them anxious. I want to go down to Miami and become a beachcomber. I'm sick and tired of being anxious coming in here. The only way I can avoid it is by being angry!"

This patient's ways of functioning as an ingratiating young man had not been effective with the analyst. Feeling threatened and impotent, he became anxious and angry at the analyst, the enemy. His anger was expressed as open, aware hostility, and also as depression (his desire to give up, flaunt his bankruptcy by becoming a beachcomber).

Another patient experienced and communicated a patently angry resistance in the form of a fantasy. At a previous session, I had made a remark about his detachment, referring to it as his "lying there cooly smoking a cigarette." The next day he began the session as follows: "As I came in this morning, I had a quick fantasy of lighting a cigarette, and of your saying, 'Put out that cigarette' and my just saying, 'To hell with you!' and walking out."

Hostility is sometimes expressed by a cold, grim determination to be impervious, by an outright refusal to engage or a determined withdrawal from engagement. One patient, a young man in analysis for three years, had been making recent excellent progress and had begun to use some of his new insight in changed behavior. As a child this patient had expressed his resentment against his parents by urinating on his toys, and he had also sought to humiliate them through klepto-mania. In therapy he had attempted to charm the analyst into fathering and indulging him.

Much fruitful exchange had occurred in the course of the prior six months. Following a particularly meaningful session, he came in and instead of getting to work was chatty and superficial, although the serious problem of impending marriage was very much in the forefront of analytical exploration. At the end of the hour I referred to his lack of engagement with me and reminded him of the many sessions in past years during which nothing had been gained except my delineation for him, at the end of the hour, of his fruitless resistance.

He immediately became serious and relived those unhappy mo-ments that had so often occurred during his analysis. "When it's hap-pening—when you do what you're doing now—I feel miserable. I really squirm. But when I leave I feel I've gotten somewhere, that I'm not afraid of taking my medicine. I feel I've come back faithfully every week and taken my medicine." He stopped talking.

I said to him, "When you're criticized, when people are deeply upset about you, you grimly sustain it and feel strong."

He then recalled a particularly kind teacher in college who had recognized talent in the patient, and had made many concessions and adjustments in order to prevent his student from getting into difficulties with the administration and flunking the course through mishandling of routine technicalities. Referring to this relationship, the patient said, "When Roberts was getting after me, when he talked to me, I'd feel sick, like going through the floor. I'd say to myself, 'I'm ruining this. I've got to do something.' But I'd never do anything to change. I'd see him trying so hard to do something about it, and I'd feel it would be weak to give in. I'd feel strong to be able to take all that and not change. I'd feel, 'I don't care what anybody says to me—I'm strong and I can take it.'"

Being impervious (see Chapter 2, pp. 53–54) not only to anger and criticism, but also to kindness—refusing to respond to any kind of influ-ence—was his pathological criterion of strength. During the past months there had been some evolution of maturity. He had had a new kind of experience, of feeling strong through his ability to be cooperative, kind, and loving. These changes had made marriage a real and imminent possibility. Now the recognition of all this change had suddenly been registered subjectively by him in his old way, as a weakening, a surren-der to my influence. The sudden switch, his refusal to engage further in the therapeutic process, was a form of "negative therapeutic reaction," a hostile, stubborn girding of his loins to recoup his strength according to the old pathological criteria.

Often during such periods of good progress in analysis we again find the patient forgetting, developing psychosomatic confusions, missing appointments or coming late, accentuating illnesses to an intensity apparently justifying cancellations, angrily accusing the analyst of tricks, remaining grimly, challengingly silent, being digressive, forgetting dreams, having no associations, and becoming depressed.

RESISTANCE THROUGH HELPLESSNESS AND DIVERSIONARY SELF-PITY

This group of waking expressions of resistance is closely related to the pseudo-conscientious forms, and is often characterized by hostility, for which it may be a facade. The helpless and self-pitying styles of resistance are, however, sufficiently common to justify some separate discussion.

A most vivid example of helplessness as a frustration of the analytic endeavor was reflected in a dream of the woman of the Induced Labor dream. Quite late in the course of her treatment, when she had demonstrated considerable capacity to observe herself clearly, she dreamed, "I was walking along the street. I walked perfectly well, but collapsed at every corner. Someone—it was you—had to pick me up." At another point she dreamed of being robbed. "I felt powerless. It was in a hotel room. Oh, hotel room, that's *this* room. What are you taking away from me—my sickness? No, I'm not powerless there—I have stopped you. In my dreams I'm always helpless, and when I talk to you I'm always so enraged and I always *say* I'm helpless. My refusal to work with you—*I've refused—that's not helplessness.*"

Depression is a condition of which self-pity and apparent helplessness are characteristics. All depressions, from the milder sulk to the suicidal preoccupations, warrant examination as forms of interpersonal practice.[17] In most depressions there can be found a refusal to engage with others except on one's own terms, a punitive retaliatory frustration of the efforts of others, a dramatization of their culpability and a moral blackmailing to compel a desired response from them. In the analytic situation depression is a form of resistance. The patient "cannot think of anything" or rails against the "slings and arrows of outrageous fortune," emphasizes the hopelessness of his predicament and the lack of understanding or compassion on the part of the analyst.

[17] This concept is expanded in the author's "Depression as a Practice—Dynamic and Psychotherapeutic Considerations," *Comprehensive Psychiatry, 1:* 194–198, 1960.

RESISTANCE THROUGH SEDUCTION

Similar to depression in its aims, although wearing a brighter and more attractive cloak, is the practice of seductiveness. A basic premise of the seductive patient is that human beings always place self-aggrandizing or pleasurable opportunities before obligations or responsibilities to others. In the analytic relationship this means that the analyst may be deflected from carefully perceiving the patient and from making demands for change upon the patient by anything that flatters the self-image of the analyst. The seductive behavior is often motivated by anxiety, often by a competitive desire to outwit the analyst.

Praise is one of the more obvious of the seductive approaches. The homosexual patient who came to analysis on the recommendation of his friend, inordinately praised the analyst and then indicated in his dream of the Hot Dog (pp. 112–113) that he wanted to seduce the analyst rather than to get somewhere therapeutically with him. The young analytic student of the Contemptible Passion dream began by exaggerating to the point of flattery his genuine respect for me, in part to fend off my anticipated demands and influence upon him.[18] The angry, battling woman of the Induced Labor dream frequently brought small gifts and flowers, almost exclusively during her most hostile periods, seeking to deflect my therapeutic demands by indicating her friendly feelings toward me.[19]

All of these patients feared the analyst as one who could deeply and seriously perceive them and influence them. They sought to neutralize the analyst's influence by lulling him into professional self-satisfaction, hoping to engender in him a reluctance to tamper with this source of his pleasure.

The seduction of the analyst is at times more flagrant than the small flatteries and gifts mentioned above. It may take the form of direct sexual invitation. Such an invitation, like any other seductive approach, is based on the premise that the analyst's desire to indulge his own appetites will ultimately take precedence over the therapeutic needs of the patient.

Acquiescence in the analyst's views is a somewhat similar form of seduction. The patient accepts the analyst's concepts and formulations and seeks to adapt his own ideas and behavior to conform with what he

[18] The discrepancy between his laudatory activity and his cynical doubts about my decency was brought under consideration by his dream of me, the night before his first session, as a figure of derogation and contempt.

[19] In a dream, Making a Play for Her, she recognized that she was trying to seduce me away from my attention to her pathology by gifts of flowers.

believes the analyst desires of him. This performance, like sexual seduction, is an effort to appeal to what the patient believes is the analyst's predominant appetite for self-aggrandizement or some other self-indulgent pleasure. The dream of the Japanese Battlefield which was described earlier in this chapter reflects this type of resistance. In the dream the patient offered his leg to be cut off by his captor, feeling "submission was the best course." The dream then progressed through successive offerings to feed his captor's (the analyst's) desire for sadistic conquest. The profundity of the resistance in this patient was reflected in the later part of the dream, in which he made it quite clear that he was confident of surviving any amount of submission and still remaining himself, unchanged. In the analytic sessions, he acknowledged and documented readily many humiliating formulations of his pathology. He worked intensely, remembered and explored his dreams. He agonized, but at the same time often thanked the analyst for astute contributions. But the patient also continued to live basically unchanged.

A subtle form of resistance lies in the patient's focusing exclusively upon his already achieved therapeutic gains. This kind of preoccupation with health or, as it is sometimes referred to, "flight into health," in part represents the patient's anxiety and fear of consolidating his gains, the fear of real change in his personality. There is unquestionably a large degree of self-deception in this activity. The interpersonal aspect of it, however, is the attempt to lull the analyst into being professionally pleased with himself and thereby relaxing his therapeutic efforts on behalf of the patient.

When the analyst does not accept the patient's high estimate of his progress, the patient's response may be taken as a measure of the degree of his resistance. Patients who are most committed to the therapeutic endeavor will welcome the analyst's more realistic appraisal.

Finally, it is appropriate to recall in this context the discussion of *insulating terms* and forms of *blurred communication* that were discussed in Chapter 2, "Feeling in Dreams." The patient who has finally recognized that he has many emotions of which he is not aware, and also that it is essential in the therapeutic process to detect and explore emotions, may appear to be pursuing his feelings without actually doing so. The analyst may be persuaded that the patient is conscientiously exploring emotions, while the patient is actually painstakingly insulating all that he detects with merely speculative phrases: "I think I get angry," or "I guess I was jealous," and the many others, some of which were clinically illustrated in the earlier chapter. These flow from the couch, producing only tentative data about the emotions, and no experientially validated facts about the patient's affective life.

In summary, waking forms of resistance are the manifestations in the therapeutic situation of the patient's usual ways of applying or warding off interpersonal influence. Pseudo-conscientious, hostile, help-less and self-pitying, and seductive ways of behaving have been classi-fied, with full recognition that there is considerable overlapping among them. Even the most benign pseudo-conscientious helpless or seduc-tive form of resistance may conceal not only anxiety but also contempt and hostility. Whatever affects are interrelated with waking resistance, their detection and mutual therapeutic pursuit are essential to achiev-ing insight into and overcoming the resistance.

The remainder of this chapter, except for the final pages, contains a passage from the analysis of a patient who experienced a nightmare in the course of therapeutic progress. The clinical interlude illustrates many of the formulations presented in the foregoing discussion of resistance.

Elevator Nightmare

The patient, a highly intelligent thirty-two-year-old married music teacher with a five-year-old daughter, had started analysis on the basis of sporadic visits, pending the availability of regular hours. She had worked conscientiously during three months of these irregular, approxi-mately weekly, sessions. She had been motivated to start treatment by a lethargy that interfered with the pursuit of intellectual interests and, even more distressing to her, interfered also with maternal interests. Her music classes, in contrast, went exceptionally well.

At the start of the session about to be reported she said nothing for two or three minutes. This was unusual for her. She appeared de-pressed, and stated that she had not wanted to come. I suggested that she say whatever came to mind while she focused upon her feeling of depression. She immediately said, "Betty" (her daughter's name), but repudiated the association by calling it a "reflex" thought: she *always* thought about Betty.

I expressed my regret that she should stoop to that unworthy eva-sion. She then began to speak her associations.

"I've been snapping at Betty so much, I've been getting so much of 'I don't like you, Mommy.' Today I waited for her to get off the sta-tion wagon from her nursery school and both of us went upstairs to the apartment. We both had to go to the bathroom but I insisted on going first and I slammed the door behind me. She ran to her room and slammed her door. In the morning she does so much whining. She says, 'I don't want to wear this, Mommy. I don't want to wear that.' And I whine back at her that people aren't going to like her if she doesn't act more pleasantly . . . that's no way to act . . . stop fussing." She said she recognized that her child had acquired this whining habit from her.

She went on, "After I told you about slamming the door to the bathroom, I suddenly remembered that I'd had a nightmare the other day." After making this association, she was again silent. I asked her if she was going to relate the nightmare. Her response was a mixture of surprised and embarrassed laughter. "Oh, do you want me to?" I made no comment, and she went ahead.

"I was riding in an elevator. There was somebody else in the elevator, very vague. Betty had come to the elevator with me and waited with me when I pressed the button for it to come. When the doors of the elevator closed, she wasn't there. I knew she had been with me just before I walked in. I kept hearing weak little sounds, sort of cries, and I saw a little bit of white like her dress, showing inside the elevator, but I kept saying to myself, 'It's all right, it's all right, she must be out-side.' Then I finally had to face the fact that I knew where she was, that she was caught between the elevator door and the outside door. I knew it was impossible for this to happen, but I had a vision of a flattened out child, and when I realized that I knew all the time that she was caught there, I felt a terrific panic at what I had done, and I woke up.

"I couldn't possibly be wanting it to happen. I woke up so terribly upset, I was afraid to go back to sleep and I held on to my husband. I got up and went to Betty's room to see if she was there. I wondered, was this dream an omen, was God punishing me because I'm such a bad person? Maybe I don't deserve to have her. I felt I'm so horrible I don't deserve to have a child."

I suggested that we look more closely at the dream. She said, "The business of knowing and not letting on I know. If I had done something right away I could have saved her. The elevator was not moving yet. I could have pushed the emergency button. I even saw a little white sticking out, like part of the dress. I'm so much more gentle with other kids. If I see this, why do I keep doing it?"

At this point I said, "In the elevator you heard the sounds of your child's cries and you saw the bit of white dress sticking out all the time. You saw what you were doing, but at the same time you didn't let your-self see. You tried to avoid the evidence and kept saying, 'It's all right, it's all right.' In the same way, you say to me that you see what's hap-pening to your child, you know your little girl is developing a whining manner from you. You notice, in an isolated way, that she slams the door after you slam the door. What you're not recognizing is that these are not isolated instances. Your continued behavior of this sort is really hurting Betty, really crushing her. The total effect of all the 'bad' things you do to her is really warping her."

Then she replied, "It must be me. I dreamed it. But I can't believe it."

There was a striking identity between her dream behavior and her waking behavior. "What you just said—'It must be me, I dreamed it, but I can't believe it,'—is an exact repetition of the dream. In the dream, in the elevator, and incidentally in the presence of that vague individual who I think was your analyst, you saw and heard what was going on, but you tried not to believe that your little girl was being crushed. Here, too, with me, you see what's happening to your child, and you won't believe it."

The existence of anxiety about her cruelty indicated the need for help in focusing upon the problem of her crushing activities. Despite the patient's unwillingness, the pursuit of this anxiety-laden area opened the only way to help her.

To maintain a clear framework of reality, and to foster her own efforts to deal with her problems, it was imperative to point out the precise evidence of the patient's unwillingness to recognize herself. I said, "Let's review how terribly important it has been to you to conceal from yourself what you are doing to your little girl. In the first place, let's look at all the evidence just in connection with this dream. First, you felt depressed and didn't want to come here today. When you lay down, you were silent for two or three minutes. That's a long time. When I said, 'Go ahead and say it,' you replied, 'I don't know what to talk about.' I said, 'Associate freely,' and you immediately said Betty's name, and then you quickly added that it meant nothing because you think of her all the time. In reply to this I said with a bit of sarcasm, 'So it's just a reflex? It's not significant? Perhaps you should talk about something else?' As soon as I made this obviously sarcastic remark, you picked it up, took it at face value, and said, 'Okay, then I'll talk about my husband.' And then you were embarrassed at having overlooked the obvious intention of the sarcastic remark, and you finally began to talk about your short temper with Betty. After reporting the door-slamming episode, you recalled the nightmare. But you still didn't tell the nightmare until I asked you to, after another long silence of two or three minutes. And then you laughed, and reported it for *my* purposes, saying, 'Oh, do you want me to?'

"After you told the dream, you indulged in self-recrimination as a substitute for interpretation. You spoke of the thoughts you had after the nightmare, the thoughts you experience again today, that you don't

deserve your child, that you're being punished. By such self-recriminations you avoided the significance of the dream. Then I interpreted the
dream, and said that you see only the isolated instances of your injury
to Betty, not the total effect, the warping of your child. When I gave
this interpretation you became confused, and said you didn't know
what I was talking about. I had to repeat the interpretation in two or
three different forms before you finally caught on that you were evading the broad significance by dwelling on isolated incidents.

"Then you said, 'Well, I see it, but I can't believe it.' When I indicated to you that your seeing it but not believing it was doing exactly
what you did in the dream—in the elevator you heard and saw, and
refused to believe—then you said acquiescently, 'All right, I believe it,
but why do I do it?' In other words, instead of looking more deliberately at your activity, you wanted to duck the issue by the 'conscientious' maneuver of examining the genesis of your behavior. When this
dodge was pointed out to you, you then responded by saying, 'You're
exaggerating my cruelty in order to have what you say take some effect
on me.' "

I stated that this succession of evidence indicated how unwilling
she was to face the reality of her crushing activity. She replied then,
"I don't really hurt her, but I omit things."

"For a child," I answered, "omission of love, tenderness, real care,
is crushing, and it is cruelty. You could fail to feed her for three weeks
and say it was only omission. The tenderness and interest are as important to a child as food, and the omission of these is as destructive to the
development of her personality as the omission of food is to the development of her body."

The patient then spoke for the first time with some evidence that
the nature of her activity was impinging upon her awareness. She replied, with real dismay in her face and voice, "I guess I really am hurting her." Then she added with a sudden access of horror, "My God,
I don't even feed the child. I give her anything that's in the house." She
was quiet for a minute, then she suddenly sat up in great agitation,
facing away from me with her fists clenched. "I can't take any more.
I've got to go."

She got up and hurried out. As she started to leave I said, "You're
frightened, aren't you?" She answered tensely, "Yes." She ran to the
bathroom and cried aloud for five minutes.

At any point in this session, from the outset, the potential value of
the hour and the dream might have been lost. With full recognition
of the importance of a patient's *spontaneous* pursuit of insight, the
therapeutic initiative was here repeatedly seized by the analyst in order

to make possible a productive use of the session. By the end of the hour the patient had begun to look at herself more directly and was in a position to deal constructively with this anxiety-laden area.

To review this session from the viewpoint of the analyst's activity: the seizure of the initiative to overcome resistance occurred at several points. When the patient entered the office announcing that she had not wanted to come, she was first given the opportunity spontaneously to overcome her reluctance. After a few minutes of silence, however, she was asked to "say it." Her protest that she had nothing to say was not allowed to stand. It was academically unnecessary to remind this patient to free-associate—she knew all about free association—but the reminder made it possible for her to engage in a process she was unwilling to initiate. (Such a therapeutic suggestion is of course useful only when a patient has sufficient willingness to engage.) The suggestion brought about the connection between the patient's depression and Betty. The importance of the analyst's initiative was substantiated by the patient's initial honesty, even though she also at once tried to cancel the significance of the association. When her nullification was sarcastically accepted (sarcasm is not advocated as a standard part of the psychiatric armamentarium) she at first leaped at this opportunity to go off on another topic. At this point it was important for the analyst to bear in mind that her willingness to engage, in spite of great reluctance, had already been manifested. In these elements of willingness the analyst finds encouragement and justification for maintaining the initiative. In this instance, although the analyst's gentle jibe was reacted to by the patient with embarrassment, she did assume the initiative and looked in the direction of the originally repudiated association. Then came the recall of the door-slamming incident. Continuing on her own initiative, the mother then reported that she had remembered a nightmare while she was telling about slamming the door.

Up to this point, in spite of the patient's enormous reluctance to look at herself, therapeutic persistence had made it possible for her to report the association and the nightmare and to approach, although haltingly, with whatever willingness and honesty she could muster, the examination of the avoided area of anxiety.

Now again the patient's spontaneous activity bogged down. When the fact of a nightmare had been reported, she again fell silent. To have left the patient at this point entirely to her own resources would have been to abandon her and to evade the therapeutic problem. When she failed to pursue the initiative, she was offered the opportunity to return to it. "How about the dream?" Her first response was elusive: she laughed. This was an inappropriate reaction to the seriousness of the problem. She began, however, to resume the initiative, managing partially to overcome her reluctance to face the frightening problem of the dream. She said, "Oh, do you want me to?" She would look at it, but would pretend she was doing this for me. I did not reply, refraining at this point from unnecessarily resuming the initiative. After a few moments, receiving no further direction, she proceeded independently to a full account of the nightmare. The patient's positive struggle for health, with watchful therapeutic assistance, was winning over her coexisting efforts to hide and maintain her pathology.

After this mother finally described the nightmare in which she crushed her child between the elevator doors and refused to accept the evidence of her own eyes, it again became necessary for the analyst to take the initiative. The patient did not follow the lead of her dream into investigation of her flagrant self-deception and cruel delinquency. Instead, she tried to give the appearance of doing so through self-recriminations. A realistic contemplation of her activities was necessary. The patient had shown some genuine capacity for engaging in the therapeutic struggle. Her real humanity was expressed, not in her self-recrimination, which was an evasive maneuver, but in her painful desire to examine her delinquency, which had already made it possible to reach this point in the session.

The therapeutic initiative was resumed by the analyst, and it was pointed out to the patient that she could not deal with her problem if she escaped into self-recrimination. An interpretation of the dream was offered, and she was confronted through validative evidence with the total effect of her cumulatively destructive behavior toward her daughter. She fought off this realization by becoming confused. Despite and because of the barrage of confusion, two or three restatements of the concept of cumulative injury were made. The patient progressed another little bit. She said, "I see it, but I can't believe it." That statement was significant. By the first part ("I see it") an increment of progress was revealed, and also a confirmation of the value of continuing the therapeutic initiative. The second part ("I can't believe it") indicated her continued resistance. The analyst then pointed out to her the parallel between her resistance during the session and her refusal to accept the evidence of her senses during the dream. The patient thereupon adopted a more subtle form of denial—a glib acquiescence. No significant resistance struggle can be abandoned easily by a patient. Her readiness to "believe it" was evidence not of genuine insight but of a continuing avoidance of the reality. It represented not a change of mind but a change of tactic. This resistance, moreover, was re-enforced by still another tactic of evasion. "Why do I do it?" One can never examine the origin of what does not exist. To the patient, the *fact* of her crushing activity toward her child did not yet exist, as evidenced by the absence of any affective response to it. The sudden interest in genesis was an attempt to outwit the therapist by a facade of conscientiousness.

The ambivalence of the patient's attitude up to this point is worthy of note. There was some extra encouragement for maintenance of therapeutic persistence both in the earlier "I see it" and in the small increment of self-recognition implicit in the grudging "I believe it," which did represent some progress beyond "I can't believe it," and still greater progress beyond the earlier elusiveness of self-recrimination. On the other hand, the acquiescent element in "All right," and the glib quality of her "I believe it," and the evasiveness of "Why do I do it?" were evidence of resistance to accepting the reality about herself and did not merely encourage but demanded from the analyst an energetic pursuit of the problem.

The patient maintained throughout the hour a state of imminent interruption and cessation of her difficultly-stimulated self-inspection. The hour showed, however, a continued progress; the analyst's unswerving attention to the anxiety area made some degree of success possible for the patient in her own struggle against resistance.

The intense anxiety and the related resistance emerged as the session developed. The exposure of the last two tactics—acquiescence and refuge in genesis—led to another slight increment of reality-perception by the patient. She said, "You're exaggerating my cruelty." Implicit in this accusation was a degree of recognition of the fact that she was cruel. One cannot exaggerate what does not exist; and she had not accused the analyst of inventing the concept of her destructiveness.

This was very tough going for the patient. She was fighting to make possible a change in her activity with her child, a form of behavior by means of which she felt functionally effective. The activity was not yet clearly defined, but its nature was gradually becoming clear. She could recognize it as something which she no longer could tolerate. She was at the same time fending off this change, which carried with it subjectively a danger of dissolution of her personality. She tried to repudiate the physician's efforts by accusing him of having a petty personal stake. She said, "You're exaggerating my cruelty to make what you say take some effect on me." This was an attack on the therapeutic initiative, and was in itself evidence of the fruitfulness of this procedure. What the patient formulated as exaggeration on the doctor's part was a subjective repudiation of the force of her new self-perception.

In spite of so much resistance, the patient had not only been willing sometimes to engage cooperatively with the therapist when offered the opportunity but also had herself occasionally adopted the initiative. It seemed therefore justified, in fact essential, for the therapist to pursue energetically measures to help the patient perceive as fully as possible the painful statement of her nightmare—that she was a crushing mother. When she accused the therapist of exaggerating her cruelty to produce an effect on her, the opportunity was grasped to cite in specific detail, with data coming from within and outside the session, how strongly she was fending off her perception that the crushing of her child was a reality.

She made another attempt to reject the fact by the formula, "I don't really hurt her, but I omit things." This was an attempt to nullify some of the distress of self-recognition, to minimize responsibility for her practices. The nightmare area was therefore pursued further. I replied that, for a child, omission of tenderness and solicitous care is crushing, and so forth.

In response, the patient finally looked directly at the problem presented in the nightmare, which had been kept in focus for her by the analyst throughout the hour, and had been painfully, disjointedly, but productively contemplated by her. The session ended with the initiative for realistic self-perception accepted by the patient. She spoke for the first time with evidence that the nature of her activity was affectively impinging upon her awareness.

The patient made rapid progress in becoming a more nurturing and tender mother during the next few months in analysis.

It was indicated earlier in this chapter (pp. 189–190) that a common source of resistance is a competitive orientation toward someone outside the therapeutic relationship. In the course of this patient's continuing analysis numerous problems became delineated in connection with the anxiety-laden area of the mother-daughter relationship. One was her competitive relationship with her husband, whose lack of affection for her and simultaneous solicitude toward the little girl led the patient to neglect and hurt the child in order to torment her husband. In addition, the patient who, as an adult, was still frustrated in her lifelong effort to elicit love from her own mother, was competitively reluctant to permit her own child to outdo her by getting maternal love, of which the patient herself had always been deprived. Finally, being a good mother represented for her a capitulation to the derogating and pious nagging of both her husband and her mother that she be more maternal. Thus a recognition of her crushing hostility toward her daughter would force her to the contemplation of her tortured feelings of personal affectional deprivation, her consequent deep resentments, and her intense competitiveness with mother, husband, and child. She felt functionally effective in all her unrecognized, covert, hostile, competitive practices. The threat of paralysis of these ways of functioning became in the course of therapy the source of anxiety and depression and the basis of intense resistance.

A complicating factor and an additional source of anxiety and resistance emerged in the pursuit of the Elevator Nightmare. This was related to an unsuspected self-concept—she was *above* having tender maternal feelings.

At the hour following the presentation of the elevator dream, she reported that when she left the analytic session in which she told her nightmare she compulsively went shopping—"Not for Betty—for *myself!*" She neither telephoned nor returned home to prepare the evening meal, and finally when she did reach home she battled by almost hysterical gaiety against the agonizing effect upon her of her child's looking like a "whipped dog." Describing this, she had the important association of her "stoicism" during the child's toddler years. While other mothers were concerned and tender toward their children, she inwardly took enormous pride in her casualness, her unworried, non-emotive, stoic manner. In reality her maternal resources were extraordinary, and in the professional framework of teaching, she did wonders with her music classes, precisely because of the close interest, the concerned, solicitous, and empathic responsiveness she experienced toward her pupils. As a mother, however, she must be above "all that sort of thing." In the maternal, nonprofessional framework her sense of self and her self-concept were rooted in emotional stoicism. She had, in effect, been horrified by the recognition of her warping neglect and at the same time frightened by the emergence of unstoical concern, and had sought to blot out this welling maternalism by the compulsive shopping and then the forced ebullience at home.

Provided with opportunity, in spite of all the anxious reluctance, the patient clinically moved ahead during the intense hour reported above. The most important problem which she had introduced in essentially noninsightful terms at the start of her analysis was her destructiveness toward the child through "stoic" neglect. It was the first anxiety-laden area to be exposed, and it became also the first area in which there was personality change.

Resistance is often interwoven with healthy manifestations. Distinguishing between them may determine the direction and outcome of the analysis. Nowhere is this distinction more important than in dealing with the patient's affection for the analyst as it develops during the close cooperation of the therapeutic effort. In the case of a woman with a male analyst, for example, the analyst is often the first individual in whom the patient has been able to place her trust, the first whose concern for her seems authentic, the first to whom she has been able to speak her inmost thoughts and to whom she has been able to expose her confused, sometimes (subjectively considered) shameful emotions— and all without being rejected. These elements in any situation outside of therapy are commonly the preconditions for falling in love. The patient's capacity to love may furthermore have become, during therapy, far greater than ever before in her life. This is a healthy development, and to "analyze" it in terms of pathology can not only seriously disrupt the patient's therapeutic efforts but also confuse and unnecessarily hurt her. It is important to help such a woman to be aware of and glad of her capacity to have these wholesome, appropriate emotions. The emotions themselves must, however, be distinguished from the *demand for reciprocation,* which may simultaneously be present. The desire for equal response is inevitable, but the *demand* for such a response is inappropriate and unhealthy. The patient does not and cannot stand in the same relationship to the analyst in his total life as the analyst does to the patient, and she cannot therefore engender the same order of reciprocal feelings. The analyst has feelings of friendship, concern, responsibility, compassion and after a long *productive* course in analysis he often has feelings of affection. The patient, in her limited and not equally reciprocated therapeutic exchanges with the analyst, does not help to make for him a qualitatively different and better feeling about himself, a greatly expanded functioning, a richer emotional life and perhaps a new kind of life in all its external and material aspects as well. There is no basis in the nature of their activity together that could realistically engender the analyst's gratitude toward and overwhelming love for the patient.

These distinctions must be made clear to the patient. Often she will feel resentment over the rejection of her unrealistic demand for reciprocal love, and be unwilling to believe that her own love is nevertheless recognized and accepted although it is not returned. Some patients fearfully anticipate this lack of reciprocity, and their love is exposed only in dreams.

In whatever way the problem comes to expression, it is almost invariably accompanied by tremendous resistance. The patient, in her disappointment, may have an upsurge of anger, cynicism, psychosomatic symptoms (including intense sexual desire), and may find herself beset by practical obstacles to continuing analysis or to maintaining the schedule. She may become withdrawn, silent, discursive, disengaged from the previously productive process. She may become extremely competitive and manifest any of the forms of resistance discussed in this or other chapters. She may feel outraged at having been subtly seduced, having been brought to the humiliating condition of declaring feelings of love, by a grandiose and power-driven professional stuffed shirt.

The development of genuine, healthy feelings of love for her analyst is the extreme degree of affectional response in a woman, and is paralleled by a male patient's equally intense love for a woman analyst. The development of healthy and strong friendship feelings also occurs with men and women patients and younger patients of both sexes. In each case there is the possibility of irrational demands for equal reciprocation of intense feeling. In each case there is the necessity for the analyst to engage the patient with him in distinguishing between the patient's healthy affection and his or her pathological insistence upon an identical response. The analyst's greatest skill is taxed in this circumstance, to maintain or reconstitute a good therapeutic working relationship, to help the patient to see and accept what is healthy, while delineating and dealing with the resistance.

Patients often do not recognize the existence of or the nature or intensity of their resistance until they can identify it through dreams of resistance. Such a dream as Fight with an Antelope, in the chapter on introductory dreams, revealed at the outset the patient's approach to analysis as "locking horns" with the analyst. At other times patients become aware of their fight against the therapist and his efforts through their response to dream material—an eagerness to blot out a dream or to avoid the area of a dream.

The central therapeutic implications of resistance involve: identifying its various manifestations; distinguishing these from healthy therapeutic activity; correlating resistance (a therapeutic phenomenon) with the patient's total personality; recognizing separately fears of and antagonisms toward the therapeutic process; persistently engaging the patient in all these pursuits.

In the process of overcoming his resistance—the anxious, competitive, and insular way of relating to the analyst—the patient engages in an extended, intense, new, and intimate kind of interpersonal experience. Through this experience of overcoming resistance his personality changes in the healthy direction of a capacity for cooperative engagement, for appropriate trust, warmth, and spontaneity.

7. *Interpretive Activity with Dreams*

THE SUBJECTIVE AND INTERPERSONAL processes connected with interpretive activity were outlined earlier, in the Introduction. Many problems of interpretation, general and specific, have already been dealt with, through both theoretical consideration and clinical example, because they are intrinsically part of the discussion of dream symbolism and of all the other types and aspects of dreams that formed the ensuing chapter categories. Interpretive processes are likewise elements of the chapters yet to come.[1]

In the present chapter some questions already referred to will be enlarged upon, and attention will be focused in particular upon the broad and crucial subject of the validation of dream interpretation.

In all dream interpretation there is a lurking danger of self-deception. It is easy to allow one's imagination to run along creating approximate life-analogues of the dream action. It is not, however, along any path of clever inventiveness that useful meanings are found. It is in the daily behavior, the deeply personal thoughts and memories, and the immediate feelings of the dreamer that source material for interpretation is found, and in the same places we find the evidence for validation. In short, validation of the interpretation of dreams is the direct,

[1] See the index under "interpretive activity" for references to the Introduction and other chapters.

affective recognition of the symbolic elements of the dream in living moments of the individual's experience. It might, in fact, be more accurate to say that we never interpret dreams—we make use of them in the process of interpreting people.

Validation of dream interpretation is the process by which the action, feelings, and attitudes initially identified in the interpretive activity are further correlated with elements of the dreamer's past and present waking experience and sometimes also with the evidence of past dreams.[2] It is through validative activity that dreams achieve their full usefulness in modifying personality. A dream interpretation (or any other interpretation) may be accurate, yet remain a mere abstraction, and therapeutically useless, unless repeatedly correlated with (validated by) personal experience. Dreams direct attention to feeling, thinking, and activity which the individual has been unaware of or is reluctant to acknowledge. When the patient acquires this recognition (through interpretive activity) and then continues to extend this recognition (through validative activity), he acquires information which can help him grope toward new ways of functioning, and he can begin to find new qualities of experience.

Validation is found in experiences within and outside of the therapeutic sessions. A fragment from the interpersonal exchange between analyst and patient may often be exceptionally convincing when it is clearly a manifestation of the same attitude that is reflected in the dream. For example, the patient of the Scared Shitless dream (pp. 114–115) saw the resemblance between her amusement in the dream at the presence of feces (symbolizing profound anxiety) on her thigh, and her smiles and chuckles in the analytic session as she described her feelings of devastation because of rejection by her boy friend. Through this correlation she gained some initial sense of her efforts to laugh off her deepest feelings.

The mother of the Elevator Nightmare (pp. 218–226) heard the cries of her little girl who was crushed between the inner and outer door of the elevator, and saw the corner of the child's dress inside the car, but continued to reassure herself, "It's all right, she must be outside. . . . The business of knowing and not letting on that I know. . . ." In the same session, while discussing my interpretive formulation regarding the nightmare, she said, "Well, I see it, but I can't believe it," providing thereby a precise waking parallel of her dream experience, and a validation of the interpretation. Correlation of the dream with the event in the session was furthermore a means of focusing still more sharply

[2] The same definition may be applied to validation of the interpretation of nondream data.

upon the problem of the dream. It helped to make possible, later in the session, a deeply emotional validation by the patient, her recognition that she had in her daily life been refusing to acknowledge to herself her neglect of some of the child's vital needs—"My God! I don't even feed her!"

The interpretive hypothesis concerning the Screwed Up dream in the previous chapter was strikingly validated by examples of the patient's behavior before, during, and after the session in which the dream was reported. It will be recalled that in the dream he was didactically reading from a book written by the analyst. In spite of his admiration for the contents of the book, the words somehow came out unintelligible, "screwed up." The validation lay in his recall of having before the dream experienced gratitude for my formulation of an insight which was to help him to stick to his dieting, and then, that same day, leaving the session and eating more than usual. During the session in which we worked on the dream he reported much crucial analytic material but, with his characteristic distortion, articulated all of it without feeling. When he left my office he unawaredly broke his diet for the second time—the insight into his resistance had been admired, but his application of it again came out "screwed up."

In the nightmare of the tiny cobras, a wife who lived as a sweet and helplessly dependent ingénue felt threatened by a public display of her capacity to be strong and venomous. This interpretation could have been merely imaginatively devised. It emerged, however, from cooperative associative and interpretive activity, and then, when clearly perceived by the patient, was spontaneously correlated by her with her behavior in her marriage. "I'm like a snake with my husband. When a snake strikes, it's right out of the blue. That's the way I pick on him. I suddenly criticize something he's doing in the midst of an otherwise peaceful situation." This validation of the interpretation in the area of her marital relationship permitted the patient to struggle constructively toward making changes in her personality and in her marriage.

The following dream with its therapeutic context will further demonstrate the process of validation, and in addition will illustrate the frequently valuable associative key first designated in the Introduction—the moment of association (p. 11).

Two Drunken Sailors

In the course of an otherwise general forward movement, toward the end of analysis, a wife and mother in her early thirties sabotaged an important holiday weekend because of annoyance with her husband. In treatment she had struggled to overcome her vindictive resentment at having been deprived of a happy childhood (pp. 183–184). Her parents had been cold to her, had neither encouraged her creative abilities nor even permitted other, less significant pleasures. She often hated her husband because she subjectively sought a parental rather than a conjugal solicitude from him, and he consistently failed her in the same way that her parents had, and aroused the same morose sense of deprivation.

Her personality had changed in analysis; she had come to recognize, and, in part, emotionally to accept, her adult responsibility for her own happiness. This responsibility often entailed her taking the initiative in the marriage relationship; it meant eliciting the best from her somewhat apathetic husband, in spite of her resentment that his best was not forthcoming spontaneously. The same requirement and conflict often applied to other relationships. Whenever she succeeded in overcoming her reluctance and accepting the necessity for her independent responsibility, she had, because of her warmth, eagerness, and responsiveness, invariably created a happy and rewarding situation.

On the weekend in question, her anger prevailed; she had bitterly resented the behavior both of her husband and of her young son (who in many ways resembled his father). She had spitefully withdrawn from both of them, thereby casting a pall over the family's holiday.

In the analytic session that followed the weekend, she evaded examination of her own behavior and blamed her unhappiness on her husband's lack of interest in the weekend. I indicated that in spite of her husband's provocative apathy she had been in a position to rescue the situation; and she was miserable therefore, chiefly because she had willfully and spitefully allowed the family holiday plans to deteriorate. As we had so often seen in the past, her anger and depression appeared to be a reaction to her once more being confronted with the necessity to take the initiative for obtaining her own happiness.

My statement reminded her of a dream (moment of association). Overcoming her depression, her resistance, her temporary reluctance to get well, she described the dream and looked for collaborative help.

In the dream two drunken sailors were in a hospital, lying on the floor. Two nurses, responsible for their care, rushed away to the nurses' quarters, took off their own uniforms, returned stealthily past the head nurse and, in their street clothes, carried out the sailors and abandoned them in the street. The feelings of "urgency and secrecy" in getting rid of the sailors were experienced during the dream.

Both spontaneously and responsively she proceeded to associate and to interpret. She identified herself with the two nurses by the characteristic quick movements with which they changed their clothes. The nurse role symbolized responsibility. She identified the two drunken sailors with her sullen husband and son. Getting out of the nurse's uniform she associated with her rejection of the responsibility for helping her difficult husband and son get back to healthy functioning at a time when they were being neurotic (drunk).

The patient recalled the dream as the analyst attributed her weekend misery to her abandonment of her mature wife and mother roles. The dream itself was her association to the evaluation of her behavior. Like any association, the remembered dream was an emotional simile (see p. 13). It was as though the patient had said, "Something in the way you described how I felt and acted over the weekend is like the way I felt and acted in a dream I had last night."

The moment of association for the Drunken Sailors dream was a creative moment for the patient, in which she brought experiential fragments from her waking life, and their symbolic expression in her dream, swiftly into connection with the analyst's expressed conceptualization. As the dream interpretation emerged, validative evidence came up, woven within it and deriving from experience within and outside the therapeutic sessions. In the dream she slid past the head nurse. Her association with the head nurse was the analyst; she felt that in some way she was seeking to avoid detection by the analyst. This interpretation was validated by the analyst's association to the start of the session; she had sought to evade the analyst by depressively avoiding the established self-exploring process. In the dream she abandoned the drunken sailors for whom in the nursing role she had responsibility; she associated the sailors with her husband and son and validated this by correlation with her weekend behavior at home when she had abandoned her neurotic husband and her son who needed additional understanding and support. In the dream she was two nurses, both delinquent; at home she escaped from her dual roles of wife and mother. Although the moment of association with the analyst's remarks about her had already begun to identify her as the quitting nurses, she further validated the identification by the subjective connection of the nurses' movements with a recognizable fragment of her own experience, her swift manner of undressing. Thus validation was amalgamated with interpretation, as interpretation emerged from the associative and interpretive activity.

The context in which any biographical item occurs to the communicating patient or responsive therapist is important for understanding such data. I have used the phrase "moment of association" for the point at which an item in the patient's awareness brings to mind a dream or dream fragment. It is thus a significant moment at which connection— affective, conceptual, or mnemonic—is made between the symbolism of dreams and material within the awareness of waking consciousness. It is one point at which the symbolic language of dreams may be observed to be linked in the patient's awareness with relevant biographical data.

Important associations to his dream may occur to a patient before, as well as during and after, the telling of a dream (see pp. 10–11). A mother's description of slamming a bathroom door in her little girl's face preceded and produced the sudden relevant recall of the night-mare of crushing her child behind the elevator door (Elevator Night-mare, pp. 218–226); both dream and waking incidents represented the mother's overall crushing effect upon her daughter. In the introductory dream of the Fight with an Antelope, the patient, during his report of the dream in which he planned to twist the animal's neck, suddenly remembered his plan just preceding the session to trap the analyst with an embarrassing verbal attack (see p. 104). The harrowing night-mare of the Crazy Woman (who symbolized the analyst proposing spontaneous expression of emotion) was a dream recalled by the pa-tient as she recounted an incident in which she took refuge from spon-taneous friendliness (see pp. 73–77).

The value of dream or associative material may be lost by a failure to note the moment of association. This is likely to happen when a patient is bringing forward in a desultory manner material which seems insignificant. Suddenly he says, "Oh, by the way, I had a dream last night." At this point the analyst may prick up his ears and feel that now, perhaps, the session may begin to be productive. He will focus his attention upon the dream. This concentration is, of course, necessary and potentially fruitful. Through the abrupt shifting of interest, how-ever, the material which the patient was verbalizing when he recalled the dream may be lost. Instead of thinking, "Now at last with the presentation of this dream we may begin to get some useful material," it may prove to be a far more productive approach to think, "Now the seemingly empty productions of this patient may begin to take on meaning through their connection with the dream." The moment at which a dream is remembered is an associative link, and a potentially crucial clue to the significance of both the dream and the preceding discourse, and also at times to the patient's indeterminate behavior and emotion.

Similarly, clues are found in memories occurring in the course of relating the dream. Some patients, sensing an unwelcome relevance, will manifest resistance by failing to report their associations during the relating of the dream. Other patients will manifest resistance by relating concurrent associations so circumstantially as to make them a means of tangential escape from self-examination. A conscientious patient, on the other hand, will include these associations as brief footnotes and return to them following the full exposition of the dream; or in some cases the patient, in order to avoid interrupting the flow of the dream, will make a mental note of such associations and recall them, stating the moment of association after telling the dream.

There are moments of association after the report of a dream that may be even more significant. A new and sometimes most illuminating fragment of a dream may suddenly spring to the patient's mind after he has given an apparently complete account. Not infrequently, this occurs in response to the analyst's question: "What was the feeling in the dream?"

There now follows an illustration of the discovery and validation of meaning through the pursuit of feeling in the dream.

Oil Well

The patient, a thirty-seven-year-old suburban wife, living in affluent circumstances, came to her session following a disturbed night of thinking and dreaming. She had been in analysis only four months and, while she was intuitive, friendly, and eager for help, she was constrained by a lifelong behavior pattern of emotional reticence. She had, however, begun to recognize the value of the pursuit of both dreams and feelings and, with a persistence of stimuli from the analyst, she had achieved a good level of therapeutic cooperation.

She reported her dream as follows: "I have to take one piece of material, a sort of cloth, and produce an object. It was an eight-sided object. I have some idea of how it would look when it was finished, but not how to loop it, or how to sew it, or whatever I was supposed to do to make this kind of object. I thought to myself that it should be a parallelogram. Then I thought, 'No, that doesn't have eight sides.' Then I had a great flash: it must be a rhomboid."

(At this point she interrupted to give an association and a description: "At the back of the house there is the beginning of a slope at the top of which Henry [husband] has made a beautiful garden, a rotation of annuals.")

"In the dream I was standing right there between the retaining wall of the flower bed and the house."

(She interrupted again with a brief association: "It was exactly where Henry and I were sitting yesterday and talking about how well the new grass had taken.")

"Suddenly that whole flower bed section began to sink. Just that section kept sinking and it went way down, with steep walls, and it formed a deep abyss. Then there was like a lake way down at the bottom and I was sure it was oil. I thought to myself, 'Oil—no one will be able to ignore this.' I had visions of machinery and trucks and men moving in to get the oil and ruining all the beautiful grounds around the house. [End of dream.]

"All night I kept getting back to this eight-sided object I was trying to make. I don't know whether I kept waking up and thinking about it or whether I kept dreaming it over and over. I wonder if all that mathematical stuff had to do with a problem my cousin had sprung on me Saturday night as we were all about to go to bed. I was up until 2:30 A.M. and spent another hour and a half on it Sunday morning. The problem had something to do with a square. We had a discussion about 'square'—the disintegration of the word—how square used to mean solid, and now it means just the opposite.

"My cousin said, 'If you can solve this problem, the rest of your analysis would be a breeze.' There was something about connecting nine dots in the square with four straight lines without lifting the pencil, without intersecting, or without going over a line. Just because the nine dots are in a square, why is it that you should have to be limited by the suggestion of the shape of a square?"

At this point a fragment of the dream came back to her as an association to the puzzle. "In the dream the object I was imagining had to be produced out of the cloth or paper material."

She then went into a discourse about the period during the war when her husband was studying to get into the Air Force, and had had some trouble trying to make sketches of an object that had to be looked at from one view and then sketched as it would appear from another. She said that on Sunday morning she had been thinking idly about these problem-solving difficulties, when she suddenly had a flash of inspiration which made it possible for her to solve her cousin's problem. She then added that during the conversation of the evening before, her cousin had spoken of some oil land in the west owned by other members of the family, who had hopes of its bringing great wealth.

She had moved along associatively from the solution of the intellectual puzzle to the memory of her cousin's remarks about the oil land, and this recall brought back another fragment of the dream as an association.

"As I looked at this oil in the dream I felt a great *dismay*."

This was her first expression of the emotion in the dream, and it offered an opportunity to get closer to what had really been troubling her during this puzzle-filled night of dreaming and wakeful tossing. I therefore said, "Concentrate on the feeling of dismay in the dream, and say absolutely anything that pops into your mind."

In a moment she said, "Sinking out of sight is the first thing I think of. Last week at the hairdresser's I fell asleep under the dryer, and I dreamed that I leaned over the balcony from upstairs in our house to call Henry and I fell. I woke up feeling a sickening sensation. I didn't land, in the dream." A momentary silence, then, "Oh—just below this slope that sank into an abyss in the dream is where they're going to start digging the swimming pool next week. Digging out oil— spoiling things in the dream—may be related to the feeling I've had about Henry's sudden decision that we were going to have a swimming pool this summer. He decided and made the whole arrangement in two or three days.

"I thought it would be fun, but I wondered really how much Henry had thought about it. I thought we had come to the end of a period of heavy spending. I thought we'd gather our finances and start a fund for all the children's college education. We've been trying so hard to plan more rationally, and we have a financial adviser—but how is he going to tell an accountant, who is trying to help us keep things in line, about a sudden, impulsive five- or six-thousand-dollar outlay? It's like confessing snitching money from your mother's purse.

"The swimming pool looms on my horizon, not entirely pleasantly. Henry said at first that we can afford it, but now he's talking economy all the time. Am I going to be reminded of the swimming pool every time we have to think of spending money for anything?"

I interrupted her and said, "How do you really feel about the swimming pool—say it right out."

She responded at once, speaking angrily, quickly, volubly, "Many things I enjoy have been spoiled by Henry in the past because of his constant reminders of their cost. I'd almost rather not have the swimming pool than be bludgeoned by Henry to use it, to have the children use it. 'Have you had your swim today?' I can just hear him—we have to dutifully enjoy ourselves, because it costs so much, and have to watch all other expenses, to be reminded of the cost of the swimming pool all the time!" And then, in a voice of unmistakable dismay, she added, "I can see the writing on the wall!"

The session was at an end, but I took a few moments to underscore the already evident connection between the dream, her specific marital difficulty in connection with the swimming pool, and some of the personality problems which were beginning to crystallize. I said, "Well, this is it—the pool of oil, the symbol of luxury [the swimming pool] is ruining your garden (your home). Now that you understand your feelings about this, its important that you talk with Henry about your feelings, and that you do it now. You need to clear the air and work it out together with him, and not try to solve it all by yourself, like an intellectual puzzle. You and Henry have the beginning of a good relationship, and he's already shown his ability to work out problems together with you. The alternative would be to go back to your old ways—herding the children to the pool to please Daddy, hating it, hating him, being cold, sarcastic, ever so sweet, and retaliating in the many subtle ways that you've already begun to recognize. You're beginning to know that your old ways have played a big part in making your husband miserable, in keeping the two of you separated, and in keeping *you* miserable."

She returned home with determination and anxiety, and inaugurated constructive discussions with her husband.

Pursuit of the *dismay* in the dream brought the meaning of the dream into awareness. It furthermore brought into focus this wife's practice of seeking, with cleverness and dexterity, to solve her marital difficulties by herself as though they were tricky mathematical problems. It was then possible to see more clearly her role in perpetuating the difficulties with her husband. During the examination of her deep resentment of some qualities in her husband which she had indulged and "coped with," many covert retaliatory activities came to light. She then, more fittingly than seeking alone to "construct her rhomboid," expressed her clearly identified feelings to her husband—in fact, she told him her dream. They were able to work on the solution of marital problems, frankly and jointly.

Each productive, collaborative, interpretive experience like the one above, particularly when it hinges so directly on the pursuit of feeling, increases the patient's ability to use dreams in the analytic relationship, to apply his insights to life problems, and to continue in the independent acquisition of insight after termination of formal treatment.

Episodic Dreams

Maintaining vigilance for relatedness and movement in all of the behavior, feeling, and conceptualization of the patient is a cardinal function in psychotherapy. In a series of dreams occurring without apparent interruption [3] the patient's sleeping consciousness formulates different aspects or different concepts of the same problem. The varying dream reflections of the same problem may show, from one episode to the next, a progression toward or a retreat from a more realistic solution or perception. Viewing parts of an episodic dream in relationship to one another is similar to reviewing, in an interrelated manner, a number of dreams that a patient may have had over an extended period of time. The correlations enable the analyst and patient to gain perspective regarding, first, the relatedness of different aspects of a problem, and, second, both evolving and shifting attitudes within the personality in the handling of a specific problem.

In episodic dreams there is an abrupt termination or interruption of one type of action and the institution of a new action. It is this sudden shift that marks the separation between the episodes. The change may involve to varying degrees any or all of the elements of the dream. Individuals may remain the same, be modified, eliminated, multiplied, or substituted. The action may have partial continuity with the previous episodes or show an utter alteration. Surroundings may become completely new, or be related geographically, architecturally, or otherwise. Time, too, may shift.

Dream episodes may or may not be marked off by alteration in the feeling, and if the transformation occurs, it may affect either symbolized or experiential feeling, or both.

Often a patient reports that he had two or three or five dreams in the past night, and it seems to him that he has been troubled by many problems. These several dreams are frequently found to be portions of an episodic dream. It is of little value, however, to press the point of formalization. Whether the dreams of the same night were or were not episodically related, the clinical problem always involves a search for possible interrelationships that may throw light on the multiple personality processes occurring within the patient at the time.

Chinese Laundry; Night Club; Restaurant

This patient married late. She had been economically independent because of a small trust fund, and had occupied herself in scientific research. She undertook psychoanalysis because she was having difficulty in dealing with the behavior of her husband, a thirty-eight-year-

---

[3] The large percentage of sleeping time that is spent in dreaming would lead one to doubt that remembered dreams actually have occurred in uninterrupted sequence. See the work of Kleitman, Dement, and others.

old engineer who was unmanly, aloof, self-indulgent, and undemonstrative toward her, although he manifested interest and concern toward others. She had been raised (after her father's death when she was two or three years old) by a maternal martyr who never remarried, who made great demands on her daughter for achievement, and then invariably failed to acknowledge it. After finishing college the daughter set up her own apartment and lived alone for several years. She dated "pretty steadily" with her husband for about two years before marriage, and during that time was more eager than he for permanency and family life. She married with some awareness of her husband's aloofness, but was confident that she could bring about a warmer, more reciprocal relationship between them through her tolerance and affectionate acquiescence. She was not succeeding, however. There was a greater affective barrenness in their marriage than she had anticipated, and she had had distressing speculations that this might be due to defects in herself. She had begun to feel deeply unhappy, impotent, and defeated in her handling of the situation.

She cooperated conscientiously and moved ahead quickly in therapy. She began to develop more independence and initiative, and made more realistic demands upon her husband. This represented greater self-respect, in contrast to her self-abasing, acquiescent marital techniques. She elicited more responsible, fair, respectful, and affectional responses from her husband, and thereby fostered in him a greater maturity and the gratifications of maturity. Her progress was nevertheless, in spite of her spouse's efforts at home and with his own analyst, an uphill climb. She fluctuated in her often lonely struggle between optimistic determination to keep striving for a good marriage and impatient rebellion against the difficulties of her position.

A little more than four months after starting analysis, she brought in the following episodic dream. Typical of many episodic dreams, this is composed of three segments dreamed without interruption and with such abrupt change in manifest subject matter that they were presented to me as "Three dreams—first dream . . . second dream . . . third dream."

"In the first dream I am in a Chinese laundry, sitting by the counter, dressed only in underclothes. It seems that my clothes got wet and I came in here to get them dried. I am on my way somewhere and I am late. I begin to feel angry at the laundryman for taking so long with my clothes. I do not feel embarrassed about sitting there in my underwear, though there are people coming in at various times—I feel that I do not care what they think, as I know why I am here. Through the back of the store I can see the laundryman's wife ironing clothes. Finally I can wait no longer, and go up to the roof where my clothes are hanging. I find that they are all bunched together on the line and I straighten them out, very angry at the laundryman for hanging them in such a way that they take longer to dry.

"In the second dream I go to a dance with a girl. I have a date with a man and I'm to meet him at the dance. The girl and I seem to be friendly and relaxed together. We go in and sit at a table. It is a big room, crowded, a large dance floor with tables around the outside. A red-headed man comes in a door at the other side of the room. He seems to be the man I have the date with. He does not see me at first, but my feeling is that he will eventually, and will then come over to me, and I tell this to the girl who is with me. My husband's seven-year-old nephew is there, and comes over and asks me to dance with him. I thank him and agree. Someone around there says we will look silly dancing together and I say I don't care, as I will enjoy being with him.

"In the third dream I'm in a restaurant with my mother [a frequent symbol for her husband]. She is taunting me and saying that I cannot get a job, a clerical job. I say that I do not have to, because at my profession I can earn more than that job would pay, anyway. Then, as we have finished the meal, she begins to stack the dishes and clean up the tables. I help a little but when she keeps on I say that is enough, and that the waiters are there to do that, and it is not necessary or fitting that she do it. She says that it's no wonder people don't like me, when I won't do things like this. I am angry, and I say that people do like me, and it's just because *she* never has that she doesn't see how other people can. I tell her I used to feel she was right, that there was something wrong with me, and people did not like me—but now I know different."

The action, individuals (except for the consistent occurrence of her recognizable self), surroundings, and feelings all change, but the problems with which the patient is wrestling are treated with continuity. Progressively, all the episodes reflect new conceptualizations of herself and her concomitant new practices struggling to emerge. In all three, she asserts independence and self-respect as a change from acquiescence and search for approval.

In the first episode (Chinese Laundry) she is angry with the laundryman (identified associatively as the analyst) for not helping her fast enough, efficiently enough, or in *her* way. She is critical of him and takes over impatiently so that her laundry (her problems) will be taken care of sooner.

In the second episode (Night Club) she is on friendly terms with a girl friend (the therapist); the patient is now a peer rather than a patron demanding service. Feeling more independent, she is also less angry and more hopeful and patient. Although she must dance with a boy for the present (her husband's immature aspect) her man will come along (her husband will achieve maturity).

In the third episode, in the restaurant, she is handling her problems with the greatest degree of independence—in fact, quite on her own. She has a good sense of her personal worth and rights, a genuine self-respect. She is virtually immune to the efforts of her mother (associatively her husband) to involve her in unnecessary activity directed toward gaining approval and buying her way.

This statement of the meaning of the episodes in the dream, although general and restricted, indicates considerable movement, a struggle for the emergence and consolidation of a new consciousness in the patient, a new conceptualization of herself as an adequate, independent, lovable person, capable of developing satisfying marital and other relationships.

The progression through the episodes, as just traced, chiefly reflects the constructive trend in the patient's therapeutic struggle. Her symbolism also, however, especially in the first episode, reflects her resistance. The course of her analysis, despite its benefits, not only represents a process too slow and unsatisfying to her impatient, controlling personality, but it also represents irrationally a competitive defeat before her therapist. She is being forced to change her personality, instead of forcing the analyst to ease her lot. Her resistance is more apparent upon closer examination of the episodes and the patient's associations.

In the first episode she immediately associated the laundryman with the analyst. "I am impatient at the slowness of progress in the analysis and blame it on you. You're not handling things in the most efficient manner. The clothes are not hung up right." With an exceptional person like herself, a short-term treatment should be possible. She is furthermore already late, having married at twenty-eight. She can't possibly have deep-seated problems, because she hasn't time for them. (Her clothes need merely to be dried, not laundered.) "Finally I can wait no longer and go up to the roof . . . I find [the clothes] all bunched together and I straighten them out, very angry at the laundryman for hanging them in such a way that they take longer to dry." It is the way the therapist formulates her problems that makes them difficult to solve.

The impatience and anger derive from several sources, partly of a grandiose, but chiefly of a competitive, nature. First, they derive from the assault on her grandiose belief that, unlike people who require long-term intensive treatment, she has difficulties capable of being handled with dispatch (her clothes need drying, not laundering). Second, they derive from the undermining of her competitive conviction that hers are *external* difficulties—her husband's problems (her clothes do not need laundering because of anything originating in her; they have merely been splashed). The competitiveness is reflected also in her feeling that she is more competent than her therapist, who is unskilled (doesn't know how to hang up his customer's clothes). And third, her impatience and anger derive from her competitive rebellion against being forced to conform to someone else's pattern and pace (she must sit downstairs in the store and wait), and alternatively being forced to take some of the responsibility herself (go up to the roof and do some of the laundryman's job).

Another source of her anger later emerged through her associations to the first episode, the association to the view of the wife ironing in the background. The patient was angry because she would like to have the analyst as a husband, and thus to solve her problems circumstantially instead of being forced to change her personality.

Resistance because of jealousy was validated through her associations to this part of the dream. It was immediately following the point at which "through the back of the store I can see the laundryman's wife ironing clothes" that she gave up waiting and impatiently went to the roof. In this connection she had a number of significant associations. She said, "I feel there is some deep, dark, important something behind all my problems. I disguise you as an Oriental—this prevents you from being someone I could be interested in personally. I have always felt, since I met you socially, before I started analysis with you, that you were the kind of man I liked in manner and appearance. I actually have felt that as to general physical type you are like my husband. Apparently I have been unable to face the implications of this kind of thinking—afraid of getting mixed up in these feelings now that you're my analyst—you cannot be analyst and man too." [4]

In general, the Chinese Laundry episode indicates the patient's resentment toward the therapist because he will not make her own efforts toward change unnecessary. In the first episode there is reflected a predominant resistance. Even in this episode, however, healthy aspects of the patient are also reflected: her freedom from false pride and her clear purpose in being in therapy ("I do not care what they think—

[4] In the chapters on sexuality and resistance, sexual interest in the therapist was designated as frequently not connected with love, but with conquest, with competitiveness and manipulation, and with opposition to personality change. With this patient, healthy and neurotic elements were both present.

I know why I am here"); and the constructive quality inferred by her taking the initiative for working out her problems (straightening her clothes) even though she is angry over the necessity.

The positive aspects of the patient's struggle toward health are carried to a progressively higher level in the next episodes. The progression indicates that there is more than a coexistence of resistance and healthy trends. It indicates the predominance of activity in a constructive direction during this period of the patient's analysis.

The Night Club episode, in contrast with the angry, impatient demand for quick service in the Chinese laundry, reveals a much greater acceptance by the patient of a healthy, independent role, a recognition of her ability for self-reliant action within restricted circumstances, and a realistic anticipation of increasing rewards and concomitant friendliness toward the therapist. She associated as follows: "The girl friend is you—I must disguise you as not a man, so that I can see you as a friend, someone to whom I can talk. The red-headed man is my husband. I seem to be feeling more sure that eventually he will be able to give me what I want and that he will see me as I want him to. I suppose that I am still disguising him because in the dream I am admitting that he does not 'see' me now, and this is still hard to swallow." The nephew, Bobby, was also red-headed. She said, "I enjoy him and the other children in the family, and I've been ridiculed for treating them as I do, instead of in the rather belittling way that many of the adults in the family treat them." Her association was to the qualities she really enjoyed in her husband and her affectionate feeling toward him. She was not ashamed to show her affection for him, although demonstrativeness was strictly avoided in her husband's family. Here was additional evidence of her self-confidence and independence in action, as well as her freedom from constraint in the face of disapproval. Instead of demanding quick solutions, she was more ready to enjoy what was lovable about her husband (his gentle and boyish self) while waiting for him to become more aware of her needs, for him to "see her." In this spirit she could regard her analyst (girl friend) in a friendly way.[5]

In this second episode she is more accepting of her emerging new personality, does not experience it as impotence or defeat, and faces more whole-heartedly and with realistic optimism the constructive possibilities in her marriage.

In the third episode (Restaurant) the patient shows further movement in the direction of healthy maturity and independence. As in the

[5] She had deleted the analyst's masculinity; the problem presented by his being sexually attractive to her had just recently come into view. Compare the dream Just Friends, pp. 148–150.

first episode, she is angry, but now it is not because she is compelled to
be self-assertive and independent. Quite the contrary, it is because of
impediments to mature living. In her sleeping consciousness she experiences anger engendered because her husband's often servile or excessive solicitude toward others interferes with their developing, as a married couple, a more self-respecting relationship with those people. She
associated, "Mother is both mother and my husband. There are times
when he treats me as my mother has, and I am just as angry and have
the same feelings toward him that I have had toward my mother. [In
the patient's personal glossary, her mother was often the symbol of her
husband when the patient was angry with him.] I am telling him that
I can be as successful, or more so, with *my* values than with *his*. I am
indicating my embarrassment at some of the ways that he is excessively
deferential or helpful in public or with strangers (clearing the table in
the restaurant) and telling him that I do not have to go along with this
to be liked—though I used to feel that I did."

The final episode reflects the farthest point of a continuous movement through three dream episodes: these symbolize an initial predominance of resistance and then progressive, constructive changes in
her conceptualizations of herself, her feelings, and her behavior.

The movement in this clinical example is also an illustration of the
evolution of health, which is the subject of the chapter to follow. Episodic dreams may also reflect movement in the opposite direction. An
example of this is the episodic dream Very Contented, But . . . , which
concludes with an episode of resistance, Holding Him Back (see p. 316).
That series was experienced by a man who had been making progress
in his marriage and was much happier with his wife, but began to pull
away when she developed more healthy independence than he was yet
ready to endure.

Other episodic dreams show no direct line of progression, either
forward or backward, but reflect disjointedly aspects of the same or
closely related problems of the patient. When, however, there is a progression, the detection of its movement toward healthy solutions or its
retreat toward pathology can serve analyst and patient as an important
guide in evaluating therapeutic achievements and requirements.

It will have been noted, in this and other chapters, that certain
items of a dream have often been omitted from the interpretive discussion. The report of the session involving the Oil Well dream contained within it a complete, brief, separate anxiety dream that the
patient recalled as an association, and which was not referred to again.
(This was the dream she had under the drier at the hairdresser's, in

which she fell over the balcony in her home.) There are many lost items, many lost dreams in the course of an analysis. If there were unlimited time, a great deal more of the valuable data of the patient's dreams could be distilled through the analytic process. This applies also, of course, to nondream material. It is necessary, however, to distinguish between loss by choice or necessity, and loss by neglect.

Whenever a patient is conscientiously examining himself, I have found it a good rule not to interfere. This does not mean disregarding dreams, but only pressing less for their priority. In the course of the few sessions reported in connection with the Crazy Woman dream (see pp. 73–77), much material from dreams drifted past unsalvaged, but the patient concentrated upon her feelings and examined with unabated involvement every bit of data she could grasp. As in that case, and in the case of the Elevator Nightmare (pp. 218–226), the decision, it must be re-emphasized, to leave something out is not made because of the potential it may have for arousing anxiety. It is precisely in the anxiety-laden areas that the patient needs most to concentrate, and needs most to be helped by the analyst (see p. 85n). When any portion or element of a dream must be dropped by the wayside, it should never be the element that carries anxiety or any other feeling, symbolized or experiential. By choice, much dream material may in fact be by-passed because of the necessity to pursue, in the limited period of an analytic session, the feeling of the dream. The wisdom of such a choice is suggested by the productive work with the Oil Well dream, where the pursuit of the feeling of dismay took precedence over everything else in the dream.

During interpretive activity there is a type of resistance that is particularly difficult to discern. The patient, quite unwittingly, is subjectively aware of himself only as the individual conscientiously exposing his personality. Despite honest and astute self-searching and communication, he is, at the same time, not acknowledging *himself* as the individual his "insight" describes. As the patient carefully elaborates his sick activities and reactions, documenting and enriching the portrayal with dreams, he does not feel the described pathology as his own. He seems to be permeated by a sense of his own conscientiousness. The phenomenon is not identifiable by the content of the patient's productions, which is always relevant, perceptive, and revealing. Its nature is a subtle aura of infatuation with the process in which the patient is engaged. It must be sensed intuitively by the analyst, and usually does not dawn upon him until he has been involved with the patient over a long period—perhaps two or three years. It is the kind of circumstance that often causes the analyst to wonder why, with all the "insights" the patient has achieved, personality does not change.

I should like at this point to develop more fully a subject mentioned in the Introduction and referred to briefly again in Chapter 2 in the discussion of the use of *insulating terms*.

The patient may plunge into the core of a dream's problem by accurately correlating associations, or by a sudden intuitive grasp but, presenting the new awareness as a speculation, he will say, if sensing his own hatred, "*Maybe* I hate so-and-so," or, identifying his fear, "*Perhaps* I'm afraid," or "*I guess* I'm conceited," or "Possibly it's connected with my being angry," or "I think," which may be padded further with "I think it might be that . . ." or even by a sort of defense in depth, something like, "Perhaps it could possibly have something to do with such-and-such." One woman began, "I think perhaps I tend to feel . . . ," although the same woman would often be utterly direct about matters she had no emotional stake in obscuring.

The insulating terms are almost always connected with the more meaningful association or with flashes of insight. The patient who is more willing to accept the reality about himself would say, instead of "Maybe I hate so-and-so," a direct, "I hate so-and-so," or a more gradual but still honest, "I'm beginning to realize I hate" or "'I hate so-and-so' is what comes to mind—let me look at that now." Or, instead of "Perhaps I'm afraid," the more committed patient might say, "I'm afraid," or "I have a feeling I can't quite identify . . . yes, it's fear. That surprises me, but it *is* fear."

The insulating term is like a pair of rubber gloves with which the patient protects himself as from an electric current in a wire he holds. He is shielding himself from the shock of reality at the very moment when he seems to be reaching out and directly grasping reality. If this subtle sort of denaturing process by the employment of insulating terms does not impress itself upon the analyst, he may feel from the substance of the communication that the patient is more deeply and more insightfully involved than is actually the case.

Such a misappraisal has further important therapeutic implications. The analyst, feeling that the patient is spontaneously on the track, may fail to encourage more intensive exploration of a problem that may be well within reach. The patient, too, may fail to pursue the problem intensively enough, feeling that he has adequately covered difficult ground. He may be pleased at having faced some problem, or perhaps glad to have "finished" with it.

From the technical standpoint, recognition of the insulating term opens an opportunity to promote sharper, more direct exploration and confrontation of himself by the patient. For example, if a patient interprets a dream by saying, "I guess it means I'm angry," it is important to say something of the nature of, "Let's not guess. It's important to know. Look at your feelings. Are you angry?" The patient's response to such an invitation to penetrate beyond the insulation can be a useful measure of his degree of genuine insight and also of his degree of commitment to the therapeutic process at the time. If the patient is sufficiently motivated toward change he will usually welcome the inquiry and look more directly at his feelings. If the "I guess I'm angry," inspected further, brings to view, *"I'm angry!"* then the patient's speculation becomes *a fact* about himself that the patient and analyst can jointly employ.

As time goes on, the more fully involved patient can learn to catch his own insulating terms and to cultivate more careful self-inspection. If the patient is less committed to analysis, he will resent the therapist's inquiry and fend it off in various ways. In connection with a dream or a waking event, he may abandon the interpretive activity with which he has been spontaneously involved. Or he may merely substitute for "I guess I'm angry" another term or insulating phrase such as "I probably really am angry," and feel that now he has given a more direct statement. He may resentfully claim that he has already expressed himself clearly. Or he may be evasive by means of a compliant change of style. If, however, the "I guess" is not picked up by the analyst, the "I'm angry"—never having registered with any immediacy upon the patient and therefore never having been integrated as a fact about himself— may be completely forgotten by him.

With either the more- or the less-committed type of patient, the recognition of the insulating terms and their direct introduction for examination as such can be extremely profitable. The more committed patient will be helped toward a more intensive and rewarding therapeutic discipline and a higher level of self-analytic activity. The more resistant patient will at least have the opportunity to comprehend another reducible obstacle to his progress.

The analyst, by his awareness of and therapeutic dealing with the insulating terms, may be able to elicit more accurate information and to appraise more clearly both the level of the patient's self-awareness and his degree of commitment to analysis.

Another form of resistance often linked with incisive, spontaneous interpretation of dreams or other material is somewhat similar to the use of insulating terms. There are phrases used to negate an insight by attributing it to the analyst, such as "I know what you will say," or "I know what you want me to say," or "I know what you are thinking." Here again it is essential to underscore the negating phrase in order to disencumber the evaluation or association that is vitiated by it. The significant fact is that the patient's association is his own evaluative connection. That the connection or formulation may also be in the therapist's mind, established there by previous interchanges, does not automatically, if at all, wipe out the significance of its associative connection in the patient's mind. On the other hand, if the patient's association or interpretation corresponds with what the analyst has offered in the past, but is merely mechanically or compliantly submitted by the patient, that is a different problem which must be determined and dealt with separately.

The use of the "I know what you want me to say" kind of phrase is the patient's way of announcing that what he is about to report can have absolutely no significance regarding his personality, and pertains only to the cerebrations of the analyst. The manner or spirit in which the patient uses or presents an association or interpretation derived from the analyst's observation in a previous therapeutic context should not be permitted to obscure the essential fact that it has occurred to the patient in the immediate therapeutic context. The patient who is committed to the analytic process will try to evaluate the significance of the interpretation that occurs to him even though it may coincide with or resemble previously expressed evaluations by the therapist.

If the patient is fundamentally battling against treatment at the time, he will resent detection of the possibly unconscious negating maneuver. He may deny it, compliantly modify it, or in some manner defend it. As with the insulating terms, the analyst's awareness of the patient's negation of interpretation offers opportunities both for appraising and enriching the therapeutic process.

There are additional unhealthy manifestations which may occur in the course of the patient's spontaneous interpretations. One of them is the presentation of an interpretation or association in its negative form. As he thinks about what a dream might mean, for example, the patient, instead of saying, "So-and-so is what occurs to me," may say, "It couldn't mean so-and-so," or "The dream couldn't possibly have anything to do with Jack, because I feel very different about him." The patient presents the thought in the negative in order to nullify it. It would be more constructive for the patient to approach the incredible implication of the dream with a remark such as, "I know I'm very resentful of the man in the dream because he's imposing on me, and I know it makes me think of Jack, but I don't think I felt imposed on by Jack. I'm always glad to do things for Jack, and I've always felt he was so considerate. I'll have to think about this." Such an approach could open the way for the patient to make fruitful interpretive hypotheses about himself from the dream. In contrast, the negation of the associative thought of Jack in the dream context—"It couldn't possibly have anything to do with Jack" —bars the way to further pursuit and eventual insight. The negative formulation, the discard of an important clue, leads to a confusion about or a total unresponsiveness to the dream or to the abandonment of the dream, or to the patient's development of plausible, contrived, and fundamentally meaningless interpretation.

There are three additional forms of unhealthy manifestations of the patient's spontaneous interpretation of his dreams. All three are frequently linked with extensive, penetrating, interpretive hypotheses, but they nevertheless basically represent resistance to genuine insight and personality change. All three are in a sense calculated to neutralize or block the interpretive activity of the analyst.

The first takes the form of what might be called an interpretive filibuster.[6] The patient presents the dream and gets to work on it with apparent zeal, often presenting significant associative and interpretive material. His activity, however, fills the sessions, with hardly a pause. If the analyst interrupts to suggest or inquire, priority ideas or associations will suddenly arise and the flood of material will continue. While many fruitful avenues to difficult problems have been seemingly courageously opened, the therapist himself has been immobilized. The patient, while associating and interpreting, has all the while managed to avoid any real crystallization of insight.

In another similar type of activity, the patient, intuitively sensing the meaning of a dream, or recognizing himself on the basis of recent therapeutic experience, hastily presents his interpretation as though beating the analyst to the punch. This is another situation wherein the substance of the interpretation may impress both analyst and analysand, while the resistant behavior becomes obscured. Beating the analyst to the interpretation is another form of resistance that is difficult to identify because the interpretation often seems so perceptive. As the therapist waits, however, for documentation and further development of the interpretive hypothesis, or as he himself seeks to pursue and elaborate it, the patient refuses continued involvement in his own meaningful and potentially more fruitful concept. The patient has placed his pertinent idea in insular form on the record before it could evolve dynamically from his exchange with the analyst, and before it

[6] This is a pseudo-conscientious form of resistance; see pp. 199–215.

could become related to the total context of his life. And then it is not pursued. He has merely competitively outwitted the therapist, while feeling and often giving the impression of genuine initiative.

The last of these three types of spontaneous interpretation by the patient which block the interpretive activity of the analyst is that of giving an interpretation and immediately rushing into a new topic. The patient reports a dream and presents an interpretation and continues talking about himself. At this point, the difficulty in distinguishing between what is healthy and what is unhealthy in the activity of the patient lies in the fact that associative material, usually so diverse by its very nature, is often quite difficult to distinguish from digression. It does not become immediately apparent that the patient is moving to a new topic. It is possible, of course, that there may be some genuine relevance that the analyst has failed to discern. (Some patients come with an agenda that insures against intensive pursuit of any single item; see Wheelbarrows dream, p. 189.) Particularly, however, with a patient who has experienced a protracted period of analysis, it eventually is likely to become clear that he is not pursuing an interpretation, but has taken refuge in digression.

When a patient is working conscientiously and has developed a significant perception through a dream, he has the incentive to pursue this perception into the realm of his waking activities. He cultivates associations, looks for validation, and welcomes help in the process. Rushing off to a new topic after spontaneously developing an interpretation vitiates the usefulness of the dream or other data.

Entirely apart from the insight achieved, interpretive activity is the heart of the curative process in psychoanalysis. In no other aspect of the therapeutic experience is its cooperative nature so fully involved. This may superficially appear to contradict the goals of analysis, and the criteria for termination, which include the capacity for independent interpretation. But the contradiction is not real. Independence does not exclude mutuality.

The cooperative essence of analytic interpretive activity necessitates several lines of interpersonal endeavor. It involves the effort to engage, during a protracted intimacy with another, in self-observation, self-exposure, spontaneous responsiveness to another, and in ready and full consideration of the responses of another. The investigation, exposure, listening, and responsiveness in this trusting interpersonal relationship is achieved through reciprocal associative activity, full communication, and the independent and mutual conceptual creativeness of interpretive activity. The complexity and intensity of commitment in such activity is among the richest, most fulfilling kinds of experience of which human beings are capable.

A long period of interpersonal experience in psychoanalysis is necessary for the patient to achieve the quality of intimacy and cooperative engagement that is an important criterion of cure. This experience generates in many patients healthy affection for the analyst. Such affection cannot be fully or sexually consummated in the professional relationship, because that relationship is in no other way totally reciprocal (see Chapter 6, "Resistance in Dreams," pp. 226–228), but it is a preparation for the patient's achievement of a fuller kind of interpersonal relationship in his private life. Nor is the patient's increasingly independent interpretive activity at termination a withdrawal from or in contradiction to the mutuality achieved earlier; neither is it a mere therapeutic severance discipline. On the contrary, it attests to a newly developed capacity for *both* self-reliance and mutuality which can be realized outside of analysis as a fuller kind of reciprocity in a context of love. In healthy love there can be no question of maintaining independence either through insularity or through domination; nor is independence sacrificed by the full trust and commitment of lovers.

Interpretive activity, then, a collaboration often first approached and developed with dreams in therapy, becomes itself an experiential basis for the healthy development of the total personality.

8. *Evidence of Evolving Health in Dreams*

D REAMS GIVING EVIDENCE of evolving health appear throughout this book; [1] this chapter, although it contains some clinical material, will be devoted primarily to theoretical and technical considerations.

Health was defined earlier as a basic confidence in one's ability to comprehend and respond appropriately to other people, and to engender appropriate responses in others to oneself. It includes a subjective certainty that an interpersonal failure, although it may represent a personality limitation in oneself, does not prove one's bankruptcy or threaten one with disintegration. The healthy individual has confidence in a continuing functional effectiveness, and enjoys a comfortable sense of self in activities based upon realistic interpersonal expectations. There is a fairly high correlation between his self-concept and his way of living. This condition is what we strive toward in the analytic process.

Personality distortions are usually expressed in activities which are calculated to *force* rather than to invite responses, to *overcome* interpersonal influence rather than to respond to it. Each failure in these distorted activities tends to be experienced as total failure of the personality, and tends to engender anxiety, hostility, withdrawal, and retaliation—all or any of these (see Chapter 6, "Resistance in Dreams").

[1] For example, in Chapters 2, 5, and 10; see also "evolving health" in the index.

253

In analysis, the sense of impending or progressing personality disintegration that at times accompanies evolving health is experienced as anxiety, and is often accompanied by intensification of cynicism and competitiveness toward the analyst. Because of these exacerbations of pathology, there is danger that the analyst may fail to recognize the signs of the simultaneous evolution of health or the danger that these signs may be undervalued. Such an error can prove particularly anti-therapeutic when the subjective awareness of change is itself the chief source of resistance.[2] Competitively the patient may be only too glad to accept the analyst's failure to discern the evidence of effective influence. At any stage of the therapeutic process, beginning with the first session,[3] persistent alertness for both personality assets and personality pathology is essential to the adequate evaluation of each. The patient learns during analysis to keep this duality in view as a guide to realistic judgments and efforts in dealing with his problems.

The duality is clearly illustrated in the following case. The dream was experienced by the patient at a well-advanced stage of treatment.

Captain-Woman

When the patient began analysis, at the age of twenty, she was a promising young pianist who had had some outstanding adolescent successes. She had, however, begun to feel increasingly tense and threatened during practice, auditions, and performances, and had on several occasions suffered such muscular tension while playing in public that she gave some of the musical passages seriously inadequate renditions. She also had experienced occasional musical amnesia, and was often overcome with indecisiveness regarding musical interpretation. She had had serious misgivings about her ability to succeed professionally, and indulged in fantasies of giving up her career and becoming a domestic servant.

She was physically attractive and was regarded by young men as an intriguing and colorful companion, although she had engaged very little in sexual play. In all her relationships she was extremely cautious, calculating, and controlling, and concealed these character-istics behind a manner that was sometimes acquiescent or helpless, or even desperate, and at other times that of a sprightly ingénue.

From very early in the patient's life as an only child, she had been groomed for musical renown. Both parents, while protesting love,

[2] Several dreams of resistance engendered by evolving health appear in Chapter 6, pp. 187–196; see also the dream Death of Husband, pp. 204–205.

[3] See discussion of the dream Contemptible Passion in Chapter 3, pp. 120–121.

seemed to her preoccupied exclusively with this ambition for her, and after her father's death, when the patient was nine, the mother had taken on the full responsibility for pressing her forward to this goal. The mother was tyrannical toward the patient, at the same time serving and infantilizing her. The patient, for the most part, played the role of an acquiescent slave, yet her frustration was apparent in her frequent infuriation and outrage.

After three years of analysis, the patient had made progress in a number of directions. Her analysis had involved, first of all, a struggle to emancipate herself from her mother. To a large extent, she had given up her unconscious professional self-destruction, which was a covert rebellion against those who sought—or whom she believed to seek—to exploit her as a protégée. Her resistance in therapy had been a part of this rebellion. She had also achieved, as therapy progressed, increasing professional self-determination and artistic integrity, and a general acceptance of responsibility for her own life, with increasing enjoyment of her activities. She had achieved some recognition of her own technique of manipulation through helplessness, and now had some success in dealing with it; and she showed a beginning of trust and a capacity for intimacy.

Despite these achievements, she had ambivalently come to several recent therapy hours declaring that she wanted to collapse or, by destructive activities, prove to herself and to me that she was helpless. The predominance of her desire to change, in the midst of this resistance, led to her spontaneous recognition and communication of these subjective but unexercised pathological impulses. At this time—so far the healthiest period of her life—she reported the following dream.

"A young man's ship is sinking, and he needs some help to save him. He goes to another ship, looking for the captain to come to his aid. Instead of finding the captain, he finds a woman who is very sexy— the movie siren type—lying on a couch. He asks her very impatiently, 'Where's the captain? My boat is sinking and I need him right away.' She says, 'I'm the captain. I'll help you.' But he refuses to believe her, acts as if she's kidding, and doesn't understand how serious his plight is. He keeps demanding, 'Where's the captain?' Finally he's convinced that she is the captain, and he has to make do with whatever help she can give him. In the stupid argument of where's the real captain, she has a sense of humor.

"They are swimming together to his ship. There is a very strong undertow that seems to drag him under, and then a big tidal wave covers them. He is panicked, but she knows how to handle this. She advises him just to keep swimming on, even if it seems that they are staying in the same place; if they give up their direction or activity, they will be overcome.

"The young man is such a jerk. He's helpless, ineffectual, whining—a weak nothing. She looks so alluring. In the water, he's again helpless, but she knows what to do. She is wonderful, capable, compassionate."

In talking about the dream, the patient said, "I hate this man. I just loathe him. He's a leech and a conceited ass, besides. He thinks he's something wonderful and strong, and he really is weak and puny." Then she went on to interpret the dream. "I feel I am both of these characters, particularly the man. I doubt if I can achieve the dignity and status of this captain-woman." Yet the conscious diffidence, ineptness, and unwillingness to mature—the "jerk" aspect of her personality—was contradicted as she went on to discuss her enjoyment of her new, constructive, independent pursuits (identified as the captain-woman aspect of her personality) stating, "My activity is what I do really like about myself."

It should be mentioned that throughout her analysis, growing up had been a frightening prospect to her—a weakening, annihilating process. Her neurotic sense of self had been achieved through covert rebellion, indicated by her muscular failures during auditions or performances, and by her fantasies of becoming a domestic servant in order completely to destroy the career her mother sought for her. In discussing this, she had once said, "This feeling of *me* has to go somewhere, and it seems to come out by wanting always to do the opposite of what's expected—not openly, but under cover. The battle is more important than what's at stake—constructively at stake, that is. Now, as I more and more *do* do what's expected of me, I feel I'm losing my *self*, my personality. I'm succumbing, I'm losing my integrity."

By "doing what's expected of me" she referred to increasingly mature and successful acceptance of responsibility for her own life. The neurotic sense of strength and self that she had cultivated was threatened with destruction as she "succumbed" to maturity. Yet she recognized that if she were to destroy her career in order to escape responsibility, she would indeed be the "jerk" of her dream. She expressed her new evaluation and repudiation of this part of her character when she said, "I hate this man. I just loathe him. He thinks he's something wonderful and strong, and he really is weak and puny." Thus the dream, together with her associations, indicated the evolution of a healthy, realistic evaluation of her pathological self as the "jerk" who fought against using her healthy resources.

In the concurrent captain-woman symbol the patient recognized and accepted in herself significant, constructive resources. Through this dream she was able to identify more sharply than ever before the real pride and pleasure she derived from healthy changes. In the ensuing months she saw more and more clearly how often and how much she wanted to collapse, to call for help, to refuse to handle her affairs independently. Time and time again she could perceive the "jerk" and take over as the "captain." She could now see retrospectively how often what had seemed to be inability was instead the obstreperously helpless "jerk" demanding outside assistance. This recognition was of particular value in the therapeutic relationship itself.

In addition, the quality of her life in general was now significantly changed, in that her pleasure in independent accomplishment was much less marred by a sense of submission. The captain became less a symbol of what was expected of her—less a model toward whom the cruel world pointed a finger with the commanding question to the patient, "Why don't you grow up?"—and more a conceptualization of herself which she spontaneously strove to fulfill. Thus while she had not yet achieved, as a way of life, the "dignity and status" of the captain-woman, the dream had focused for her, for the first time, a goal of maturity, independence, and womanliness—a goal which her already achieved growth made it possible for her to envision.

The clarification of the patient's goal through recognition of its partial achievement opened the way for her to recognize and attack new problems, which she had before only dimly sensed. For instance, although there were great attractions in being a "captain" she felt threatened, for, she said, "I feel that to be strong is to be unlovable." This distorted conceptualization of lovability was a major problem which could be perceived and dealt with only as a result of the crystallization, through the dream, of her increasing healthy independence.

Thus the dream evidence of evolving health, associated with real gratification from healthy functioning, can sharpen the goal of therapy, making it the patient's own and not that of the therapist or others. The patient's therapeutic efforts take on a clearer direction and become more productive. Moreover, such a dream can provide incentive to the patient by marking more clearly the connection between his gains and the therapeutic struggle. And finally, the discernment in dreams of evolving health crystallizes achievements already made and opens the way to the perception and pursuit of new problems.[4]

The evolution of personality is essentially synonymous with evolution of consciousness. Changes of personality are basically changes of

[4] See illustration and discussion of the contributory role of an insight in the perception and pursuit of new problems in Chapter 2, pp. 98–99.

consciousness. What is the process of change of consciousness that takes place in a successful analysis? We know that intimate collaboration is a basic feature of the curative process, and that intellectual, emotional, and behavioral changes in the patient are inaugurated by this collaboration. Engaging in a healthy interpersonal way with the analyst gives the patient a new kind of experience. This comes slowly, with confusion, with risk, with fear, with hostility. It comes interrupted by counterinfluencing activities on the part of the patient, but slowly it does come. Through clearer perception of his own role in the failures he has had with other people, through the new kind of experience—cooperative interaction—through the new perceptions and conceptualizations (including an increasingly realistic self-concept) that he achieves while working together with another human being, the individual gradually changes the pathological kinds of activity that have distorted his personality in the course of its evolution, and a new kind of personality, of consciousness, slowly develops. A healthier functional effectiveness evolves, the individual derives from this new activity a healthier sense of self, and this, reciprocally, augments his capacity to function healthily.

Throughout this volume there has been consistent emphasis on the crucial role of interpersonal activity in the therapeutic process. In this activity, the value of attention to feelings has again and again been stressed and clinically illustrated.

An aspect of the interaction which has received relatively little attention is the *intellectual exchange*. The analytic relationship develops and is sustained mainly through verbal communication—report, formulation, speculation. What is the role of this exchange of ideas? Can an intellectual practice really bring about a new awareness of self? If it does, can the acquisition of this new awareness significantly modify the personality? What is the role of the clearer, more accurate, more realistic view of the patient—the so-called "intellectual insight"—in changing the patient's personality?

Traditionally, in the various psychoanalytic orientations, there has been a tendency to denigrate the role of intellectual insight. It is true that the patient's spontaneous intellectual comprehension, or his grasp of the analyst's formulation, do not necessarily lead to significant behavioral change. But neither do they necessarily remain sterile. Intellectual grasp becomes a potential basis for new experience. Throughout therapy one must recognize the degree to which the patient does and does not employ the new knowledge as the basis for new behavior and consequent new self-observation; one must search for and deal with the ways in which the intellectual insight, the conceptual change, becomes sterilized by the patient, isolated, somehow kept from behavioral, social, and interpersonal experience.

An examination of the conceptual change which occurs during introspection and the exchange of thought raises two questions. First, what precisely brings about the changed conceptualization of self? Second, what determines whether this changed conceptualization will lead to changed behavior and, eventually, to a changed personality?

The brief consideration of a clinical case will serve as a suitable point of departure in the search for answers to these theoretical questions.

The clinical material comes from a young man referred to previously (pp. 123, 169, 188), about thirty years of age, a social worker, married, a father, and in analysis for a few sessions. The patient's manner was quiet, soft, and friendly. He had a capacity for putting others at ease. In the initial interview (about two months before the beginning of his analysis) a crucial aspect of his personality had been brought to light—a consistent, forceful imposition of his will upon others, a tyranny almost utterly obscured by his outwardly genial manner. The new characterization came as a complete surprise to him.

When he returned two months later for the start of treatment he reported his dream (Analyst-Chauffeur).[5] It will be recalled that the discussion of the dream, which revealed a dependent orientation toward the analyst, crystallized to some extent another new view—that his "dependency" was one of his techniques of tyranny.

The following session, a week later, began with the patient's statement that the intervening days had been anxious ones for him. At home he had found situation after situation in which he was behaving exactly as he had always behaved, in spite of having gained what he felt was a great deal of insight in the course of the first two sessions of analysis. Through our exchanges he had recognized that in his relationship with his wife he had been operating with bland disregard of her needs and rights and that when this quiet tyranny was challenged by her criticism or complaint, he had responded with tension, anger, and sarcasm. In disciplining the children, while his manner was one of soft paternal reasonableness, he nevertheless manifested intolerance of any deviation on their part from the kind of behavior he required of them. In his professional operations, when colleagues did not agree with him, his pseudo-amiable humor served to whip them into line or to punish them. He also had begun to realize that he felt fury when his supervisor made

[5] In the dream the therapist was assuring the patient of cure, and taking care of him in a very special, friendly way, voluntarily conducting sessions at the patient's home and chauffeuring him about the city.

demands which prevented him from managing the job in his own benevolently despotic way. The varied manifestations of his pattern of tyranny began to impinge upon his awareness. It also began to dawn upon him that he could not dissipate his pathology or acquire a changed personality by the simple process of coming to analysis and gaining insights from session to session. He would have to exert effort—independent, deliberate discipline—to modify his behavior in accordance with his new insight.

This brief presentation tentatively answers the first theoretical question. The change in the patient's conceptualization of himself was initiated in the very first session by his willingness to examine seriously a new idea incompatible with previously held important ideas about the nature of his personality. Through his independent exploration of the relevance of the analyst's hypothesis to his way of living, and through the impingement and integration of consequent more accurate perceptions, his consciousness was modified. He became a man with a new awareness of himself.

What determines whether this new awareness will lead to a qualitative change in the patient's spontaneous interpersonal behavior? The brief presentation above does not answer the question; it does, however, indicate the direction of the answer. The patient did not withdraw, or become depressed, or attempt to procrastinate by rationalizing that the process must be a very long one. Instead, the recognition that he would not change without his own effort, in spite of his anxiety, was accepted as a challenge.

The process of healthy change of consciousness can for convenience be examined in a somewhat rough progression and separation of phases. In each, there are many possible ramifications. The acquisition of each insight into the patient's behavior opens up, for example, the further problem of exploring the patient's stake in maintaining his neurotic behavior. Different stages may take lesser or longer periods. Each stage may simultaneously involve several elements of the personality, and insight may be restricted by failure to recognize the existence or the nature of other elements, or to perceive the connections between and among these elements. The infinite complexity of personality change makes any structuralization necessarily an oversimplification. Still, it is possible to make some tentative formulations of stages or elements in the process of personality change during analysis, and to clarify to some extent the role of intellectual exchange in the total analytic activity.

As the process begins, the patient, either spontaneously or in response to questioning, reports to the analyst biographical data. These data reveal the attitudes, feelings, values, and practices of the patient in many ways—by direct statement, by his selection of incidents, and by his emphasis, emotional reaction, and inflection during the presentation. In response, the therapist formulates a new hypothesis regarding some aspect of the patient's personality.

Provided the therapist's formulation is close to reality, the hypothesis establishes a potentially crucial point in the therapeutic experience of the patient. It becomes crucial—that is, leading to change of consciousness—if the patient honestly examines the hypothesis. If he does, he responds to the hypothesis with associations—the spontaneous awakening of relevant memories (see pp. 12–13). This involves a willingness to experience and define feelings, and a deliberate, disciplined effort toward greater understanding of the attitudes related to these feelings. The patient who is predominantly unwilling to experience and define feelings and to examine attitudes, may develop confusion, be uncomprehending, or become involved in any of the resistance maneuvers discussed earlier in Chapter 6. To the extent, however, that the patient is determined to change, he gives the hypothesis tentative consideration and then, with disciplined concentration, engages himself in the activity of retrospective empathy, diligent introspection, and definition of his evolving and recalled affects. He re-evaluates the data he has presented as well as the new associative memories.

On the basis of his re-evaluative work with the analyst's tentative hypothesis, he may find that it has some validity. Sometimes he may constructively modify the analyst's hypothesis. The re-evaluation carries him beyond a hypothetical new view of himself to a new recognition of himself. He may resolve to institute or discontinue certain kinds of behavior. If this initial consideration of the hypothesis extends over several sessions, data from new experimental behavior may play a role. The new recognition, however, may have been derived within the therapeutic situation exclusively, through the activity of exchange of ideas between the analyst and the patient, and through the resultant introspection.

This change of consciousness makes possible another phase of intellectual activity, which is an extension and intensification of the re-evaluative process. There is a prolonged period of documentation, outside of and within the therapeutic sessions, of the patient's new conceptualization of himself. Through persistent inspection and constant searching recollection, and through the impact of sporadic, tentative, experimental behavior, the individual becomes aware of many thoughts, feelings, and actions which he had been interpreting unrealistically and which he now perceives freshly and more accurately.

The patient begins to see that what happens to him is at least in part a consequence of his own activity. Achievement of clarity is sometimes retarded by an overwhelming preoccupation with his past and present disappointments, frustration, anxieties, resentments, and sadness, and therefore considerable assistance from the analyst is required to maintain the focus upon the patient's specific responsibility for his own unhappiness. With deeper understanding of the correlation between the nature and the consequences of his own behavior, he has achieved a more fully integrated insight. He may still, however, be struggling vigorously against any fundamental modification of his interpersonal behavior.

Instances of healthily altered behavior may spontaneously follow deepening insight, sometimes even without the individual's awareness. More often, though—in spite of the patient's conviction of the necessity and benefit of change—determination, self-discipline, and courage are required in order for him to make indicated modifications in behavior. Now that he recognizes some of the practices that constitute his pathology, he sees that he must stop doing those things and start doing something different, and that it cannot be accomplished by glib resolution but only on the basis of long-term commitment. This is difficult, because even if he has had some experience along the new lines, he is not certain of the results of new practice, or the outcome of giving up familiar, even though recognizably sick, functioning. He feels anxiety, a threat of destruction of his personality (see p. 169). This does not apply to each and every instance of new behavior; changed behavior that has developed from new insight may be recognized by the patient only in retrospect. The struggle, the resolve, does nevertheless initially precede most incidents of changing practice.

Through repeated experiences of this kind, the patient moves toward spontaneous and established new behavior. Intensification of the process occurs from time to time as the result of the phenomenon of speculation. The individual begins to imagine himself relating to others in the manner of happier people he has observed, and enjoying better consequences. He begins to sense the possibility that he can become a different kind of person.

The patient gradually reaches major qualitative changes in personality—consistency and spontaneity in his new practices. The changed behavior is no longer merely stylistic or mimetic, nor is it maintained by self-discipline. It has grown out of a new, deeper understanding associated with changed values, new feelings, more spontaneously pursued healthy goals. It is sustained by the gratification inherent in the new behavior.

Through these experiences, the patient develops an expanded view of the possibilities of his life, together with a recognition of his real limitations. His self-concept has become more realistic. In the course of acting, feeling, and thinking differently, he makes new perceptions of the environment, achieves more understanding of himself in relation to the environment.

Instead of feeling like one who has lost his identity by changing, he feels an increased sense of self-integration and satisfaction. He feels like a new kind of individual. This experience increases his confidence, makes his desire and search for health more spontaneous and optimistic, and strengthens his determination, when required, in repeating all the previous processes on a higher level. In the therapeutic session his new consciousness, new conceptualization and practices, and new feelings, enable him to struggle with increasing success to change his personality still more.

These phases or elements in the change of consciousness are set forth in an attempt to define in greater detail the process of cure, the healthy change and growth of consciousness.[6] Naturally, all of the phases in the patient's changing relationship with other people take place also in his relationship with the analyst. He works on this relationship with the analyst, changes his behavior in that relationship, and has further personality change from his new experience with the analyst as well as from his new experience with others.

It must be kept in mind that people who are not and have never been in analysis can experience similar growth through life experience, through being forced by new circumstances into new kinds of practices. The analyst's role in making new hypotheses about an individual's activities may be filled by friends, a spouse, a relative, a teacher, even an enemy. If the individual who is criticized undertakes realistic self-examination, the above schematized process of changing consciousness can be initiated. In therapy, however, there are three unique and favorable conditions: the commitment of the patient to change, the psychoanalyst's skill, and the persistence of the analyst's efforts, over a long period of time, to initiate and foster the process of change.

As healthy personality change occurs, there is a phenomenon with profound therapeutic implications which sometimes arises: the occasional occurrence of *feelings of unreality*. This experience of opera-

[6] See B. S. Robbins, "The Process of Cure in Psychotherapy" in Paul H. Hoch and Joseph Zubin, *Current Approaches to Psychoanalysis*, Volume XIV. New York: Grune & Stratton, 1960, pp. 96–108.

tional and emotional disorientation, as patients report it, sounds alarmingly like a schizoid phenomenon. It is often as disturbing to the analyst as to the patient, and presents, therefore, a serious problem of technique. The uneasy therapist may desist from all therapeutic demands upon the patient and, even worse, may attempt to "support" him with "reassurances."

There are very definite and identifiable differences between schizophrenic panic and the feelings of unreality during healthy change. The schizophrenic, as he panics, loses his orientation to the world, no longer knows who he is, why he is doing what he does, what has gone before or what is ahead.[7] The patient who has feelings of unreality in the course of healthy change has become more related, better integrated with reality—his feelings, practices, and thinking have rather suddenly become more rational. What appears to be a feeling of unreality is a subjective sensation of his own personality being unfamiliar. New spontaneous behavior and new emotions are flowing from new insight, and they feel strange because the connection with insight is concurrently not identified. What such a patient has basically in common with the panicking schizophrenic is some degree of not feeling like himself. He differs crucially, however, in the direction in which his whole life process is moving. The panicking schizophrenic is experiencing a disintegration of personality; the patient with somewhat sudden emergent health is experiencing a greater integration of personality.

Whether or not there is accompanying anxiety—and there often is not anxiety, only the "unreal" feelings—it is important to delineate clearly with the patient the existence and nature of the healthy changes and their relation to his feelings of unreality. If, instead, the therapist desists from further demands, thinking that the patient is at a dangerous brink, the patient—especially if he senses the analyst's withdrawal—may not know how or where to proceed, and for him there is only one place to which he can retreat—to the familiarity of his pathology.[8]

If a generalized supportive "reassurance" is given, the patient may take superficial comfort from the analyst's interest, but basically he is more confused. He is being offered "support" at a point where he dimly senses an increment of strength. An opportunity is furthermore being lost to call the patient's attention to the *real* gains he has made. Except

[7] For an excellent description see Doris Bartlett, "Schizophrenic Panic," *Psychotherapy*, 1: 109–120, 1956.

[8] The analyst's withdrawal in this kind of situation has the same implications as therapeutic withdrawal from any anxiety-laden or potentially anxiety-laden area (see p. 180).

for the analyst's early speculations that his own skills combined with the patient's probable assets and necessary efforts are likely to be productive, genuine reassurance can occur only when there is evidence of change in the patient. The analyst, by underscoring this change, enables the patient then to experience newly or more strongly a sense of assurance regarding his established and emerging inner resources. It would be unfortunate to let the therapist's empty authority be substituted for this solid and healthy experience.

One further drawback of misplaced "reassurance" is that, for both patient and analyst, it fosters a subjective and objective dichotomy in the therapeutic relationship, as opposed to the practice and feeling of collaboration. When the analyst points to achieved progress, he is calling the patient's attention to the fruit of their joint effort. A merely "supportive" reassurance emphasizes to the patient his dependence upon the analyst for strength, and vitiates his contact with his own resources. For the analyst to deal with the patient in such a way is inappropriate in a framework in which the cooperativeness of the activity is itself the major force engendering personality change.

Emerging health sometimes brings manifestations of resistance in the form of sadness or gloom over the dying state of pathology. This cause of regret is invariably misinterpreted by the patient. An individual who is making progress and pointedly documenting his insight into persisting problems may sigh and say, "I am sad about seeing these sick things still there in myself." This may be wholly true. But when it is only partially true, and if the sadness reflects a weary reluctance to give up the neurotic way of life, it is essential to help him to delineate and document that reluctance.

The feeling that the improved situation "will not last" or that "something is going to happen" is another manifestation of this subtle reluctance to persist in therapeutic effort. It usually represents the patient's refusal to accept responsibility for his gains, and consequently for their continuance. The gloomy prediction is an attempt to establish for himself the conviction that coming events will depend entirely on external forces—not on what he does. This almost invariably foreshadows the patient's return to his former pathological way of functioning. He subjectively, not critically, senses the sad consequences of such a regression.

Regret may occur cloaked in a preoccupation with gains. A male patient, who had progressed far in developing independence, one day gave me a fully documented account of how well he was doing, but there was a discrepancy between the cheerful facts and the heaviness in his voice. I interrupted his report of new, mature, independent, and successful activities with the suggestion, "Let's try to detect in all these experiences the feelings of hesitation, the reluctances and fears that you've had to overcome—the elements of dependency you still have to contend with."

This was a moment of association, and he replied, "I had a dream the other night. It's kept coming back over the last few days" (Mother Just Died). It was these "last few days" which he had begun the hour by describing in a spirit of subdued cheer.

"Some woman said what a shame it was that my mother just died. I knew in the dream she was dead six years, but I went into another room and cried, and in the dream I was looking at myself crying and wondering why I was crying. It shouldn't have brought the tears, but when I went into the other room I really broke down. Still, I could sense that it was not a tragedy—I could get along."

In the dream, his attachment to his mother represented his problem of dependency, which he was in reality overcoming: health was not really a tragedy—"I could get along." He was "wondering why [he] was crying." He had thought he was dedicated to becoming manly and independent, and did not know how much he mourned the passing of the boyish dependent way of life. Pursuit of his feelings and his dream helped to clarify both the emerging health and the more obscure obstructive regret.

The evolution of health occurs, then, at all stages of analysis, and in the context of the pathology from which it is emerging. It is essential to detect the forms and interrelationship of the healthy and sick elements, as they are manifested in the patient's dreams, in his activity in the therapeutic sessions, and in his everyday life. For the patient, the evolution of health occurs in a struggle against the maintenance of a familiar but restricting pathological integrity. During the course of analysis, he learns the constructive techniques with which to struggle, and becomes increasingly more skillful and more committed to concurrent and future effort.

The influence of new, more gratifying and subjectively liberating experience is ultimately the most convincing and effective incentive to striving for health. Something of this conviction was expressed in the language of one patient's dream.

"Somebody was enclosed in walls. No one knew about it. He was closed in, and couldn't break out.

"I was the one inside, suffering in this closed area—and I was on the outside, too, struggling to let me out. I finally did it, and it felt so good."

9. Occurrence of the Analyst in Dreams

In a dream a patient was driving her car. A blue-eyed policeman whom she described as attractive and friendly stopped her and cautioned her not to go in that direction.

In the analytic session she soon became aware that her direction in the dream reflected the irrational course she was pursuing in her waking life, but she had no idea of the identity of the blue-eyed cop. When I hypothesized it might be me, her immediate response was, "But you don't have blue eyes." "Neither am I a cop," I said. She responded with laughter, in which I joined. She had not known how much she felt I policed her life, nor how warmly she responded to me in spite of this; nor was she aware that she had any response to my masculinity. With the dream as an introductory and symbolic statement, she then began to dare to examine her feelings about me.

How frequently is the analyst an individual in the dreams of a patient? Why does he appear? In what forms? In what kinds of action? In what kinds of relationship? Associated with what emotions?

The analyst appears in most of the dreams used in this book, not because of any intention or selection, but because the analyst occurs in a majority of each patient's remembered dreams. (See also the discussion of the dynamic concept of the dream, pp. 4 and 7.) Considerations of why he appears, his forms, actions, relations, and the accompanying dream feelings, have been explicit or inherent in past chapters.

The frequency with which the analyst, in human, animal, or inanimate form, appears in his patient's dreams is not surprising when all the reasons for his appearing are considered. A primary reason is that all of the patient's interpersonal problems become manifest, in one way or another, in the therapeutic interpersonal relationship. In addition, the analyst is an intimate participant in the examination of these problems. He is involved also in all of the patient's struggles to maintain pathological functioning, and in all the patient's struggles to change this functioning, to achieve new and healthier conceptualizations, feelings, and behavior. The analyst, then, is related to all the patient's old and new problems of feeling, thinking, and practice, and is recurrently woven into the substance of the patient's remembered dreams.

One basic premise underlying the examinations of the role the analyst plays in the dream life of the patient is that *the dream role reflects the patient's relationship with the analyst himself, not with the analyst as surrogate for somebody else.* It is, furthermore, a relationship of the present, not of the past.

Transference, the supposed transfer to the analyst of affects applicable to some other person, is an obscuring rather than an illuminating concept. The misperceptions, the distorted conceptualizations, the neurotic goals, the angers of frustration experienced toward the analyst, may be, for example, the result of a warp in the patient's personality that developed in the relationship with his father. The patient has, however, throughout his life been reacting with this warp in his personality. When he irrationally hates the analyst in the same way he hated his father, a parallel response has occurred. But he is a person spontaneously reacting with hatred in the immediate circumstances; we have no basis for assuming that this emergence of hatred in the analytic relationship is or can possibly be a response to someone outside the immediate interaction, a response which is then transposed to the analyst. To assume such a mechanism directs attention away from the patient's evolved and totally functioning personality.

The clinical problem is to investigate the kind of personality the patient has today, to seek out precisely what he is experiencing in reacting to the analyst, and to discover the elements of the immediate interpersonal situation which are engendering the irrational hatred.

The concept of transference has historically served two useful purposes: first, it calls attention to irrationality in interpersonal feeling and activity; and, second, it focuses upon the genesis of the irrationality in the patient's past, in the history of his experience with people. Both the irrationality and its genetic perspective can, however, be more fully explored and comprehended if unencumbered by the dubious concept of affective transposition.

Examination of the past, besides lending perspective, makes possible a critical distinction between the unmodifiable conditions of childhood and the potentially modifiable conditions of adulthood. Through his childhood memories the patient can examine the interpersonal matrix in which his personality developed. His practices sprang into being in response to specific situations, the responses arising without subjective awareness that there was any other choice. What the patient did was distorted, but it was the best he could possibly do as a child in an adult environment. Now, as an adult, he has a choice: he can make the choice to change, and he has the power to change. Sitting behind the couch, one may say with sympathy and conviction: "Thank God you were a little bitch then—it kept you from sinking under. You put up a nasty fight for some of the things you wanted and needed. You hit back, you pushed people off. You forged some kind of strength. You stayed alive."

It is equally necessary, however, to look at the angry, lonely, hardbitten, sometimes self-pitying patient, and to say more. "Yes, thank God you were a bitch then, *but it's not necessary to be one now.* Being a bitch kept you alive then—*it keeps you alone now.* You fended off your parents and your older sister then, but now, by acting the same way, you drive off friends, you drive off men who might want to marry you. *You are beating off everyone, including your analyst.*" [1]

The patient who dreamed of his small son performing fellatio on him (pp. 133–138) had been raised by a powerful father and a bullying older sibling. During his childhood, he had often experienced impotent, vindictive, and retaliatory rage because he could not force from his father a greater paternal interest. In his third year of analysis, at a time when considerable healthy change in his personality was manifesting itself, the patient became infuriated that he was still impotent to force the analyst to a paternal rather than an appropriate interest in him. The rage he felt toward me was the same *kind* of rage, but it was not a transference of anger actually felt toward his father and merely *expressed* toward me. It was *felt* toward me because of the nature of

[1] Irrational demands in the present engendered by deprivations in the past (transference distortions) are illustrated in relation to a husband in Chapter 6, "Resistance in Dreams," in the discussion of the dream Death of Husband, pp. 204–205.

the current interaction between us. It was the rage that this patient always felt toward people he could not manipulate.

It was at this time that he dreamed of using his helpless, passive child for sexual pleasure and for indulging himself in a sense of utter domination. Quite explicitly he said in the session, "I'd like to get you in the position where Henry was in the dream—where you're helpless, where I'm using you, degrading you."

The distortion in this man's personality was manifested in two ways—in his rages (or their psychosomatic equivalents) and in techniques of making people passive in his hands. He became that kind of person initially through the experiential molding effect of responding to certain kinds of treatment from his father. Treatment from others in the present, which may be similar, or which he interprets as being similar, engenders in him *freshly* in the present the same kinds of emotions.[2] His emotions are personality manifestations which arise under given circumstances, toward children or toward women, sometimes toward other men, often toward his analyst.

If one says to the patient that he is really angry at his father, not at the analyst, one deflects his attention from an intensive examination of his activity and feeling in response to the current situation, one comforts him by assigning blame to the past, and relaxes the urgency of his responsibility for the present. The patient must deal with himself as a creature of the present in the life of the present.

Interaction with the analyst is the focal interpersonal experience in which the distinction is made between the restricting child status of the past and the powers and possibilities for change in the present and future. It is potentially liberating to the patient to make this distinction. The sudden recall of a childhood experience comes not because of the intrusion of a past emotion but because of the identity in the nature of present and past emotions.[3] It is helpful to orient the patient in some fashion, such as by saying, "The feeling you experience now reminds you of the way you felt and the way you acted then, because all of these feelings and actions are much the same. But there are crucial differences between the conditions then and now: You had neither knowledge of people nor freedom of movement then—now you have both.

"We can discover what your behavior is producing now with others, and also with me, and what different possibilities there are for

[2] See B. S. Robbins, "The Myth of Latent Emotions," *Psychotherapy,* 1: 3–30, 1955.

[3] For discussion of emotional similes, see p. 13.

you if you use your capacities differently. If you discern and discontinue those elements of your behavior which contribute to unhappy consequences, you will have new experiences and new feelings in relating to people."

The frequency with which the analyst occurs in his patient's dreams can give rise to distortions in the analytic process, sometimes introduced by the patient, sometimes by the analyst. The failure to identify or acknowledge the analyst as the individual in dreams is a common form of resistance. Even if a character in the dream brings the analyst to mind, the resisting patient will discount his own free association. He may say, "I *automatically* think of you as a possibility," or "I think it's you because *you* always think so." At other times the patient privately makes these or similar rationalizations, stubbornly neglecting to verbalize the occurrence of the therapist as an association. The resistance is sometimes the patient's resentment at the importance of the analyst in his life. More often, however, an adverse reaction to the frequency of the therapist's presence in dreams is only incidental, and the resistance relates more directly to the specific problem of the dream.

The analyst, on his part, may introduce distortion by being automatic and arbitrary in assigning himself a particular role in the patient's dream. Such glibness in interpretation tends to stimulate or re-enforce, if not to justify, the kind of resistance just described. The mistake in interpretation may arise as follows: the analyst recognizes in the dream an interpersonal problem; the patient is having this difficulty not only with the analyst but also concurrently with another person; the analyst identifies the individual in the dream as himself—the dream, however, refers specifically to the relationship with the other person, perhaps a husband, son, neighbor, or parent. The analyst's suggestion that the difficulty pertains to himself is out of harmony with the emotional and experiential matrix of the patient's associations. An artificial framework for exploration is constructed by the analyst. Perhaps, in addition, a false issue is created between him and the patient—the analyst believes the patient is resisting, whereas the patient is really talking about a different part of his life.

Sometimes a problem that the patient formerly had with the analyst, but which he has worked out, comes up later with a new person. For example, a patient may have struggled with the problem of acquiescence in his relationship with the analyst and may have had substantial success in overcoming this difficulty. Months later, in a relationship with a girl friend, his old problem of acquiescence again arises, and he comes into the therapeutic situation with a dream. The problem is in the patient's relationship with his new girl friend, but the analyst is not aware of this. The patient may not yet associate the disturbance reflected in the dream to his relationship with the girl, but he may nevertheless reject intuitively attempts by the analyst to make acquiescence toward himself the problem of the dream. The analyst would be quite wrong to say, "Ah, I guess the old problem of acquiescence toward me is still alive." The patient may even say, "I thought of you in connection with this dream, but I still don't think that acquiescence toward *you* is the problem." Indeed, by such an assertion the patient would be virtually demonstrating that acquiescence toward the analyst was *not* the problem. If the analyst at this point should interpret the patient's disagreement as resistance, he would be introducing the following distortions into the relationship with his patient: (1) He would be acting against the cooperative nature of the therapeutic process. (2) He would be blocking the way to investigation of the problem of acquiescence toward the girl friend. (3) He might be robbing the patient of a valid sense of achieved progress in his dealing with acquiescence in the analytic relationship. (4) The patient would sense something arbitrary in the analyst's interpretively assigning himself a central role in the dream; this would cause him to doubt the analyst's self-identification in subsequent dreams where the occurrence of the analyst is authentic, and would interfere with investigating the nature of the patient-analyst relationship.

When such an initial therapeutic mistake has already occurred, value can still be derived from the dream. In the hypothetical case above, even after the therapist had misidentified "the old problem of acquiescence" toward himself, he might, in deference to the patient's honest disagreement, have said, "Well, I may be entirely off the track; let's go ahead and see what associations you have," or, "Do you have a different hunch about the dream?" With this, there would then have been a good opportunity to get to the associations about the girl friend and to an eventual recognition of his disturbing acquiescent practices with her. The total therapeutic movement could then have been productively evaluated for the patient in somewhat the following manner: "You've come a long way in dealing with your problem of acquiescence. Certainly your progress in overcoming your acquiescence with me has made analysis more productive; in this hour, by refusing to acquiesce to my ideas, you've made progress possible in several directions. You've made it possible for us to get much more out of the dream, to examine other areas in which you are still acquiescent, and to see how this is interfering in your relationship with X."

It has been repeatedly emphasized how similar the patient's ways of relating in interpersonal experience with the analyst are to his ways of relating with others. There are nevertheless several somewhat unique features which color the therapeutic interaction and its reflections in dreams.

The perpetual requirement of trust—the necessity for the patient to reveal himself utterly in the analytic relationship—is one of the factors that distinguishes it from other relationships. The amenities and all the aggressive and defensive social maneuvers of everyday life which preserve insularity are strongly subjected to nullifying influences in the active analytic milieu. Whatever problems the patient has in relating intimately (for example, cynicism, competitiveness, anxiety) operate in analysis just as they do in other interpersonal contacts. In analysis, however, trust is a basic assumption of the activity into which the patient has voluntarily come. There is a pressure and a necessity to lay bare his mind and emotions; the requirement, as well as the patient's limitations in this area, are held constantly in focus. His failures in trusting seem disproportionately large because of a pressure upon him rarely equaled in other relationships.

A second factor in the therapeutic interpersonal relationship which causes it to differ from the patient's relationships with other people is the patient's *continual subjection to the analyst's intense influence.* Such exposure to another's influence complicates the problem of the constant required trust.

In previous chapters I have discussed the cultural forces producing a "western man" whose personality develops through social experience to function in a competitive, manipulative, and counterinfluential manner. Underlying these emotional, conceptual, and behavioral distortions is the conviction, usually unaware, that interpersonal relations always involve either power over others or subjugation to them, and that therefore the goal of interpersonal influence is always to gain competitive advantage and dominance.

All human interaction consists of mutual influence. The influences we give or receive may be aware or unaware, and may be salutary or destructive. The evolution toward health includes the development of the ability to *discriminate* between salutary and destructive influence. In the analytic relationship, the patient must struggle early and intensively to overcome the impulses toward *indiscriminate* application of his counterinfluencing techniques, and he must expose himself voluntarily to a constant interpersonal influence—one which he needs but can benefit from only to the extent that he is able to commit himself to it. Unlike his other relationships, in analysis he must strive to permit the influence, to collaborate with it, and to do so constantly and across the total span of his personality.

Eventually, of course, the patient evolving toward health by means of this collaboration comes to recognize that he is engaging in the development, with another person's help, of new kinds of independent functioning. In the course of this process of change, however, while the patient is wrestling with the pathological problems of influence and counterinfluence, his competitiveness may be re-enforced by certain pathological perceptions of the nature of the analytic social dyad. Some actual advantages of the analyst are perceived by the patient as sources of threatening competitive advantage in the interpersonal exchange. The therapist often has economic or educational advantages, or both. He has professional status. He may have the advantage of age over youth—or sometimes of youth over age. In our culture there is the real advantage of male over female; whichever way the sex of the analyst varies from that of the patient, the variance is almost certain to provoke and re-enforce the competitiveness of the patient.

Competitive response by the patient to the analyst may not be due entirely to the patient's misperceptions. There may be real problems of competitiveness, culturally shared, in the personality of the analyst. The analyst's problems may relate to any of the status factors just listed, or may be of a personally specific nature.[4] Commonly involved is the analyst's carefully and competitively guarded emotional reticence.

The patient's competitive orientation toward all people is, then, intensified by his uniquely exposed position and by the uniquely continuous and pervasive exercise of the analyst's influence. Furthermore, the cultural forces at work in the analyst and in the analytic situation may additionally engender the patient's pathological reactions to influence.

Associated both with the need to trust and with the patient's competitive resistance to influence is the problem of his *cynicism* (see pp. 64–86), a third factor that is uniquely accentuated in the analytic relationship. In undertaking analysis, the patient is committing himself to an intimate relationship on the basis of a premise to which, in most cases, he cannot yet subscribe. The patient tries to believe that the analyst will not misuse his professional position, will not harm or use the patient for the gratification of personal desires for power or glory.

---

[4] For an unusual and valuable discussion of the occurrence of the patient in the dreams of the analyst, see E. S. Tauber and M. R. Green, *Prelogical Experience,* New York: Basic Books, Inc., 1959. For another rich source of meaningful observations on the therapeutic interpersonal process, see Frieda Fromm-Reichmann, *Principles of Intensive Psychotherapy,* Chicago: University of Chicago Press, 1950.

He tries to believe that the analyst will keep the patient's welfare as the constant focus of their activity. But he does not yet have a real belief in the analyst's sincerity, and therefore, as a result of the unusual pressure to trust and his intensified competitiveness in the analytic situation, there will arise a correlative accentuation of his cynicism, which is then reflected in the dream representations of the analyst.[5]

You Hold Me Close

The young woman who dreamed of the analyst as a crazy woman (pp. 73–77) had many other dreams which indicated that her limited capacity and great need to trust made the perpetual intimate contact of analysis, simultaneously frightening and tempting. The problem of her fear and cynicism showed slow, agonizing resolution, reflected over six years in the changing symbolism[6] of the recurrent analyst in her dreams. Early in her analysis, her desire for closeness and her simultaneous aggressive cynical defense against it were expressed in her dream of a paternal kindly senator. In this dream she at first felt toward the symbol of the analyst a type of filial warmth, which soon turned to disdain as she became seductive and he leered.

The Crazy Woman dream occurred two and a half years later, and was followed by five months of intensive pursuit of feelings in dreams and in daily experience, carried out in the captive intimacy of analysis. During these painful months she was anxiously risking a great trust. A vivid nightmare (Parachute Dream) revealed her deep uncertainty. She dreamed of taking a plunge toward intimacy—jumping from a high window at the urging of an unidentified "trusted friend" who had given her a parachute to make the attempt safe. She landed with a great crash because the trusted friend had tricked her by sewing the parachute to keep it from opening.

After these five months of analytic progress she continued her struggle during the summer vacation, and returned with a dream that, in its total context, demonstrates both her difficulty with intimacy and its unique accentuation in the analytic relationship.

The patient came in for her first session after a ten-week summer intermission. She shook hands firmly, showing as much intimate warmth as she had ever dared and at the same time revealing her characteristic

[5] See, for example, Parachute Nightmare, Contemptible Passion, Token Kindness, Kindly Senator. For a discussion of the reciprocal relationship between competitiveness and cynicism, see Chapter 2, "Feeling in Dreams," p. 95.

[6] See discussion of changing symbolism in Chapter 1, "Symbolism in Dreams," pp. 45–46.

tendency to shrink away from contact. She sat down on the edge of the couch, exchanged a few words about vacations, and thanked me for the card I had sent her. Then she said that she would like to get to work. She lay down, and started: "I've had several dreams about you during the summer. One of them I recall very clearly." She was silent for a few seconds and began breathing heavily. "I'm choking to death—but let me get this over." She forced her way on. "The dream—and I shall tell you *exactly* how I feel in this dream, everything—in this dream you physically put your arm around my waist and physically hold me close. [Pause of a few seconds.] A number of emotions *violently* come upon me. They are very conflicting. First emotion: I feel good. Second emotion: I feel a terrible discomfort and fear. Third emotion—no, it's a thought, and it's the thing that preoccupies me in the dream: How am I to interpret this action? How am I to think you reason? Either you're a bastard and teasing me, or you're doing a nasty, a bitchy thing, but you don't realize it and your intentions are good. Or, you're doing an *ordinary* thing and it shouldn't bother me at all. You are not raping me. It's very usual and normal and it's very wrong of me to get upset.

"By the way, in this dream, while you're holding me this way you point out that inside it's comparatively dark and outside it's light. You're showing me the light.

"All this is how I really do feel. I haven't wanted to feel all these feelings about you. It's upsetting. But it all comes out in the dream, and it's the way I feel."

I asked her if there were any sexual overtones in the dream, whether I was excited.

She answered immediately, without undue emphasis, "No—it all looked very innocent. I'm puzzled about my feelings. I want you to depuzzle me." She was silent, waiting for me to explain.

I said, "I can't choose from these feelings and tell you which one to reserve as your exclusive feeling. I can't really 'depuzzle' you, but there are a few things that occur to me. It seems to me that in this dream and in your waking feelings there are elements of the Parachute nightmare. In that nightmare, you remember, you were deceived by a trusted friend. *I* was your trusted friend, and I showed complete treachery. You've come a long way since then. There is actually now more trust—you experience trust close to someone in the dream, and you feel trust in your waking moments, the way you act toward me now. You have some doubts about my motives, but my threat to you is slight compared to the cataclysmic destruction in the Parachute nightmare that you had last spring. There you were persuaded to jump and then found the parachute sewn together, and you had the feelings both of being deceived and of being dashed to pieces. In this dream, and in your feelings today in telling me the dream, elements of your fear and distrust are present, but the degree of trust and the degree of sureness about your positive feelings and your sense of security and comfort while you experience these emotions, is tremendous compared with how you felt when you dreamed about the parachute."

She said, "I wanted to believe you were innocent in the dream—either that it was nasty but well intended, or ordinary and normal and well intended." Then she continued, "I guess I *can* answer it. Emotionally and logically I want to believe that you do the right thing—but no, it doesn't—I'm sorry, it can't—I still emotionally believe you're being very nasty to me, but you're innocent and don't realize what you're doing. I guess that's a step forward in the dream, as well as consciously. I want to believe that you are innocent in your intentions, but I can't believe your behavior is nice, even though your intentions may be.

"The thing is, though, *I've got to believe.* Do I have to believe everything you do is all right? Maybe we can still work together. I suppose you feel it would be a good sort of exercise for me to feel close to you—as practice. From your point of view, it doesn't mean anything. But from my point of view it's playing with TNT. To you, it's all so casual and easy."

I said, "I certainly do not take your fear and your struggle lightly, and I would not synthesize warmth to give you something to feel warm about. It would be disrespectful, and would never help you."

She went on exploring the problem. "What is this TNT? I don't want to frustrate myself. To love makes me *want* love. And that would be very impractical. It's worse than just not having you. If my life were more satisfying than it is, it wouldn't be so bad. My frustration isn't just plain frustration, but terrible, *torturous* frustration. I guess that's what the TNT is. I'm not clear. No, I *am* clear. That's why I don't want to be a reasonable amount of warm and friendly to you, because it's teasing to me. I'd rather have nothing."

I interrupted in order to attempt clarification. "I don't think that you would really rather have nothing. Furthermore, you can't disown the feelings that you actually have. I think it would really be easier for you to face your loving me than to feel it and try to deny it. Enjoy your loving me. It is a feeling you have now as a woman, not as a little girl, and it's a good feeling to have.[7] You've told me when you've hated me, and feared me, and distrusted me. You've acknowledged those feelings and suffered with them. Now enjoy your feelings of love, even

---

[7] See discussion of the patient's love for the analyst on pp. 226–228, 290.

though you can't have love in return. To deny any important feeling that you have is to become disoriented about all of your feelings. But if you acknowledge your feelings of love for me, you can be sure of what you are and who you are, something that has been so hard for you to achieve."

She responded at once, "Maybe I might be more willing if my feelings could be a secret. But I have to tell you. I don't want to talk about these things at all. If I didn't have to talk about them, then our relationship could be warm. I want to say, 'To hell with that, let's not talk about that.' Then I could feel it here. Then it wouldn't be so threatening, and I could be friendly. That reminds me of my mother. I really believe that she is friendly to me, but she just won't show it."

It was the end of the hour. Her initial anxiety, the heavy breathing and inner struggle on the couch, had all subsided in the course of the session and were replaced by some quiet tears. She sat up, looking a bit shaken, but she was able to look at me directly, which required some courage. She appeared more sure of herself and less lost than on so many previous occasions. With quiet directness she asked for an extra minute to wipe the mascara streaks from her face before she went out.

A reflection of achieved health and progress toward trusting was this patient's representation of the analyst in a clear, realistic dream portrayal of himself—no longer a crazy woman or a homosexual sister, not leering at her like the kindly senator nor destroying her with a defective parachute like the untrustworthy "trusted friend." In the dream You Hold Me Close the analyst was a real man showing warmth and affection. Her feelings of trust had finally dominated over fear, cynicism, and competitiveness. The prospects of fulfilling her desire for love and intimacy in the analytic relationship were gloomy, but the prospects were now brighter outside; this was indicated when she stated that, as the analyst held her intimately and closely, he was pointing outside and "showing me the light."

To offer much more than you can hope to receive and at the same time to maintain trust in the interest and concern of the loved person (especially when you are paying him for his professional services) is a difficult interpersonal test for anyone.

A fourth factor that is uniquely accentuated in the analytic interpersonal relationship is the *constant stimulus to anxiety residing in the effort to trust, to collaborate, and to change.* In his daily life outside of analysis the patient may be able to adjust to threatening situations or to avoid them; unexpected workability of his pathology, or the appearance of unsuspected healthy resources, may serve to carry him from situation to situation despite anxieties. In analysis, however, the commitment to conceptual, emotional, and behavioral change is like a perpetual promise of anxiety-laden situations, both in and out of treatment, all directly related to the activity of the analyst.

A fifth and final aspect of the special interpersonal framework of the analytic situation is the *involvement of the analyst with the spontaneous search for and enjoyment of healthy change.* The analyst is not always the threatener and the antagonist. The patient in the You Hold Me Close dream felt that there was, on the part of the analyst, a warmth and a desire to help her. Sometimes the patient, appreciating the analyst's unremitting efforts, regrets his own obstruction. The patient who walked on the road (Holding Him Back) blocking the way was not anxious or angry, and in the dream he knew that the person he was obstructing was a good friend. Similarly, one woman, married a dozen years and with several children, had a very brief dream (No Intercourse Yet) the night after she was told by the analyst that although she had worked conscientiously on some problems, she had managed for nearly two years to avoid going deeply into the subject of her sex life. Her dream was: "My husband made a comment to the effect that here we'd been married a whole month and hadn't had intercourse yet. I felt very badly because I'd been so thoughtless." For the patient at this time the prospect of change through her work in analysis had, like marriage, the promise of a new life. The analyst was represented as someone to whom she was not responding adequately, and to whom, without accompanying dread or anger, she felt very close.

He's Not So Bad

The following dream of beginning change and enjoyment of change associated with the analyst reveals a considerable range and transition of feeling. The patient was an unmarried, attractive, creative, thirty-five-year-old woman who had been brought up to feel superior to other people. Her regal grandmother had objected to her playing with the "common" children on their street. Her mother disdained sewing, and so the family's sharpest term of derogation was "Dummer Schneider!" ("Stupid tailor!"). The patient had kept herself somewhat aloof from analysis during her first year, but had tried hard to be friendly.

"I go into a room where my grandmother is shouting vituperations at a man in the window of an apartment across the court. I take over and shout at him, but I realize my heart is not in it. I really have nothing against him.

"Later in the dream he is helping me to hem a dress. He's not so bad after all. He's very skillful.

"He does not do it all, but leaves some for me, and I don't resent this."

She immediately associated to the dress she was wearing and said, "I never could bear sewing. This dress has been in my closet a long time because the skirt was too long. Finally I altered it.

"The person helping me with the skirt was you."

She described her grandmother as "imperious, tyrannical—part of the policy that I was too good to play with other children on the block."

In the dream, her grandmother was an individual representing the patient's "imperious" attribute, something that made her angry with the analyst, whom she had kept at a distance, "across the court." Then, as she took over in her more realistic form, she found when shouting at him that her "heart is not in it." She brings the analyst in closer, into her home, working with her. He is in the contemptible (for her) role of a tailor, yet she admires his skill and feels "he's not so bad." Futhermore, she accepts his bringing about her cooperation, thereby indicating the beginning of the resolution of her struggle against his influence: "He does not do it all, but leaves some for me, and I don't resent this."

This dream and the patient's interpretive activity together reflect the patient's germinal acceptance of the singularly influential and intimate role of the analyst in the healthy alteration of her personality.

The analytic relationship, then, is unique in that it makes necessary an almost inordinate degree of trust, subjects the patient to constant and intense interpersonal influence, provokes the most isolating defensive cynicism, is the most persistent source of anxiety, and is also, more than any other relationship, the source of welcome change. The analyst, the participant-agent in all these interactions, recurrently pervades the waking and sleeping consciousness of the patient.

10. Terminal Dreams

Terminal dreams may be roughly defined as dreams that occur during the last few months of a predetermined, mutually accepted termination of analysis. The term may also refer to dreams that occur during the period leading to a discussion of termination, during the period of discussion, and afterward. "Terminal" refers here to the planned conclusion of productive treatment, and not, by and large, to circumstances of arbitrary or unavoidable interruption.

Consideration of dreams from the terminal phase of analysis is basically a consideration of the criteria and problems of termination. To evaluate the patient's assets and handicaps is an intricate task for both analyst and patient during this difficult time. The patient may wish for termination, or he may wish to avoid it. There may be healthy or unhealthy reasons for his desire to continue.

His feelings toward this long-standing relationship and its intense, vital activity are likely to be mixed. The patient's terminal dreams and waking activity occur during a period of more rapidly evolving health, a more actively advancing process of personality change, than ever before experienced. In this new context, all of the analytic problems already considered continue to arise; they are now, however, more readily and more competently dealt with by the patient because of the therapeutic gains he has achieved.

The patient will have developed more meaningful, friendly, noncompetitive relationships with others and a greater capacity to give and to receive love; he will be less cynical, more spontaneous and genuine in his emotions, more realistically self-confident, and more realistically aware of his limitations. He will have made significant inroads into the solution of his major personality difficulties. He will have established a good beginning toward the fullest use of his intellectual and emotional potential. These are the positive accomplishments.

Some of the difficulties of ending analysis are related to the patient's erroneous expectations when he entered analysis; he may have entertained the notion that termination would coincide with a cessation of all his painful problems—that he would have developed great skill in "operating" socially, or would have transformed himself in some way that would make him universally acceptable, or perhaps that he would have rid himself of all the constraints, angers, anxieties, and other feelings that had complicated his interpersonal activities. Remnants of the unlikely expectation—that through analysis he will surmount all problems—distort for the patient the meaning of termination. He may cling, reluctant to abandon hopes of fulfilling the "ideal" and unreal condition; or he may be eager to terminate prematurely, because of a reluctance to commit himself to the new ways of dealing with life problems if the early "promise" of analysis is not to be fulfilled.

In contrast with the patient's fantasy of "cure," successful termination takes place instead when the patient can spontaneously approach his continuing or new problems in a rational, constructive fashion. He combines independence with cooperation, and employs all the skills acquired in analysis, including free association, the exploration of feelings, and the use of dreams.

The following brief presentation—a dream and the patient's dealing with it in his analytic hour—demonstrates both the patient's ambivalence [1] and his highly developed capacity to apply rationality and analytic skills relatively early in a terminal phase of analysis. (A detailed discussion of specific criteria for termination, and further clinical illustrations, will follow.)

THE PRINCIPAL'S OFFICE

The patient, who had hated the influence of his family and then of his analyst, was approaching the end of three years in analysis. He was the young man who had earlier experienced a dream in which he had enjoyed remaining coolly unresponsive to the efforts of an old woman (analyst) who was trying to arouse him (Old Woman Mastur-

---

[1] Ambivalence during healthy change: see Captain-Woman dream, pp. 254–257.

bating Him, p. 148). About two months before the session to be reported, we had had a discussion in which it had been agreed that his
progress justified our seriously considering termination at the beginning of summer. His healthy development had accelerated during the
two months, but his course had nevertheless been characterized, as is
so often the case, by alternations of therapeutic advance and retreat.
The advance had flowered in an increasingly mature love relationship,
and the patient had begun to think seriously of marriage. The retreat
was an increasing pathological resentment of the constructive changes
that were becoming obvious in his personality.

At this time he dreamed about returning, in his adult state and
"spoiling for a fight" with the principal, to visit the public school of his
childhood. He was provocative and insolent, and said to the principal,
"What a jerk you are! Who told you you knew how to educate people?"
Then, "The principal was about to reply and I got frightened and left
before he could get started."

The patient immediately identified me as the principal. When I
asked him what his feelings were toward the principal in the dream,
he lay silently on the couch for a long two minutes, then suddenly announced, "I started to go to sleep." (As in the dream, the patient did
not want to hear the analyst "get started.") After further association to
the "dumb bastard" principal, he recalled that at the exceptionally
fruitful previous session, during which he had explored his feelings
about his girl, he had "wanted to find out what you thought of my
getting married to Shirley. . . . I wanted to use you as an excuse to
get out of it. I was [and he elided back to the dream] . . . laying for
the principal, provoking him. I thought he'd tell me what a brat I used
to be back in public school."

I interrupted, "Let's leave the dream and pursue your feelings
toward *me*."

He replied, "I'll tell you what's really annoyed me: the last two
times I've been here it's been very gratifying and I haven't wanted to
believe it. I'm getting well and I'm changing a lot. But I've been trying
to believe that I've really just been putting something over on you. I
want to feel it's not really happening."

He paused a moment and suddenly said, "Now I know what the
dream means. I made you into a jerk. I said you don't know how to
educate people. Then you were just about to say to me, 'You *were* a
brat,' and I didn't want to hear—because it meant that I *used to be*
something that *I'm not any more*. I haven't wanted to believe I've
changed."

His feelings about termination were strong and mixed. He had nearly five months of analysis ahead, and was moving in a way that he found "very gratifying." Yet in the dream he was putting on a consoling charade of being in the same state as when, in elementary school, he derived his sense of self from functioning as a rebellious "brat." At the same time in the dream he had anxiety, because insight, actively part of his sleeping consciousness, encompassed his personality change.

The patient worked well in the session. He responded coopera- tively to the stimulus of the analyst, pursued his own feelings, and also tackled on his own initiative the problem reflected in the dream; in this manner he reached the meaning of the dream. He was afraid and angry because of the interpersonal influence that had effectively acted upon him, and he was simultaneously "gratified" by his awareness of the results of this influence. In the dream he ran away to avoid hearing of change. In his waking state, too, he wanted to run from the recogni- tion that he had changed. But his healthy efforts predominated.

Criteria for Termination

The patient's fitness for termination must be considered from two standpoints. One is retrospective—the measurement of his progress in the correction of his most crippling personality pathology; this progress must be substantial, although the potential for improvement may vary with different patients. The other standpoint is current and prospec- tive; it is the evaluation of the individual's readiness to terminate the formal clinical process and to carry his gains forward without assist- ance from the analyst.

There are *five criteria* for evaluating the individual's readiness. The first is evidence in the patient of a high degree of *awareness,* both of the changes that have occurred in his personality and of his persist- ing pathological attitudes regarding these changes. Either denial or exaggeration of change indicates inadequate preparation for dealing with persisting problems.

A second criterion is spontaneous, intensive, direct *communica- tion* in the analytic situation. Communication at termination must in- clude correlations the patient makes between the new ways he relates to others and the new ways he relates to the analyst. This correlating process tends to dissolve the dichotomy between analysis and "life." It makes the analyst more of an ordinary human being for the patient, and it makes the patient feel more like a unified ordinary human being in his relations with all others, now including the analyst.

A third major criterion for terminating is evidence of genuine *commitment* to continuing independent work on problems.

Fourth is the patient's initiative and spontaneity in the *use of the tools acquired in analysis:* free association, pursuit of emotions, and the ready intensive employment of dream material, with particular emphasis upon validation through experiential documentation.

The patient's achievement of a capacity to *function independently and at the same time with the analyst's participation* constitutes a fifth important criterion for evaluating the patient's readiness to end his formal analytic experience.

ROYALTY COMING TO AN END

The following presentation of a dream with its clinical context demonstrates another patient's progress toward fulfillment of the criteria for termination. The patient, a kindly, soft-spoken physician, had come into analysis for training. Nothing was accomplished during the first year, beyond a minimal impingement upon him of the fact that he was often unaware of his feelings and that, like other mortals in analysis, he needed treatment. In the course of everyday living, this patient often became angry with his wife and children for not showing sufficient affection and deference. His patients, his friends, and his staff members of lower rank, on the other hand, all bowed to his kindness and wisdom, and he behaved toward them as a benevolent father. Gradually over the next two years he made progress in demanding less deference, in beginning to live a more companionate life with his wife, and a less lordly one with his children. His relationships in general became warmer, his professional life more productive. These ordinary successes, however, were cold comfort compared with his former grandiose satisfactions. As he improved, he dreamed once of living in Siberia, where, in addition to the chill and the barrenness of the setting, his family and others failed to praise the food he prepared as they camped along the way: "They don't show a great deal of enthusiasm for what I have cooked up for them," he sadly related, interpretively.[2]

Three months before termination he came in with the following dream, which he said was vague in detail but clear in essence. "Royalty was coming to an end in the United States. There was no lamentation, but an intellectual concern. What adjustments would we have to make in the process of democratization? I had some anxiety over what would happen now."

He tried to recall more, failed, and began to comment. "It's ludi-

[2] This is an example of a patient's independent interpretive activity—initiative in the use of tools acquired in analysis.

crous. It seems I'm making fun of myself in the dream. I laughed at it as I woke up."

I said, "Laughing at it on waking up is not the same as laughing at it during the dream. In the dream you experienced some anxiety." I then reminded him that he had often denied anger by laughing it off.

He accepted the challenge and began to look seriously at his problem.[3] His first association was his ten-year-old son. "Arnold's become quite sharp in his criticism, now that I've stopped cracking down on him. I gave him a little lecture about there being no more royalty in this house, something about more democracy." The patient expanded a little on the parental problem of discipline.

I interrupted to comment that the focal problem was that of "royalty" and not that of raising children with adequate discipline. "You've been royalty with your wife, too," I reminded him. "With regard to the children, some of your difficulty arises from a confusion between normal paternal responsibility and maintaining a regal role in your home."

He picked this up.[4] "I remember now, when Arnold stamped off to the bathroom to wash, as I had instructed him to do, I was concerned. I was thinking to myself, 'How can I be a *good* king?'"

He followed immediately and spontaneously by turning to his marriage and profession, and exploring these areas within the emotional framework of his kinglike attitudes and demands.[5] He said he had just finished writing a paper. His wife had been very reasonable in not objecting to his taking time away from the family for this work. Then, continuing to make fair appraisal of her, in contrast with the old complaints about her not giving enough recognition to the importance of his work, he said, "But I think she objects to my not being able to relax with the family when I'm *not* working. It's hard to settle down. There are so many things I want to do at once. I don't seem to accept my limitations. My grandiose goals continue. I was glad to get this paper finished, yet I resented having to spend so much time, instead of being able to do a good job effortlessly.

"Maybe I have a stake in keeping a lot of work ahead of me, to maintain my importance—my head-of-state position. People are waiting for the work of the great man. Maybe this is the royalty.

"I straightened out a metal strut of my little girl's bicycle fender and she said, 'Daddy, you're so strong.' I used to cultivate that in them.

[3] This is an example of the patient working independently and at the same time collaboratively with the analyst.

[4] See preceding footnote.

[5] This is an example of validation through experiential documentation.

So I made a long speech about how it was nothing, any Daddy could do it, I'm really not stronger than a lot of people, etcetera, etcetera."

He paused a moment and I interpolated softly, "A grandiose speech of self-effacement?" He burst out laughing and then said, "It's so hard to give it up!"

Then, becoming entirely serious, he spontaneously pursued the theme of the dream. "I know I was not making fun of myself in the dream—I really *am* concerned about giving up royalty. I get a feeling of annoyance when I don't get recognition from the children. I feel my kingdom has been taken away by analysis, so I'm still trying to be chief in some of the lower courts." [6] He paused, then added, "I'm still looking for respect."

I felt that his final sentence was a slight retreat into unclarity after a very honest self-confrontation and communication. I therefore concluded the hour with a reclarifying comment: "Respect for you from the children is important for *them.* Just keep it respect, not awe. When you're respected by them, it's not because you're a king, it's because you're a man, and a father."

Throughout the session, the consistency and intensity of the patient's awareness and searching, and his readily communicated documentation, conveyed his commitment to continuing independent analytic effort.

THE SPECIAL GUN

The male social worker who, early in analysis, had the Analyst-Chauffeur dream was at termination still struggling, but now struggling successfully, with the problem of his dependent tyranny and with a related problem, his sadism.

In the dream, "I had a very special gun. It could be set in two different positions. In one it gave off a ray that had healing, curative properties; the second position was for killing. I was using it in a healing way, but I was afraid of the second notch into which the mechanism could slip.

"I was getting pleasure using the curative position in the dream. The gun had a rechargeable battery. I was worried that I didn't know enough about how to use it, but felt I could go ahead and use it to help as long as I needed to, and it wouldn't get lost or used up.

"Then I was showing someone how it could go into the killing position. I end up being attacked and shooting many people, like the ending of 'A Connecticut Yankee in King Arthur's Court.'"

[6] This whole passage indicates awareness of gains and of persisting problems, and also demonstrates straightforward communication.

The patient had opportunity for only a few interpretive statements, as it was the end of the session. He wasted no time. "In the dream I don't know where I got the gun. It was from a different culture—that makes me think of you: you've handed me understanding—something I can use to help or to hurt. That you 'handed' it to me denies that I got it from our working together.[7]

"My increased awareness and understanding of myself and of other people—I can use that to be more skillfully destructive than I was before. I don't think I have done this."

He made a spectacular "killing" at the end of the dream, "like the end of the Connecticut Yankee." This was in keeping with his long history of good-natured sarcasm, his witty undermining of friends and family. It was true, however, that his greater awareness had come to be used predominantly in a constructive way.

Several weeks later he was "feeling good about progress and able to do more. I've moved more and more toward feeling Doris' [wife] and the children's needs, and instead of wiping out my awareness I've been acting on it, more and more." [8] But also, he said ambivalently, on another day, "I'm trying to wipe out cooperation with Doris."

His difficulty continued, with anxieties and rages, toward his wife and analyst. But his recognition of the problems became continually sharper, his self-appraisal more accurate and quick, and his independent and cooperative attack on his neurosis more consistent and effective. The cooperative work on his sick behavior was pursued not only with his analyst but also with his wife. (Among married people, development of this latter capacity is an incidental but often important criterion for termination.)

The same patient's readiness for termination, measured by the criteria of his orientation toward persisting pathology, was reflected vividly in another dream and his handling of it, a few weeks before the end of treatment.

MADMAN

The patient described a burst of anger at his wife. This was caused by her assertion of the independence and equality he had been struggling with himself to permit, and even to encourage, in the marriage. Unlike the many years before analysis, however, instead of using withdrawal and depression, threats of retaliation, and verbal lashings as

[7] This is an example of the patient's awareness of persisting pathology: his unwillingness to yield dependency and to accept responsibility for his own growth.

[8] An example of the patient's commitment to independent pursuit of problems.

clubs to beat her back into line, he confronted himself with his feelings and his behavior, genuinely apologized to his wife, and, with her, rationally tackled their difference. That night he had a very disturbing dream.

"There was a madman, a psychotic, sitting at a table outside a mental hospital. I was sitting opposite him and there was a vague third person also present. The way this fellow was talking showed he was obviously sick. He looks at me suspiciously with narrowed eyes and says, 'Now I know you're the cause of it all.' I was frightened, and actually heard myself wake up with a strangled cry, but the dream continued. This madman's attention is deflected by the other person, and I walk around the table to come up behind him and give him a rabbit punch. But I realized you can't treat sick people this way. Besides, I knew the third guy was quite capable of taking care of himself if any difficulty arose. In the end, we tackled the disturbed guy together; we pinned his arms back and took him to a ward.

"I woke up and felt very anxious, very frightened—I heard every noise in the house—I started to associate:

"The patient is me. The dream and the anxiety are my reaction to analysis, and to yelling at Doris at supper time. I'm afraid of my own destructive potentialities—that's the madman. I've been having dreams about my destructiveness all through analysis, starting with that tiger.[9]

"I got anxious—then I asked myself, 'Do you really think you're not going to be able to deal with these destructive tendencies?' And I realized it wasn't so—even what I'd done that night, yelling at Doris, doesn't mean it's going to go any further than that—that I can't cope with these potentialities and tendencies. I did apologize to Doris—and felt it. I didn't sit and sulk. I felt *rotten* about what I'd done, and I did something about it. I went to the room she'd gone to, and I apologized. And I changed the whole way I'd approached the self-assertion of hers that I'd gotten into a rage about."

The patient, on his own initiative, was looking at his feelings and actions, and was changing his behavior in the most sensitive areas in accordance with his growing insight. He was using the techniques gained in analysis and was communicating to his wife and his analyst. He worked on the dream independently and saw himself in it as still sick. He knew he had a long way still to go. He realistically evaluated the evening's pathological incident, not letting it overwhelm him, nor

---

[9] Earlier the patient had dreamed of a tiger that had not been adequately fenced in by the man in charge (analyst). At that time it was the analyst's exclusive responsibility to handle the patient's problems.

exaggerating his capacity to handle the problem (with a single, swift effort like the rabbit punch). In the dream he pictured himself meeting the challenge and collaborating with the analyst. This independence and collaboration were reflected in all of the remaining sessions.

Patient's Reluctance to Terminate

The general problems of evaluation of a patient's readiness for termination of a productive therapeutic experience have been stated and illustrated. There are, in addition, a number of common difficulties which can be usefully examined. One group that may be examined collectively are the patient's efforts to *avoid* termination.

Not all reluctance to terminate is pathological. Genuine affection, gratitude, and enjoyment of the relationship has grown to some degree out of the camaraderie and personal growth experienced in the jointly undertaken long-term activity. There have been significant changes wrought in the patient's way of living, and life is more valuable than it was at the start. The meaningfulness of the friendly, communicative contact with the analyst is even greater in the case of a lonely patient, still unmarried, and without enough nonpathological time behind him to have cultivated enduring intimacies. Some have no family, or no potential in the family as presently constituted, for emotionally re-warding experience. The factor of healthy warmth toward the analyst, a prizing of the contact, must be considered at termination in the same way as when it occurs earlier during the course of therapy (pp. 226–228). For the analyst to mistake for pathology this fondness, which is based upon a hard-won capacity for affection and intimacy, will produce at termination the same kind of hurt and, more serious, the same emotional confusion. What is more, the opportunity for resolving such a therapeutic mistake may not occur if analysis is terminated. The healthy reluctance to relinquish a meaningful relationship must be recognized, respected, and welcomed, and placed for the patient in the perspective of his increased prospects for greater and more fulfilling intimacies than are realizable with the analyst.

Apart from this healthy reluctance, the struggle to avoid termination means resistance. There is no new element of resistance, but it is occurring in a new context: the intensification and acceleration of personality change are greater at termination than any yet experienced. All the resistance problems of evolving health are correspondingly intensified. If the resistances are not understood as accompaniments of rapidly evolving health, there is risk of unjustifiably keeping the patient in treatment, or of fostering unnecessary discouragement, or of depriving the patient at the time of discharge of the clearest and fullest sense of both his progress and his capacity for continued progress.

The patient's progress must be kept in view, but his resistances must nevertheless be dealt with. His struggle to avoid termination is often his unwillingness to undertake a fuller commitment to the changes already achieved, and a fuller personal responsibility for carrying on the process of change. This phenomenon is similar to what occurs at the termination of a therapeutic year, when some patients withdraw from the imminent demands for independent analytic effort during the summer separation.[10] During the course of treatment, whenever the patient has "slipped back" he has had the assistance of the analyst in the identification of the problem and in the recovery of a rational, constructive direction. Termination necessitates his mobilization for increased vigilance and effort, to deal independently with his irrationality.

Some patients manifest an exacerbation of old pathology in order to convince the therapist that it is too early to terminate. The dream, earlier in this chapter, of the Principal's Office demonstrated vividly the patient's desire to make the analyst believe that he was as sick now as at the start. The patient's progress had, however, been kept fully in focus, and because of that he anxiously fled the principal in the dream before the ruse failed. Bridling against his accelerating gains, which by then had brought him to the verge of a good marriage and to an unusual academic success, he said, "I think *you* feel I'm not ready to get married," indicating that *he* was not ready to terminate and to take on alone and more intensely the problems of living. At times he almost pleaded to be released from responsibility, instead of being encouraged to assume more. On one occasion he declared provocatively, "I want to avoid love and marriage—I want to remain a son-of-a-bitch, I want to make people kow-tow, I want to keep on screwing around!" Such exacerbations of rebellion and withdrawal were constantly related for this patient to his familiar pathology, such as his competitiveness with the analyst, his grandiosity, his unwillingness to be tender. The patient was constantly engaged by the analyst in making the correlations between his outbursts of resistance, the gains he was achieving in his personal, academic, and analytic life, and the subjective sense of danger that he experienced while consolidating these gains. His participation in this kind of correlation, illustrated by his spontaneous and clearly communicated interpretations in the session to which he had brought the Principal's Office dream, indicated his growing qualifications for termination.

[10] See discussion of Wheelbarrows dream, p. 189.

A competitive conceptualization of human relationships [11] militates against the patient's healthy acceptance of the completion of therapy. The patient's sense of competitive defeat, because of his having changed, will become exacerbated; it may be experienced toward the analyst, toward some other person in the patient's personal life, or toward both.

A patient who has reached a point in the ambivalence of evolving health where the healthy change predominates will recognize, communicate, and deal with this unbearable, irrational sense of a final victory for the analyst. The patient of the Principal's Office dream had in a major fashion overcome his destructive activities with others, and had become essentially consistent and spontaneous in rewarding forms of interpersonal behavior. One day, two months before his last session, he made an angry complaint. After recounting distinctly self-motivated new behavior, he wailed, "I'm so sick of being good, of being told what to do!" While he constructively handled and communicated the problem, this statement exquisitely demonstrated his irrational outraged sense that his new behavior was being caused by the domination of another person.

Similarly, the young woman of the Captain-Woman dream (see pp. 254–257), as she terminated, had to fight off a fantasy of her analyst having the feeling that, "he did it, he can rub his hands with glee! So much has been set in motion, I don't think I *could* stop completely. He won. May he never have another patient!"

A patient may be equally unwilling to allow his changed behavior to benefit someone other than the analyst—perhaps a spouse or a parent (see Chapter 6, "Resistance in Dreams," p. 189). Such an adversary, in the patient's mind, does not deserve to have the thorn in the side removed, much less to have life enhanced by the patient's growing health. "Defeat" seems even more humiliating because these antagonists are now immune from the patient's attacks and counterattacks; they are free to remain neurotic and seem thus to be confirmed in their criticisms of the patient. (The *patient* was wrong because *he* was the one who had to change.) "Mother is getting what she wants," complained the patient of the Captain-Woman dream. "She remains as horrible as ever and gets what she wants. *I* have to work and change. May she *never* have pleasure from anything I do—*ever*. She made me a monster, a bitch. I worked and worked and tried so hard to change, because *I* couldn't stand it. I didn't change for *her*. Yet she gets the benefit of *my* work. I can't *bear* it!"

[11] This was discussed previously in Chapter 2, "Feeling in Dreams," pp. 86–87, and also in Chapter 9, "Occurrence of the Analyst in Dreams," p. 273.

Revenge, the competitive attempt at correction of this "unfair" price for health, was dramatically reflected in another dream of the same patient.

THE RABBIS' CURSE

"There is a group of rabbis just leaving my apartment, but there is an awesome atmosphere about this departure, like Israel leaving Egypt. Yes, they'll leave (and *they* are part of *me*) but in leaving they will call down the most, *most* venomous, hateful, vengeful curses. The rabbis are at the door leaving and I stand within, shoulder to shoulder with [analyst], but still I am with the rabbis in spirit. I, the 'I' within the door with [analyst], am just horrified, shaken to the core and frightened at the sight of such undisguised hate and revenge."

She interrupted, "All right, I give up. I can't *act* this way and still live, but I call on the fates—I, the rabbis, call on Jehovah, the avenging God—to do my dirty work for me. Can these people go unpunished? Is there no justice? But I hate with such a passion. I can't bear to give up the feelings of hatred and revenge. If I could only arrange this with the fates. If I could only hurt without hurting myself—but *I don't want these feelings to get in my way.* I want to be a captain [12] and live well. This captaincy is still so new and so precious that I hate the thought of losing it. I hope I don't try to corrupt it into a new power and weapon— except I *can't,* and I wish I could give up *trying.*"

Despite the intense competitive vindictiveness, there is here a predominance of health—a complete acknowledgment and communication of all feelings and a firm choice by the patient to prevent feelings of revenge from being destructive to her.

Irrational difficulties concerning "dependency" [13] are also commonly associated with the struggle to avoid termination. A "dependent" inclination toward the analyst may be dealt with quite adequately without employing instinctual "parent surrogate" concepts. As with the other emotional problems throughout this book, dependency is tackled in terms of what I believe to be its essential nature—characterological. Even a symbol such as mother's nurturing breast (for an example, see p. 294 below) may reflect the insistence upon being served of the *experientially* evolved demanding personality.

Proportionate to its lifelong severity, this is a problem that tends to intensify as completion of analysis approaches. After a productive

[12] This is an example of the patient's personal glossary; "captain" referred to her most healthy, womanly, mature self. See Captain-Woman dream, pp. 254–257.
[13] See discussion of dependency in Chapter 6, "Resistance in Dreams," p. 183n.

psychotherapeutic experience, the patient is actually further from either real or irrational dependency than ever before in his life. What he is seeking to maintain is the practice of dependency, which has been a weapon in his competitive conflict with others, including the analyst. Losing this major interpersonal technique evokes irrational rebellion and compounds his sense of defeat from being forced to change.

The vindictive young woman of the Rabbis' Curse and the Captain-Woman dreams had lived in great "dependency" on her mother and other people whom she had compelled to decide for her, encourage her, pack her suitcase, choose her dress. In order to achieve a self-reliant posture toward life she had first to face and to get beyond her feeling that the analyst would "rub his hands in glee" at "forcing" her to become independent. Eventually she was able to say, "I really have to be a woman, use my own judgment and act on it—and not be a little girl who throws herself on others' mercy. I can't leave the satisfaction of my needs to other people. I have to—*and I'm afraid I can*—take care of myself."

The patient of the Analyst-Chauffeur dream had a terminal dream in which he ambivalently sought out an old prostitute (the analyst) who had too high a price and flabby breasts. He associated to a childhood scene and said, "There was a real contrast between my mother's flabby breasts and the full breasts of the neighbor who was nursing her child—it makes me think of being *chauffeured* around by you.[14] All you've offered me has been a flabby breast, compared with what I want." His very next association seemed to express a symbolic reversal of the situation, in retaliation for his ungratified "dependency": "I had to start writing out the check for you four or five times—there was no ink in my pen." He had failed to force me to take care of him, to let him be "dependent" with me; instead he felt forced by me to write out checks, pay for services, act like a man.[15] Here again a familiar problem was revived and intensified in the terminal context. Therapeutically it was correlated with the patient's first dream in analysis (Analyst-Chauffeur) as a persisting problem which was now substantially less incapacitating, one which he would deal with on his own in the future. He was well prepared to handle his dependency by himself

[14] This is an example of a patient's personal glossary; see Chapter 1, "Symbolism in Dreams," p. 32.

[15] One patient associated the reluctant yielding of dependency with a profoundly witty "song title" once announced by a comedian: "I'd love to stay in your arms forever, but put me down now, I have to go to work." This title has occurred usefully more than once as an association of the analyst.

because of the personality changes and new skills he had developed through his analytic experience.

DANNY'S CLIMB

The following dream vividly reflects the ambivalent, painful conflict over giving up dependency. It is designated as terminal because it occurred two months before the conclusion of a long period of analysis. The patient, however, decided to return for further analytic work after a few years of professional success but insufficiently meaningful personal life.

In the dream, "Danny, an eight-year-old boy, is in a car or tricycle, going up a hill. For one reason or another, he can't control the car. It may be that he can't drive, or it may be that there's something wrong with the car itself. The car swerves to the right and to the left. It rolls back. It circles around completely.

"At last he succeeds in getting it under control, and gets it up the hill. There he finds his mother waiting. His mother has been on top of the hill all the time, watching Danny's struggle, and waiting for him to make it. Danny gets out of the car and bursts into tears—feeling, in addition to relief at having survived the trip, terribly angry and irritable, especially at his mother for having permitted him to go through the agony he has just gone through."

He spoke of the admiration he consciously had for the real mother of Danny. In waking life he knew her to be loving and firm; unlike his own mother, "she loves Danny very much and holds on to him with open hands, not clutching tightly."

He interpreted: "Danny is me, the mother is you. There is some unconscious respect for you, for your uncontrolling concern for me, which I don't allow myself to register consciously. This becomes even more important in the context of the dream. The car is my life in general, analysis in particular. The wavering, swerving, etcetera actually describe my own wavering during the last couple of months, and especially during this past week. I've been making fitful progress in one area and regress in another. That the car makes it up the hill is both a reflection of the fact that over all, during this period, I did succeed in the struggle—as well as the fact that I really want to succeed."

In this case his "really wanting to succeed" was what brought him back after a few years for further work, which then made it possible for him to deepen his personal commitments and rewards, and to move into a larger and more meaningful work area wherein to use his human and intellectual capacities. Even at the conclusion of this first experience of analysis, however, the patient demonstrated in his competent, responsible, and independent handling of the dream his readiness to terminate and to deal with his problem of dependency on his own.

Consistent with the cooperative basis of the whole process of analysis, termination should be openly and jointly contemplated. The discussion is often, with great value, taken up long in advance—months, a year, or even two years. Thinking about it provides an opportunity for evaluating progress, and sets a marker from which to measure further gains. An analyst may be extravagant in judging the effectiveness of his own efforts or the potential of the patient. The patient, too, may err in estimating his degree of change or of commitment. The patient's progress may show unexpected fluctuations before he consolidates his gains. For any or all of these reasons, it may become necessary to revise the plan for termination. The revision would then derive from application of the criteria suggested early in this chapter—chiefly the patient's awareness of his persisting problems, his independence, initiative, and competence in tackling them, and the predominance of healthy motivation.

Until the final session of analysis there almost always remains some of the patient's struggle to restore pathological integrity. One woman expressed it this way: "I feel I never want to give it up. I've kept it all my life—it's the dearest thing I have. What is this 'pearl beyond compare'? It's *me!*" The sense of "me" has come from functioning in familiar pathological ways for many years. The healthy patterns achieved during analysis have been exercised for a much shorter time. The patient, in his new consciousness, now has more conviction, more confidence in being able to handle his problems and to mingle with and relate to people, but nevertheless in his new personality he has considerably less experience. He leaves analysis with mixed feelings, but with an overall realistic optimism.

The essence of the subjective experience of termination is well reflected in the following dream.

DYING AND BEING REBORN

"I was on my way to visit some relatives. They were able to sense I was sick, and I realized I was dying. As I got to the group I died. Everybody was crying. But I wasn't crying. I could just feel I was being reborn over. Right in my dying, I was being reborn again. I felt good about it. I knew I was going to be happier. I knew I had to die and I had to be reborn.

"Somehow the dream wasn't gruesome, not at all like in some of my other dreams about death. This had mostly to do with being reborn. I felt good. I was emerging from some other kind of life, and entering *this* life."

11. Working with Dreams in the Therapeutic Session

OTHER PERIODS FROM ANALYSES have already appeared in the foregoing text. Chapter 2, "Feeling in Dreams," it will be recalled, included a series of dreams involving the induction of a man into the realm of his emotions. Chapter 3, "Introductory Dreams," included a review of the first few weeks in analysis of the man who approached therapy with the plan to manage on his own (Straight and Narrow), to fool the analyst (Faking It), or to lock horns with the analyst (Fight with an Antelope). Chapter 5, "Anxiety in Dreams," included a tense period of a couple of weeks near the middle of analysis of an extremely isolated and cynical young woman (Crazy Woman; Shit Piles Up).

This final chapter contains a series of dreams representing a six-month period midway in the analysis of a depressive man. The material is not treated exhaustively; I have tried to select material that conveys a sense of process in the emergence and handling of personality problems, and the role of dreams. This series of dreams demonstrates many of the dynamic, technical, and theoretical considerations presented in the foregoing text. The reader will continue to find emphasis placed upon feeling and therapeutic collaboration.

The patient had entered analysis one and a half years earlier, at the age of thirty-nine. He was married, had two children, and had been through a fifteen-year succession of economic failures, a record utterly inconsistent with his demonstrated ability during the initial phase of each undertaking. While his manner was affable, his credo was to keep his deepest feelings to himself, and this had been a serious obstacle in the course of analysis. He often *acknowledged* feelings which were betrayed by his dreams, fantasies, manner of speech, or even by his outward behavior, but he almost never fully or spontaneously discussed or explored his feelings and was therefore limited in his knowledge of them. He had, however, in this first year and a half of analysis, begun to acquire a broader concept of and approach to his feeling life.

In the course of analysis he had started a new business and was making good progress, although he resented starting near the bottom after his years of experience. He had lived all his life under the domination of two much older cousins who had moved in with the family to "rescue" the mother when the father died during the patient's eleventh year. Actually the father had been a cypher in the family. The mother had been a hard business woman, a dominating matriarch, and she soon took over the two cousins. The older cousin, although he was under the domination of the patient's mother, became a kind of substitute father for the patient, with an enslaving paternalistic oversolicitude. Against the two dominating figures in his life (the older cousin and the mother), the patient had subtly retaliated with vindictive failures in all the projects in which they supported him. The mother had died several years before the patient entered analysis, but the two cousins, particularly the older one, had maintained the same enslaving paternalistic relationship, to which the patient had continued to react as always. This relationship was conducted under the mutually self-deluding aura of fraternalism.

The three men and their wives cultivated tight family ties almost to the exclusion of significant social relationships outside the family circle. The patient was the constant recipient of large and small handouts, ranging from resort vacations, restaurant checks, and theater tickets through new and almost-new clothing.

At this stage of his analysis he was no longer seeking handouts. He had asked the cousins for a substantial loan with which to consolidate his new business on a more secure basis, and was quite certain to repay the loan by means of his own present and future efforts. Such a loan would mean an acknowledgment of their respect for his ability—a respect for which he had striven, and which he could never receive along with the handouts. He was always to them the "beloved" incompetent kid.

At the time of the dream about to be presented (Spilling His Guts), he had been extremely depressed because he had not secured the needed loan through his cousins, although he had succeeded independently in arranging for one elsewhere. In analysis he had talked merely about his efforts to get the loan, but had not revealed his depression. He had kept up a bold front.

He started the session by describing a long telephone conversation that he had had with his older cousin on the evening before the dream. This had been a final heart-breaking attempt to get some recognition in the form of the substantial loan—not a handout to cover a grocery bill, an insurance premium, or even rent, but an amount that would carry him for six months or a year. The older cousin had flatly reneged on a promise of the week before, simply unable to see the essence of the patient's request—his desire for independence.

The patient then presented the dream: "I was walking about in the street of a summer resort town. There were great crowds on the street. Everybody was very happy, very gay. People were going in groups to different parties. I'm not with anybody, and I'm not going anywhere. Then I'm standing on top of some steps watching people going by. Arnold, a guy I like very much that I grew up with and whom I see once in a while, is there with his camera. He's signaling to me, wanting to take a picture of me. A man seemed deliberately to be standing in front of me and I say to him, 'What are you doing there?' He turned and I see it's another old friend, Timmy, a guy who committed suicide a few years ago by jumping in front of a subway train. Then Timmy and I stand next to each other. He just wanted to get into the picture. Then Arnold begins to back up and to get me into focus. As he backs up he suddenly seems to be in the remote distance. He's up on some platform trying to focus and suddenly he falls.

"I screamed and ran to him. He seemed to fall from a height. As I get to him I see his guts are splattered around. His eyelids fluttered. I cried, I groaned, I wracked myself with grief. I call out, 'Call an ambulance, get a doctor, get someone! He's still living!' There weren't too many people around. There's a bench right there and on it there's an older sister of the guy who committed suicide. There's another sister beside her. While I'm frantic to get help and shout to get someone, this older sister turns somberly and quietly to the other sister and says, 'What happened?' The other one says, 'Can't you see?'

"And I'm crying, 'Please God, save him!' and I look and his eyes are open and looking at me and his guts are no longer splattered. I woke up with a feeling that he was going to recover and I felt so relieved and glad. I woke up crying fearfully."

He was quiet for a few moments and then said spontaneously, "It could have been me that was lying there and encouraged that everything was going to be all right."

He became silent again and I said to him, "Say what you're feeling."

In response he burst into tears and continued sobbing as he talked. "Jesus, I don't know what's happening to me—I'm *scared as hell*." I asked what he was scared of. He replied immediately, "Nothing, just scared—of the future." He lay there silently struggling to regain control of himself.

Seeing his efforts to master his anxiety, my first association was to an element of the dream. I said, "I think you're scared of spilling your guts.[1] You've been trying to get yourself in focus like the guy with the camera in the dream. I've been urging you for so long to say what you *feel*. I think you have all this anxiety because you're scared you'll die if you spill your guts, if you really start to express your feelings."

He replied after a moment, "During this last week I've been particularly depressed. I got very depressed at the end of last week. I had it in mind to tell you about it. Then I arranged a loan, and now I feel better about it."

Now, having a second association with the splattered guts, namely, the friend who had jumped from a subway platform, I asked, "Have you had any suicidal fantasies?"[2]

"No, not at all," he responded quickly.

"The guy who obscured you while you were trying to get yourself in focus for the picture was a guy who committed suicide," I reminded him, adding, "and he also had a wife and two children."

He replied at once, "That's why I told you about his suicide—I was thinking about that. Many times I feel, 'What the hell is this all about?' Just the other day I was telling my best friend Alex, 'I'm over forty and I'm not a man yet.' I'm too much of a wordy guy. I talk, I blab, I analyze, I rationalize, I convince myself, I convince others—but the real accomplishment isn't there. Yet I know that's not altogether true. I know what I've got and I know what I can do."

"You feel pretty alone, don't you?" I interpolated.

"*All alone*. Some people think I'm quite the guy—they look at me with envy."

I asked, "Who were the two women on the bench in the dream?"

He replied, "I don't know. They were older women. There were

[1] This is an example of an associative process transitional to interpretation; see p. 19.

[2] See preceding footnote.

two women, sisters of this guy who committed suicide. When I heard her say, 'What happened?' it was so obvious, I didn't even bother to answer."

"What does this remind you of?"

"What do you mean?" he asked, puzzled.

"What are you reminded of? The young fellow has just fallen and lies there with his guts splattered all over, and this older woman is siting there, callous, with no comprehension of his distress, of his need for help?"

"That's the way she was. That describes her perfectly." He remained silent for several moments.

I said, persisting, "Who's it like?"

Angrily he shot out, "My cousin!" Then he went on with intensity. "Alex is a real friend. He thinks those cousins that have supposedly done so much for me are selfish, lousy people. He's been saying this for years, but I always felt he didn't understand them." Only then did the patient recall, "As I was walking here this morning, I was thinking of my cousin, and how I finally had to—and how I finally managed to get a loan from somebody else. I was thinking to myself, 'He must hate me.'"

It was the end of the hour and I made a few final remarks. "It seems to me that you show in the dream a healthy concern for yourself and a confidence in your survival through your own efforts instead of trying to survive by getting the old woman, your cousin, to respond and save you when you spill your guts. Sunday night you spilled your guts to him, and like the woman on the bench he showed no real concern, nothing but callousness and lack of comprehension. You had to manage some other way—and you did. I think this is a very hopeful dream. We have to look more at your real feelings about your cousin, your real feelings of self-confidence, and we also have to look at your loneliness."

The patient came in two days later and filled the hour with a spontaneously honest, affectively communicated, and detailed story of his boyhood feelings toward his castrated father and about his mother's scorn both for himself and for his father. He spoke of his hatred of the cousins under whose domination he grew up. "I was in fear of my mother and cousins. They represented authority."

He talked without any further stimulus from me about his isolation and loneliness. "I never had any close friends. Every time I'd try to be with a group I felt a sense of not belonging. Once they tried to organize a social club. It was going to cost ten cents a week. My mother didn't know what I was talking about and I couldn't join. I wanted to be friendly with them and I never could. I guess it was more me than them. I never gave of myself. When we moved to Queens I could turn on the charm and make friends, but inside myself I was always reserved and aloof."

He recalled the great pride he used to have in his ability to charm people, and he remembered saying to his mother: "We moved from Brooklyn to Queens and then we moved from Queens to Manhattan, and I always made friends, and if I moved somewhere else, I guess I wouldn't miss them." He added at once to me, "I guess I felt bad, but I acted boastful. I've always been able to make friends, but never close. When I was about twenty, I used to talk with a nice girl in the neighborhood. I wasn't in love with her, but we used to talk together. I was telling her my impressions of the world, of women, and so on, and suddenly she started to cry. She said, 'I feel so sorry for you, the way you talk.' It hit me on the head. I realized I'd been telling her that people didn't mean anything to me."

His isolation, diffidence, and cynicism are understandable in the context of his childhood home: "Father was just a removed character"; the mother was a matriarch whose affection he doubted—"I was supposed to be a girl—all the goddamn secrets"; and the older cousins helped him only at the price of his own enslavement.

The dream and the work of the two sessions that followed it bring to view some of the ambivalent elements of evolving health. That the patient's success in life would depend on his own efforts, and that he possessed the requisite personal resources, had just been "brought home" to him by his successful negotiation of a loan in his own name and through his own initiative. A pathological component of his reaction to this constructive product of more than a year and a half of analytic struggle was a depressive resentment, bringing in its wake memories and dream representation of a friend who committed suicide by jumping off a subway platform.

His determination to stand on his own feet in the new business represented the abandonment of his familiar way of functioning, his previous dependent way of life. This precipitated anxiety in the preceding session during the report of his dream, particularly when he interpreted the final portion as a representation of himself "encouraged that everything was going to be all right" in a situation where he had stopped demanding succor from others. This commitment predominated over both depression and anxiety and was again reflected in the following hour, when on his own therapeutic initiative he faced and communicated his feelings.

Interpretive Activity

This dream in its clinical setting offers a particularly good opportunity to examine the interpretive activity of both patient and analyst. Interpretation was not only spontaneously initiated by the patient but it was also, notably for him, pursued with affective genuineness.

The interpretive activity flowing from this dream will be considered, first, in connection with the associations and interpretive hypotheses of the analyst. "Spilling your guts," a common phrase, was the analyst's association, stimulated first by the vivid description of the dream character whose "guts are splattered." It occurred a second time when the patient, surrendering his usual emotional control, sobbed and verbalized his fear. The open display of deep feelings reenforced the potent imagery of the dream and brought to the analyst a reiteration of the associative phrase.

The phrase may not have represented the patient's conceptualization of the dream image. Nevertheless, the introduction of "spilling your guts" and the interpretive hypothesis in connection with his expressing emotion was relevant both to the immediate moment and to what was going on in the patient's life outside. The interpretation fostered the tone of affective openness and honesty that the patient had already spontaneously set.

The analyst's association to the dream from his own life (the phrase "spilling his guts") and his memory of the patient's report, at the start of the hour, of the angry, frustrating telephone conversation with the cousin, led to an interpretive hypothesis. This was not explicitly offered, but it formed the basis for questioning the patient. The questions led to an area of difficulty suggested by the dream. The recognition clearly depicted in the dream—that his cousin was callously indifferent to his needs—was one that the patient until now had been reluctant to acknowledge. At this point the constructive elements in his ambivalence achieved predominance and the recognition was spontaneously and feelingly expressed.

The analyst had a third association to the patient's life in response to the dream image of splattered guts. (The first was the patient's emotions manifested in the session, the second his outpouring to his cousin on the telephone.) The third was the friend who had killed himself by jumping off the subway platform and under a train.[3] This suicidal

[3] The patient is represented in the dream by three individuals—the photographer, the friend who committed suicide, and his clearly identified self. See discussion of individuals as attributes, pp. 4–8.

friend, it will be recalled, was a character in the dream who obscured the patient when the photographer tried to get him into focus. After the patient became anxious and wept in the session, and the analyst re-emphasized the importance of expressing feelings honestly and fully, the patient then reported a depression he had concealed during the previous week. At this point the analyst recalled the friend who committed suicide. The patient's report of his concealed depression and the subway suicide character of the dream combined to form an idea—that the patient might have been experiencing suicidal fantasies. The patient was asked this directly and denied it at once. But the hypothesis had important connotations, particularly for an individual who traveled to work (and to analysis) by subway! Working out his problems, getting himself into focus, was the opposite of killing himself. But the suicidal man "seemed deliberately to be standing in front of me." It was the suicidal friend (like the patient, a married man with two children) who got in the way and interfered with the patient's getting himself into focus. It was while this self-analytic self, the photographer, was *backing away* into the "remote distance" to focus upon the suicidal *alter ego* that he suddenly fell from a platform and had his guts splattered.

It was important to bring the patient back to view himself at close range and to pursue the hypothesis that he might be entertaining suicidal impulses. When asked directly if he had had such fantasies he abruptly backed away (as in the dream); he replied quickly, "No, not at all." However, when the analyst explained the basis of the hypothesis (that it was because the person who obscured the picture of himself had committed suicide leaving a wife and two children) the patient at once indicated that he had had the same association as the analyst: "That's why I told you about his suicide—I was thinking about that." This was followed at once by an expression of hopelessness: "Many times I feel, what the hell is this all about?" and then by the recall of expressing disgust with himself recently to his best friend: "I'm over forty, and I'm not a man yet."

It is important to delineate and emphasize for the patient the signs of evolving health. This is particularly true when it is—as frequently happens—accompanied by depression. False reassurance at almost any time is harmful, and probably never more harmful than when a patient is depressed: he believes he is powerless, and false reassurance obscures his genuine resources instead of mobilizing them. False reassurance is doubly inappropriate when the depression is a reaction to therapeutic progress, because it sabotages the patient's constructive powers when these are expanding.

Authentic reassurance also may be rejected because, when he is depressed, the patient is partly in the grip of an unidentified angry recalcitrance and consequently does not readily welcome any recognition that carries with it an inherent commitment to intensified therapeutic effort. The depressed patient is particularly unready to achieve a *spontaneous* recognition of his own evolving health, but is nevertheless, in his ambivalence of change, more than usually accessible to a proffered delineation of his positive resources.

The patient's first words when he finished reporting the dream were: "It could have been me that was lying there and encouraged that everything was going to be all right." His spontaneous recognition of the optimistic content of the dream and his willingness, in spite of his depression, to *initiate* interpretation, were both evidences of health. These considerations, in addition to the emotionally affirmative conclusion of the dream, appeared in the analyst's view adequately to attenuate the danger in the suicidal implications. The analyst nevertheless had to maintain the initiative to further explore the positive aspects of the dream. Consequently with the patient's *immediate* interpretations and with his ready expression of feeling after interpreting the dream (feeling "scared"), the analyst interpreted the patient's representation of a photographer ("It could have been me . . .") to be the patient seeing himself as someone who tries to get things in focus. The patient acknowledged in the dream terminology that he was trying to look at himself honestly. The analyst also pointed out at the end of the hour that the patient showed a genuine concern for himself ("Please God, save him," and later, "I feel so relieved and glad") and, even more, had confidence in his survival ("He was going to recover"). And, above all, the patient's confidence in survival existed on the basis of looking to his own resources ("His eyes are open and looking at *me* . . .").

Altogether, the dream offered evidence that the patient was moving toward giving up his dependency and his irresponsible destructive depression. He was developing confidence in his future, based upon self-reliance. The essence of this concept of the patient's status and movement was derived from the combined interpretation of patient and analyst.

The second approach to the dream is from the standpoint of the validation of interpretations. There was significant confirmatory activity of the patient within and outside of the therapeutic experience. Caught in a difficult financial situation, he had turned for the first time to his personal outside resources instead of insisting that his cousins rescue him. When in the past he had been in a tight spot in an enterprise backed by them, he had often been "self-destructive." He would go into a depression and ignore his responsibility for the investment the cousins had already made. They would then be forced to rescue him in order to rescue themselves. In this way his irresponsibility had functioned as a tyranny over them, and as a vindictive punishment of them for patronizing and infantilizing him. It was a circular process in which they never respected him as a man and he retaliated by not acting like one. Both sides in this mutual enslavement and mutual retaliation covered their destructiveness with exaggerated fraternalism.

When the patient began to be independent and manly, the cousins found this unbearable, but their intolerance was, as usual, covert. When he now needed substantial assistance, they did not refuse outright—they made humiliating excuses and offered humiliating pecuniary compromises which ignored the patient's real needs of both a financial and morale nature. This was the "callous indifference" of the dream. The patient was tempted to act in the traditional pattern but, perhaps because he could not retaliate by bankrupting the cousins' project (since this one was his alone), he was stimulated to fantasy a more desperate measure, suicide. He was ambivalent. He was depressed, *but he nevertheless acted effectively in his own interests.*

The ambivalence is clear in the dream. He screams to the callous old woman (his older cousin) for help, but nevertheless achieves without her a *healthy restitution* (". . . eyes open . . . guts no longer splattered . . . he was going to recover"); there is a sense of self-confidence and hopefulness as the dream ends. This affective experience in the dream may be readily correlated with his remark after telling the dream, "I got very depressed at the end of last week. Then I arranged a loan, and now I feel better about it."

A significant waking confirmation of the interpretation of the dream was his speculation, on the way to this session, that his cousin must hate him. This speculation, whether accurate or not, was courageous, since it carried with it the implication of his standing alone.

The self-confidence was more significantly confirmed later during the session when he said, "I know what I've got and I know what I can do." In addition, there was considerable honest expression of his feelings during the session, and increasing honesty and independence in the sessions immediately following.

Here was ample validation of the healthy restitution in the dream, from the patient's activity outside and within the therapeutic situation.

There is also confirmatory activity to be found in that part of the interpretation concerned with the patient's resistance to change. He had avoided communicating and examining his depression during the previous week in therapy and had failed to open the immediate session with the revolutionary formulation that he had made on the way to it, namely, that his cousin must hate him. As in the dream, he had in these ways *"backed away" from getting himself into focus.* But his depression was the aspect of his activity that most clearly validated the negative aspects of the dream interpretation. Discouragement is a normal response to adversity. Depression, however, is always pathological, hostile, and ultimately self-destructive. His response of depression, associated as it was with memories of his suicidal friend, was in the direction of self-destruction and in opposition to growth.

There are, then, as the patient's total behavior within and outside therapy is observed, evidences from his activity which are validative of both the negative and positive elements formulated in the interpretation of his dream.

Anxiety, as well as depression, is associated with this man's progress. Although Spilling His Guts was not an anxiety dream, anxiety developed in the patient *following* his interpretation of the dream. His waking fear during the session ("I'm scared as hell"), after his spontaneous positive interpretation, is comparable to the anxiety that sometimes develops in sleep during dreams of evolving health (see Growth Pills, pp. 187–188). His anxiety was related to the basic sources of pathological anxiety: fear of the bankruptcy or imminent bankruptcy of a crucial technique of living (see p. 157). This man had taken a big step toward independence and had already broken away from his older cousins to a degree that made it extremely difficult for him to succeed in the old way (through coercive dependence). In the framework of further paralysis of his dependent form of functioning, the increasing self-reliance was a frightening prospect. The depression, a seeming passive relinquishing of constructive efforts, was an unconscious but active trend toward nullifying his commitment to change and a movement instead toward business failure or even suicide. In the pathological framework, depression guarded against a loss of dependent control. In the framework of emerging health, however, this suicidal threat to himself was reflected in the dream as a source of wild dismay. Anxiety, however, did not develop until a further waking commitment.

In the dream he was "relieved and glad" over the restitution to health and the prospect of continuing life. It was in the session, when he realized that he had really committed himself to a self-directed and self-sustaining life, that he burst out crying and felt deep anxiety. The *fear* developed on the couch when he made the identification, not only of his own restituted self, but of his gladness to be healthy. This combination was manifested in the peculiar elision of his interpretive statement: "It could have been me *that was lying there and encouraged*

that everything was going to be all right." In the dream he was separate from the injured man, while in the interpretation he fused his
onlooker's experiential feelings with his symbolic self (his clearly identified self). This more solidly identified the recovered man as himself,
and also more solidly identified the feeling of encouragement over the
prospects of continuing in a life of self-reliance. At this moment of relinquishing his only familiar way of functioning effectively, this moment of commitment to a new way of living which was not yet firmly
established, he got "scared as hell." An accentuating factor was, I
believe, the fact that, while this process was taking place, his pursuit
of independence was reaching its fullest and most frightening expression right there in the waking collaboration of the analytic session.[4]
His therapeutic efforts had brought about the evolution of a healthier
personality, about which he felt encouragement but also profound and
anxious doubts.

The relinquishing of pathological goals is slow and difficult. Patients often paradoxically expect the fulfillment of a neurotic goal as
a reward for renunciation of it. With all his growing independence,
this man had continued to harbor the hope of achieving his cousins'
acceptance and respectful support.

By continuing to see them more realistically, he finally faced the
fact that there was a direct connection between his self-destructiveness
and his cousins' thwarting of his efforts to elicit their respect. He was
able to recognize many evidences of this connection during the following months. Over the years he and his wife had often been peremp-
torily invited to various expensive social functions, and there humiliated
in a style of genial patronage. Many summer vacations had been spent
as guests of the cousins in a captive atmosphere of synthetic family
unity. In retrospect the patient recognized these degradations and con-
strictions and correlated them with frequent sulking and deeper depressions and occasional vindictive irresponsible losses of irreplaceable
money borrowed for betting. He was later able, after conquering his
unwillingness, to identify the *current* irrational sources of sullenness,
tension, insomnia, and self-destructive impulses, and sometimes he was
able thereby to modify his actions. At other times his insight came out
of hindsight. Eventually he grew to recognize quite consistently his
immediate negative feelings, motivations, and rationalizations surrounding these family interchanges. He achieved progressively a more

---

[4] When pressed for the object of his fear, he replied, "The future." Fear of
future developments in the midst of an encouraging trend is, especially in depres-
sives, often a sense of the danger of their own destructive, sabotaging potential.
This was probably a contributing factor in this patient's anxiety.

equal footing in both the business and social relationship with his cousins. With the older one the predominant course was a clear separation, which required firmness on the patient's part. With the younger one, however, greater and greater equality developed in their exchanges. For the first time in his life the patient began to be the social host and sometimes even the business advisor to the younger of the cousins.[5]

As is common in dealing with dreams reflecting the emergence of health, the work with this dream led to mutual attention to a new problem.[6] The analyst, stimulated by the introductory portion of the dream, himself raised the question of the patient's *loneliness*. (The start of the dream included: "Everybody was very happy, very gay. People were going in groups to different parties. I'm not with anybody, and I'm not going anywhere.") The analyst's recognition of the patient's sense of isolation from people did not of course come from this dream fragment alone. It came as a growing awareness in the analyst while the patient sobbed in his anxiety, and particularly as he observed the patient's efforts to recover composure, to wrench himself from the intimacy with the analyst. A sense of the patient's loneliness continued to evolve during the discussion of the depression he had concealed the week before the dream. This depression became associated, at least after the dream, with the old friend who had committed suicide. The sense of the patient's loneliness finally crystallized as he painted himself as a "wordy guy. I talk, I blab, I analyze, I rationalize, I convince myself, I convince others—but the real accomplishment isn't there." This was a seriously self-critical description of the tactical facade of sociability which divorced him from meaningful relationships, a description stimulated by the discussion and reaction following the telling of the dream. There was a note of healthy optimism ("I know that's not altogether true. I know what I've got and I know what I can do"). Yet in the main it was a picture of an isolated individual. When I said, "You feel pretty alone, don't you?" his answer was immediate and feelingly expressed: "*All* alone." And thus *the important new problem emerged.* The patient pursued it most effectively by himself in the next session, when he gave, with more intimate emotional detail than ever before,

[5] The problem of independence, focused particularly in this long history with his cousins, was not eliminated with the insight crystallized through working with this dream. From then on, however, it was overcome more effectively and at a faster pace. After consistent slow growth, a crucial advance in independence occurred again six months later. At that time a related anxiety developed in connection with his son's growing independence (dream of the Lost Son, below).

[6] See Captain-Woman dream, p. 257. "I feel that to be strong is to be unlovable," was the expression of the new problem emerging for her.

an account of his childhood, his loneliness then, his sense of minimal status in the family, and the building up of his proud insularity.

The problem of loneliness had turned our attention toward his marriage. Three and one-half months elapsed before the next session, and during the interval he had been involved in intensive exploration and beginning change in the problem of his previously unidentified isolation from his wife. A major difficulty was that of overcoming his competitive subjugation of her. Because of his nurture under the dominance of a most subtly and successfully manipulative matriarch of a mother, the patient had to overcome a profound reluctance to give himself with any generosity or confidence to a woman.

He came in to the session and started to talk about having taken a dancing lesson with his wife the night before. For years she had wanted him to take dancing lessons. He would become angry when she started to teach him, or he would walk away, or he would jokingly avoid the whole situation by refusing to dance, saying that he had tin ears and two left feet. Now he at last had taken a dancing lesson. Several times during the lesson, when his wife had tried to correct him, he had restrained himself from exploding or dropping out angrily. It was the first time that he had ever allowed her to correct his dancing. He had gone through a whole lesson. His wife had been very grateful, and had been very affectionate to him when they returned home.

He went on to say that he had recognized how very competitive he had been with his wife. This problem had come up a week before, and he had thought about it a good deal. He said, "I guess I'm competitive with others, too. I must be 'top banana' all the time. *That reminds me,* I did a lot of dreaming last night. I can't remember it all. It was very complicated, but I remember three parts of it [Three Bedraggled Cats].

"In the first part there were three cats, and somewhere in this dream the three cats were lost. They strayed away or something. A couple of days later they came in through the window, one after the other, bedraggled, hungry, tired. It was very odd to me that a cat could find its way back. The minute they came in, two of them were somewhat vague, but one of them was very clear and came and snuggled up to me like a human being in its happiness at being back. I thought it was silly that a cat should act like a human being.

"The second part [The Unkept Date] was much more complicated than I can remember, but I know that I was with a woman who was not my wife and I made a date with her which I know I never kept.

"In the third part [No Destination] I was racing along the highway in my car. I was all alone and seemed to have no destination."

I asked him what his feelings were in the dream, and he said that in the last two episodes the predominant feeling was that of frustration. He was unable to keep up with what was happening. It was "like things were twirling me around." But in the first dream "the feeling was warm. I marveled at the cats' instinct to come home. I knew dogs did. There was so much more to the whole dream."

"What association do you have with cats?"

"There was this one particularly, the way it purred and snuggled after it came through the window. I have no use for cats. Yet in the dream I felt relieved at their coming home."

"What was your association with the snuggling and the warmth?"

"I was just glad they were home."

"What in your life at present is like that?"

"The way my wife was warm and comforting and snuggling last night. These last few weeks she's been beat and frustrated ["bedraggled"]. Last night she wanted to talk over summer plans, and the children did, too. They wanted to know about whether they would be going back to camp, or just what. We've been under a great strain financially and I don't know where the money is coming from or what I can promise them. The three of them were like the three cats. The cats were almost human. I get discouraged." [7]

I interrupted: "The two following episodes in your dream suggest your flight from intimacy in marriage."

He said, "Am I a conceited guy? How smart can I be? I can see myself as overbearing and dominating."

I said, "The outstanding thing in the dream is the feeling you have about the cats in general, that they want human warmth from you. Even though they come in, as you say, 'bedraggled and hungry,' they do not rush to the kitchen for food. They do not jump onto a couch and snuggle up on a pillow. This cat, the one that stands out, is not looking for shelter or food. These are the material things that because of your financial problems you are finding it difficult to provide for your wife. But this isn't what she wants. She comes and snuggles. She wants human warmth from you. But you want to get away from this, to solve

[7] It should be noted that this patient at first proved reluctant to associate with the snuggling and warmth. This had been a very difficult problem for him. He had always tried to avoid giving warmth to people, and particularly to his wife. Recently he had begun to develop responsiveness in his relationship with her, as exemplified by his going through the dance lesson which, I then learned, was one of several they had already attended successfully. He was able to feel more sympathetic with her interests and needs, and therefore more cooperative in developing dancing as one of their marriage pleasures.

your problem with some date, somebody outside of your marriage, who makes no demands for human warmth. Going in this direction, you try again to get away from all human contact. You are speeding along by yourself on the highway, and you have no destination in mind—just to get away."

He said, "I don't have an answer."

"You mean you don't have the warmth to give?"

"No, that's not it. I've begun to give warmth. In the dream I'm relieved and amazed. I thought that cats could get along by themselves. I'm glad that they came back."

I asked, "How did you respond to this cat in the dream?"

"I petted her, just the one. She looked at me with hungering eyes. I petted her, which is the last thing I'd do to a cat. This makes me think immediately of all of the affection and warmth that I've been withholding from my wife. I recognize I'm giving her something now that I've been withholding all this time, something that I now feel, wanting to satisfy her, a conscious wanting. I've had the knowledge all along that I wasn't doing it, that there was something I wasn't giving, but what I wasn't recognizing was how much I was holding back. Before the marriage the boys always used to say, 'satisfy your wife.' Of course, in their minds sex was predominant when they said that. I know now it means satisfy her emotionally too. But I must have fallen down badly. I blamed my wife for being frigid and unresponsive, but it was me. For a long time sex was an ordeal and a task for her, but lately her responsiveness has been so intense and quick. It could have been that way for a long time."

The *moment of association* that produced the recall of this dream was vital to a grasp of the underlying problems. The patient had talked about overcoming the strong competitive feeling which had existed between him and his wife throughout their fifteen years of marriage. He had always kept her out of his business, out of his intimate thoughts and feelings, had derogated and patronized her. During the two years of his analysis, he had gradually begun to give her a fuller place, and in the past year had not interfered with her taking on a time-consuming community activity outside the home. She had been most successful, and was now admired in the community. When she considered continuing for another year, he began to exercise pressure against such a choice by using all kinds of noble rationalizations. "Why don't you live in your own home more, why don't you have more home life?" Besides, in his annoyance he found it impossible when she was away to concentrate on the office work which he brought home.

In reviewing all of this material from previous sessions, it became clear that his feeling was a competitive one, that he couldn't stand the acclaim his wife was getting through her own productivity rather than through her association with him. As indicated, he had begun to overcome this competitiveness; he had not only acceded to her desire to take up some of the new social dances with him, but he had actually taken criticism from her in the learning of the dance.

But doing this had entailed a struggle. As he reported his feelings of competitiveness toward her, saying *"I must be top banana all the time"* (moment of association), he suddenly remembered the three dream fragments (i.e., episodic dream). He started with the first, the Three Bedraggled Cats, in which there was the most intense feeling. In this dream his competitiveness, and his conflicting desire (his "conscious wanting") to fulfill her emotional needs, stand out in sharp contradiction. Will he respond to the entreaty in the cat's eyes, and the snuggling, or will he move away? Will his wife get what she needs from him, or will he succeed in keeping her at a distance? His association preceding the thought of the dream led to our joint interpretation of this conflict.

There is emotional movement within the episode: he begins by representing his wife as a cat (and he cannot stand cats) but he discovers he has no revulsion, marvels over the animal's human quality, and is surprised by his own gladness at her return.

In the succeeding episodes the conflict that has arisen between his desire to respond with human warmth, and his desire to escape from this kind of situation, is again illustrated. He seeks first to substitute a casual date for the warm relationship with his wife, but he does not keep the date. Again, in the third episode, he seeks to get away, this time by taking lonely flight, but he is aware in the dream that this solution leads nowhere.

This dream reflects very clearly the evolution of the patient's compassionate recognition of his wife's need for human warmth. It illustrates also, in the succeeding episodes, his flight from this compassion and the resultant loneliness, the evolving responses to a conflicting problem through the transitions in an episodic dream.

The conflictual problem was pursued during the next two weeks, at the end of which time came the session now to be reported.

The patient had for some time recognized that his wife loved him genuinely, and that he had never accepted more than a small amount of what she offered him in the marriage. He had in addition prevented her from realizing her socially creative abilities. This thwarting of her ability was something of which he was totally unaware when he entered analysis.

He did, however, have some capacity to recognize the needs of others and to nurture their capacities to grow, attributes which, before treatment, he had cultivated almost exclusively in his relationship with his children. These qualities had begun to play a part in the relationship with his wife, and he was achieving substantial constructive change in his marriage.

The ensuing dreams occurred at the beginning of his third year of analysis. Two weeks before, he had mentioned that his wife was running for re-election as president of a community center, a position in which she had already had a very successful year. The patient objected to this activity on grounds which he had persuaded himself were sound. A second year of presidency for her would interfere with the development of home social activities which, he felt, were important for his growing business. The irrationality of his point of view had been discussed; there was no necessary conflict between her public activity and their social program—the two activities were in no sense mutually exclusive. At that previous analytic session he had given the impression of accepting the desirability of his wife going on for another term. The issue had not again been referred to during the intervening weeks.

He came in and started the hour in a glow of well-being, saying, "I had a very contented dream [Very Contented, But . . .]. I was standing somewhere viewing vast fields. They were so green, so luxurious and fruitful. The land was scattered into many farms. It was all so productive. I had such a contented inner feeling as I viewed it. It was all sort of flowing with food, and good things growing.

"But there was a *discordant note*. It was not all complete. There was a disturbing element. It was completely unclear what this disturbing element was. It was all a matter of feeling. I could feel all this as I was sleeping.

"Then the scene changed completely [No Time for Cousins]. It was like another dream. I was in a public place like at a gym or something with my two older cousins. I heard Bert say to someone, 'Get three tickets.' I asked him what that was for. He said, 'Three tickets for a show for you and me and Al.' I said to him immediately, 'I'm sorry, I'm doing something with Marge [his wife].'

"Then I was in my bedroom at home [What Are You Doing Here?]. I was with George—you know, the guy who got me started in my new business. I dreamed he was sleeping in my bed. I was already up and I said, 'Come on George, it's time to get up. What are you doing here in my bed?'

"Then I was walking in the street [Holding Him Back]. I was right in the middle of the street. George was in a car driving right behind me. I wouldn't let him pass. He was very nice and friendly and kept going along very slowly behind me and calling out to me, 'Hey, come on, let me pass.' But I kept right on and wouldn't give way. He was laughing and good-natured about it. I kept walking slowly. I was very determined; I was refusing to get out of the way. I knew I shouldn't be walking this way, holding him back. There was no room. He couldn't get around me."

This was the end of the four-part, typically episodic dream. The patient went right on to talk about the fruitful aspects of his life. He talked about how well his daughter was doing in school, and what a joy she had been at home. He talked about two friends, both of whom had completed analysis. The wife of one had been telling my patient's wife that he, my patient, would "slip back. You'll see, you'll see." He went right on to say, "Of all the people I've known who have gone to analysis, only one of them has changed. Even she is pretty rigid as a person, but I can see that she is trying hard. I think it's a question of luck, what kind of analyst you go to. I might have wound up with somebody else and lost out.

"It's funny how all these things are working out. I had a wonderful evening last night at the dancing lesson. Marge is so happy. It's been something she has wanted for so many years, and I'm not even forcing myself. I'm enjoying it. Marge wants to go out dancing, and we will, as soon as we've had a few more lessons. If anybody had told me two years ago that I'd be taking these lessons I'd have told them they were nuts.

"There was a fellow at the affair the other night. We got talking and he told me he was an atheist. He said he became an atheist when he read Freud and found out that sex was the center of everything. I told him that I had thought that once, too, but that I felt now there were other goals just as enriching."

He continued without interruption, looking at the green fields. "I was telling Marge the other day how much I felt I had gotten out of analysis. I told her that what appealed to me was your warmth. I said, I couldn't have lain down and talked to a cold person. I would have been talking to a person like myself. I would have been exuding coldness, and receiving coldness."

The hour was over. As a parting comment I told him that I felt he showed increasing self-confidence and optimism about himself, and that he seemed to be taking inventory of his gains during his two years of analysis. I added that there was, however, some hidden problem very clearly indicated by the "discordant note," and that we would have to explore it so that it would not impede his getting to that fruitful country. Furthermore, in the last episode of his dream (Holding Him Back) I suspected that he was walking along interfering with his analyst's progress in the work we were trying to do together. He chuckled as he got to the door and said, "I knew that was you in the car behind me. I knew George was you."

At the next session five days later, he immediately started talking about the dream of the green fields. He said without preliminaries, "I've been making Marge's happiness my primary objective. Everything in the dream was laying itself out in a better pattern, but something in the situation was not good."

I asked him, "What was all the fruitfulness in the dream?"

He said at once, "I've gotten myself on the right track. I can plan a future, not dream a future. I feel that in the next period of time I will succeed, that I'll really be successful, but this interlude right now is something that I just can't skip over." He paused and sighed. "I can't deny it. It's a depressing situation and it's bothering me all the time. I've gotten a good start and I've laid the groundwork but it's tough being without ready money and I'm not going to the cousins. I want money for the house, I want money for Marge, I have to get money for the insurance premiums, I'm holding everybody off. It gets depressing. That's the discordant note."

At this point I said to the patient, "So often you have taken refuge from an emotional problem by emphasizing your financial difficulties, trying to attribute to them all of your frustrations and depressions. We are both quite aware of your financial difficulties and we are aware that they can make you unhappy and *discouraged*. But getting depressed about them is something different. When you get *depressed* and start elaborating financial burdens it has always turned out in the past that there is some other emotional difficulty that you're trying to avoid looking at."

The patient immediately said, "That night I had another dream." (I noted the moment of association.)

He went right on. "That night, after the last session, I mean, I had another dream [Incorrigible Wife]. I just want to tell you something that happened before I tell you the dream. Marge had been shopping with the kids in the car and she had asked them to help her up to the apartment with the packages. Libby [his daughter] acted up. She just walked away into the house without carrying anything. I told Marge that if I had been there I'd have actually spanked her. Marge disagreed with me but at the same time she told me how she had screamed at Libby and then she told me that she was afraid that if she spanked Libby she'd just lose control of herself." He added, "I've never laid a hand on Libby. Maybe that's been a mistake. Maybe she needs some physical discipline.

"Anyway, here's the dream I had that night after Marge told me what happened. I came into an apartment house lobby. Marge was there with Libby and began to complain to me about Libby's behavior, how Libby was impossible. She couldn't get her to do anything. I said to Libby, 'You come right upstairs with me.' She refused.

"Then I was in the elevator with *Marge*. Marge was saying she wouldn't come upstairs with me. I said she would so, and a violent argument started between us. There was another person in the elevator and I was embarrassed.

"Then we were in our apartment and we were having a serious talk about getting a divorce. A second cousin of mine was there—he's a real no-good stinker. His father and mother were there, too, although his father is really dead. He was talking to his mother with a lot of feeling, saying, 'I work hard mornings to get you a mink coat.'"

At this point the patient lay silent for a few moments. Then he continued, "On the other side of the room Marge had a canasta game going, and I was angry because she had a canasta game casually going on when we're in the midst of a serious talk about getting a divorce. Then some people come in from the community center, and Marge insists that they stay."

At this point the patient again stopped talking. He was under severe tension and blew a long stream of air out through his taut lips, a sort of angry, quiet snort. He continued silent, sighed a few times, and writhed tensely on the couch.

I asked him to say what he was feeling.

"I don't know. I feel mixed up. I'm mixed up emotionally. I don't know. It seems to be something connected with religion. I don't know. I'm just mixed up."

Without pause he continued. "Marge is going into this thing to-night, as I knew she would. Once she decides she really goes into things. We're having a big party next week, a mob. I have a need for a lot of people, and I've invited a lot of them, and she's handling it in a big way." He began going into details about the people who were coming to the party and the arrangements that had been made. Then he talked of some minor activities with the children.

I interrupted to bring him back to the dream. "Let's get back to the dream. I noticed that after you described your cousin telling his mother in the dream about working mornings to get her a mink coat, you stopped and were silent for a few moments."

"When I heard that guy say it, I realized that the work he did mornings was ultimately to be free of his mother, to give her the mink coat, and that was it. That guy's a failure, a get-rich-quicker. All his life he would have a job—he would get a good start, and he would show a lot of promise. Every time he got a job he would start in sweet as honey, and soon he knew more than the boss and he'd try to take over and he'd land on his ass. He never succeeded in anything."

I interpreted directly, "I guess you recognize he's a stand-in for you."

The patient immediately responded, "*I know I don't want to look at this. I could have worked out this dream, but I didn't.* Why not?" [8]

I said, "There's something in the dream involving your feelings about your wife. Perhaps some of your attitudes toward her resemble those that you had toward your mother. Your second cousin, who is in some ways so much like you, is reminding his mother how much he is doing for her."

"Why am I talking of divorce? We were at a party last night. Marge was the prettiest one there. Over the years people have said to me, 'How can she stand living with you?' Marge isn't stupid. What is her need for me, except that she must love me. How is she like my mother?"

I replied, "Marge isn't like your mother. As a matter of fact she is quite different. *Your attitude* toward your wife, however, is very much like your attitude toward your mother. Your mother tried to enslave you. You don't distinguish this from Marge's efforts to win your love in response to her loving you.

"It seems to me that there are two important attitudes toward your wife that come up in this dream. One is an attitude you had toward your mother. You kept a distance from your mother, but you did give her the externals of filial concern. The externals are like the mink in the dream, which to you meant freeing you of further obligations.

"In the dream your cousin spoke about 'working hard mornings' to get his mother a mink coat. In reality you have had considerable business success since you started working mornings in analysis. You

[8] The moment of association for the dream was my statement: "When you get depressed and start elaborating financial burdens, it has always turned out in the past that there is some other emotional difficulty that you're trying to avoid looking at."

give Marge the external benefits derived from your work here, but you won't give her yourself.

"The second attitude toward your wife that comes up in the dream is like your attitude toward your little girl when you're angry with her. You remember, when you and Marge were talking before going to sleep, you thought maybe Libby needed a little 'physical discipline.' You were exasperated and you wanted to beat Libby into submission. In the dream, there is an immediate substitution of Marge for Libby. First you insist on Libby going upstairs with you, and the next moment you are in the elevator with your wife, insisting that *she* go upstairs with you. *She's got to.*"

It was the end of the hour and I made the following interpretive summary for him to carry away with him. "I believe it is this problem that represents your depressed feelings, the discordant note in that Very Contented dream. It is connected with your relationship to your wife, not to your financial difficulties. I think the discordant note is comprised of the two elements that I mentioned. One of them is this superficial fulfillment that you're trying to get Marge to settle for. You'll give *things* to her, you'll work hard mornings in analysis and bring her a more polished guy, a greater success in business (the mink coat) instead of really giving yourself to her. And the other element is your coercive approach to her, your insisting that she behave a certain way, like a little girl who is supposed to have the proper attitude toward her daddy. In other words, in your dreams it was your attempt both to have Marge settle for a 'mink coat' and to force her to 'come upstairs with you' that kept you distant from that fruitful countryside. In your waking experience it's your distant and coercive attitudes that keep you from having all the fruits of a good marital relationship and a good life. These two factors comprise the discordant note. Let's pursue this problem and these feelings further."

The fuller interpretation of this dream was limited by the restrictions of time, and was postponed until the next session. There it was augmented by a supplemental dream expressing the same unresolved problem.[9] The patient came into the next session two days later looking, acting, and feeling very depressed. After a few sighs he recounted a dream of the previous night (The Child-Woman).

"I was in a large movie house. I was put in charge of doing something minor like collecting tickets while the manager took a nap. I

[9] The phenomenon of continued expression in new dreams of an unresolved problem in which the patient is deeply involved is well demonstrated in this serial development.

was sore, because how the hell could I watch the movie if I have to be taking tickets?

"A woman slipped on the marble in the lobby and I sat her on a seat. A crowd gathered around her and she was concealed by all these people. She said she was all right.

"Much later I was standing in the street and I see her walking with a fellow, and I start to ask her how she feels and I see she's not a woman but a child. She walked away. She was all right."

As usual, I asked, "What was your feeling in the dream?"

"I was disappointed when I saw it was a child, not a woman." He laughed. "I was just thinking how last night Marge was telling me about [a movie star]. Marge said this star has the body of a woman but the emotions of a child. So in the dream I was disappointed when it was a child and not a woman. I'm disappointed in myself, too. *There are a lot of things I should be doing, and I'm not doing them.* I should be working harder, doing a lot more. I've stopped trying to build my business by studying in the evenings. I haven't had enough incentive."

The pursuit of his dream feeling of disappointment at finding his wife a little girl instead of a woman had brought him to his feeling of depression and his lack of incentive to fulfill his own role as the husband and the breadwinner. A few weeks before this dream he had mentioned casually that he was no longer staying home and working on weekday evenings, as had been his custom. Since he had been in the new business his studying had been valuable. But now that his wife was working hard for the community center, he had been going with her and waiting around on the periphery of her activity, doing chores, escorting her home. This suggested the ticket-collecting in the movie in the dream; his feeling of being assigned menial tasks seemed to refer to his wife as the manager of the movie house. At the previous session we had discussed her probable re-election at the community center; she would be running the show.[10]

In connection with his reported lack of incentive I replied to him, "You haven't been working here either for the last two weeks. You've been fighting me."

He answered incredulously, "I have?"

"Yes. You've been getting depressed, and you've been avoiding any initiative in working on your dreams. Who is the woman who fell in the lobby?"

[10] It may have referred also to the analyst placing upon him, at the previous session, the responsibility of working on the dream. The patient had to work on the relationship with his wife as exposed in the dream—his scolding her, the talk about divorce—and he had to work by himself, while the manager (analyst) took a nap!

"I don't know."

He then remained silent for nearly a minute until I asked the obvious question, "Who comes to mind?"

Angrily, begrudgingly, and impatiently he shouted, "Marge, it's got to be Marge."

I asked how he felt toward her in the dream, and he replied, "I was worried. I was afraid she'd hurt herself. I felt good when she said she was all right, but she really took an awful spill. Maybe she said she wasn't hurt because she was embarrassed."

"In your last dream, the action also started in a lobby."

"That was the lobby of my house."

"Your little girl Libby was there. You were scolding her and she turned into Marge. You were scolding your wife in the elevator in exactly the same spirit in which you were scolding your little girl in the lobby and telling her to come home upstairs. In this movie lobby dream, the woman whom you identify now as Marge, in the reverse order of your other dream then turns into a little girl. Your deprecating association to the little girl, who had been Marge, is a woman's body with a little girl's emotions."

He laughed with somewhat good-natured and embarrassed recognition of the correlation.

At this point I asked him directly, "Did Marge stay in the running for the presidency of the woman's section of the community center? You spoke about your resentment of this two weeks ago, and then you indicated to me an apparent reversal, an acceptance of her right to be engaged in such activities."

"Yes. I told her it was okay with me and that I felt my attitude had been wrong, and she stayed in the running."

"But you didn't tell *me* that you'd done anything about it. You never referred to it again. I believe you've been sore at Marge for these last two weeks, ever since you agreed to her going ahead. I think that, to you, wanting the presidency is having little-girl emotions. I think the movie house may be the community center, and I think you're exasperated with her and insist that she come home, just as you yell at your little girl to come upstairs in the elevator in the last dream. I think that because Marge has continued to want an independent life, a framework in which to express her social abilities, you've been cold to her, and that this is represented by the discussion of a divorce after you get her upstairs in the dream. Throughout your marriage you have punished her most by withdrawing, by sulking, by walking away, in effect by divorcing yourself from her whenever she would not act in slavish accord with your desires. Her fall in the lobby may even indicate that if she goes on with this presidency stuff you hope she falls and breaks her neck, so to speak. This unwillingness on your part for your wife to fulfill herself (as she has begun to do more than ever since you've gotten healthier)—this unwillingness represents the *discordant note* in your 'very contented' dream. As I said last time, it is this which keeps you at a distance from the fruitful lands. I think it is your reluctance to face this immediate problem of your trying to dominate your wife that is represented by your walking in the middle of the road and blocking the way for your friend in the car behind you. He is the guy who was responsible for your starting a successful career in business, and who is a stand-in for me, who has helped you in other ways to make use of your abilities both in business and in your family relationships.

"I think," I went on, "that a very subtle process has been going on in your development. I think that you've been gaining a great deal of enjoyment out of your family life and out of the increased companionship, in which you've helped your wife to express herself and to achieve some of her own goals in the marriage. Only a short time ago you spoke glowingly, in connection with the Very Contented dream, of the happiness that you had in finally going in for dancing lessons and contemplating social dancing with your wife, who has been wanting this throughout the many years of the marriage. I think that in a subtle way you have been trying to use these healthy changes also as a means of seductively getting back the old control—to dominate her and compel the same slavish compliance that you used to enforce with coldness and divorcement from her. Her cultivating genuine independence infuriates you. When you get upstairs from the apartment lobby, and try to bring her into line by talking of divorce, you are exasperated by her going right ahead with her activities, which are represented by the presence of the people from the community center who are in the canasta game.

"There is no question but that you've come a long way and have a much happier life and a much happier marriage, and you recognize the fruitfulness of the changes in your personality. But you cannot use these changes to beat your wife into submission. I think you are depressed by the loss of this possibility. I think the strained consequences of your efforts in this direction, efforts of which you have been unaware, represent the *discordant note*. Your wife is not a little girl. She is a woman. By treating her as such you've had your greatest satisfactions. Your depression is not lack of money, it's your fighting me and angrily fighting to maintain your old dominant role with your wife."

The work with this series of dreams illustrates the analyst's persistent initiative in pursuing the dream material in the face of the patient's definite resistance. The productiveness of this approach is indicated by the patient's substantial cooperative response, in spite of his resistance.[11]

The analyst's persistence here is prompted also by evidence of evolving health in the dream material. The Very Contented dream indicates a happy outlook on a new way of life. The fourth episode of the same dream (Holding Him Back) indicates a recognition of the friendliness of the analyst which surmounts the patient's resistance. Likewise in the third episode (What Are You Doing Here?) the patient regards the analyst, despite the why-are-you-getting-so-much-into-my-life attitude, as a friendly "bedfellow."

This brief series of dreams and the therapist's insistent attention to their interpretation in the face of the patient's resistance,[12] led soon to the healthiest and most productive period in the patient's life. This progress was preceded, characteristically, by an intensification of recalcitrant despair, a final holding action in the form of depression, as set forth below in the report of the following session. Then the patient got to work on his business affairs and plunged ahead. He included his wife in confidences about his business in a way that he had never done before. He accepted her winning of the presidency, and during the ensuing weeks both their social and sexual life became more meaningful and companionate.

Many of the dream elements were not pursued point by point, symbol by symbol.[13] But in the development of the interpretations the patient took an active and not a compliant part, although he required considerable therapeutic stimulus. Even in the prelude to the angry dream of the Incorrigible Wife the patient started the hour with spontaneous collaboration. He did this by taking the initiative in interpreting the episodic dream of the previous session, the dream ending with the determined resistance of the patient in holding up the analyst in the car. Regardless of what other dream data were left unexplored, it may be observed that feeling was emphasized throughout.

It is of significance too that the analyst's comment in connection with the patient's return to this dream was the trigger or moment of

[11] Compare Elevator Nightmare session in Chapter 6, "Resistance in Dreams," pp. 218–226.

[12] See discussion of interpretive activity of the analyst alone in the face of the patient's resistance, pp. 22–23. This is an example in which such activity is concurrently productive.

[13] See unexplored dream data, pp. 245–246.

association for the Incorrigible Wife dream. When the patient, instead of continuing the spontaneous examination of the episodic Very Contented dream, started off on the tangent of depression over financial affairs, the analyst pointed out to him that he frequently took refuge from emotional problems in this way. In response to my comment that he might be rationalizing about the source of his unhappiness, the patient remembered the new dream.

This series of sessions continues now (after the Incorrigible Wife dream) without a new dream but with the focus coming even more sharply on the hostility and derogation of his wife depicted in the Child-Woman dream.

The patient came into a fourth consecutive session of the two-week period that began with the Very Contented dream. He looked very unhappy, lay down, and was silent for a full minute. Then, impatiently but quietly, he said, "Shit." After a silence, "I feel all ugly inside." Another silence. "I've tried to figure out what's the matter and I can't."

I said, "You've learned free association—use it."

He replied at once. "I've been trying for days. I feel mean inside. I'm frustrated. I feel angry, but it goes inside instead, not against anyone."

"That's unlikely," I said. "Maybe it does go against someone."

"Not against my family, anyway," he answered quickly.[14]

"That's your first association," I pointed out.

He tried to back away. "If I associate, I begin to imagine things. I feel pressure in the back of my head. It's all a blank wall." (This is an example of psychosomatic confusion.)

I said to him, "Let's face it—you don't want to get past the wall."

"Because I can't see anything beautiful on the other side," he parried weakly.

He was resisting, but with a transparent lack of conviction. This was a familiar pattern in his analysis. He was stubborn, but he wanted help.[15] I said, "Let's look at what's been going on here. You've had a number of dreams during the past couple of weeks, and you've refused to look at them adequately. I left you at the end of the last session with a very important thought to pursue. You feel something—a discordant

[14] This is an example of a patient's resistance by the presentation of an association in negated form; see Chapter 7, "Interpretive Activity," pp. 249–250.

[15] As in the episodic dream of twelve days before (Holding Him Back), he was walking in the middle of the road and not letting the analyst get ahead, but he was at the same time well aware of the good will of the analyst.

note—that you don't want to talk about. You know how to work in analysis, you know how to work well. I'll bet your evasiveness right now is more humiliating and painful for you than facing your problem would be. You left last time with the important problem that you continue to resent your wife's independence. You like her competence, but you want her to use it in your service, and not for her own enjoyment of herself. While you've achieved a great deal in your marriage, and have a much better relationship with Marge and give a great deal more to her, you still have a strong desire to keep her subservient to you." I then spent some time reviewing the dreams of the past three sessions and the interpretive hypotheses that I had formulated in the face of his resistance. I referred to the positive gains, but I also emphasized the negative forces in his marital relationship, which were the basis of his present anger and depression.

When I concluded the recapitulation of the dreams of the last few sessions he was silent only a few seconds. Then he said, "I apologized to Marge the other night for my attitude about her re-election to the presidency." But then, with an immediate reversal, he added resentfully, "Just the same, when she's rushed and under pressure she screams at the kids."

I said, "She screams at the kids, it seems to me, when she's under pressure from *you*."

Ignoring my comment, he now brought up and repeated some earlier rationalizations with which he had defended his opposition to her renomination for the presidency. He wanted and supposedly needed her to make entertaining at home a "full-time job."

Then he vacillated: he praised her superior abilities as a hostess and homemaker, and then petulantly criticized her as "stupid" for some minor indecisiveness. This led to his reporting an incident of the evening before when his wife had prepared dinner for the family and an old friend who was visiting. She had come home a little late, but there was no need for any formality. Yet, as he put it, "She was so nervous, showed such lack of poise. I tried to calm her down."

After this last statement he was silent for a few moments. When he spoke again there was a change in his voice. "Do you think she's nervous because she feels some kind of pressure from me?"

Finally, dimly, for essentially the first time in nearly two weeks, a willingness to take the initiative in honestly examining his own feelings and behavior in his relationship with his wife had begun to take hold. This willingness emerged with the compassion recalled and seemingly re-experienced when he said, "I tried to calm her down."

In the spirit of his own inquiry, I asked, "What do you think?"

His immediate response was to bring out the contrast between her intense nervousness when she prepared an informal supper with one friend as a guest, and a recent large dinner party for over twenty people which she had carried off with grace and efficiency. As he put it, "She wasn't at all nervous then, and she said later that she'd expected me to put pressure on her. She said how good she felt about my not doing that and how nice it was."

I immediately suggested to him that his question, whether his wife was nervous because she felt pressure from him, seemed to be answered by his own association to the big dinner party. She was happy and efficient and managed beautifully and was grateful when he didn't put pressure on her. With this evidence, supplied through his own valida- tive activity, it became clear that it was not the presidency of the com- munity organization that would lead to her nervousness, her "stupid- ity," her lack of poise, or her yelling at the kids. It was the pressure from him. He had finally begun to face this, and to recognize his in- tense desire to constrict her, to make her become a person exclusively occupied in his behalf, rather than someone developing and enjoying herself in her own right as a wife and a mother and a member of the community.

The patient left with no further signs of depression and his prog- ress for the next two months until the summer intermission was fairly consistent.

The material of the dreams and the therapist's persistence in bring- ing it forward in the face of the patient's resistance was responsible for the ultimate resolution of this important period of the patient's fight against change.

The analytic hour next to be examined occurred two months later, and concludes the six-month period beginning with the dream Spilling His Guts.

For three weeks the patient had been discussing some rather dramatic events which had involved the greatest degree of business initiative he had ever taken. The chief difficulties had already been essentially resolved, and while the whole project was not yet fully con- summated as planned, it had represented a considerable success for him. During the course of negotiations and planning, he had shown his independence and initiative not only among those with whom he was negotiating but (more significantly in the framework of his emo- tional development) also vis-à-vis his older cousins. During the three weeks of these negotiations he had enjoyed a great deal of self-respect.

At the present session he started to speak in a subdued spirit.

"I want to tell you a dream that I had about two weeks ago. It's been hanging over me ever since [The Lost Son].

"I was on a very crowded subway platform. I had lost David. The station platform was very crowded and the people were in groups all along it. I was running down the station going from one group to the other, yelling *David, David!* (That frantic feeling—*David, David!*—has been persisting for the last two weeks.) I was anxious and distraught and very worried. I was worried what would happen to him. I woke up feeling upset."

Spontaneously he went on to interpret the dream. "Maybe I was getting scared of losing David already. He's getting a little older. I can see definite changes. He's beginning to have an adolescent maturity.

"I always said and I thought I really believed that kids should be encouraged to be independent and now it's coming to the test. Even when he was an infant I always loved to be with him. I used to love to give him his bottle at night. I bathed him and diapered him. I used to carry him over to my mother's with a valise full of diapers and bottles.

"I've tried not to think about it, but I've often wondered how I'd feel if he ever said, 'You go with your friends, and I'll go with mine.' I always wondered, when that day came, and come it must, what I'd do."

He went on to recount an incident, characterizing it as illustrating the very problem he had been fantasying. "Sunday a widower who has a nineteen-year-old son was over. The boy was with a group of his friends, nineteen- and twenty-year-olds. I was talking with the father about Father's Day. He said his son had looked forward to Father's Day and they were going to spend it together. Then came Father's Day, and some friends of the boy called up and without any thought the boy went off with them.

"What a Father's Day card Libby [daughter] wrote to me! Talking about Libby, I don't have the same feeling as with David. I feel she'll always be there. It's just a feeling."

At this point I spoke for the first time. "In the dream you were yelling for David in a frantic way. Perhaps you were not so worried about David as you were about yourself. The way you describe yourself in the dream, it sounds a little like the kid getting separated from his parents in a crowd at Coney Island—getting lost."

"I don't want to be lost from him!" he answered at once, and emphatically. "I don't know why I should feel this way about him. *Nothing special happened.*"

But a good deal *had* been happening, and I stepped in at this point to focus and correlate. "Something special has happened. All your life you've been bound by strong *artificial* ties to your cousins. During these

past big three or four weeks in your business you've declared your independence from them more definitely than ever before. I think you
have sensed emotionally the fact that *artificial bonds can be dissolved.*
Now, about you and David—you have given him a great deal of paternal companionship and genuine love, but there have been *some* artificial bonds by which you have held David close to you. For example,
for years you prevented him from sleeping overnight at the homes of
his friends. You made him feel bad if he didn't want to spend time
with you. You have always felt that if you did not bind him to you by
indulging and praising him, and by sulking when he displeased you,
that you would not have a strong relationship with him.

"It's very important for you to distinguish between these artificial
bonds and the real affection. In your relationship with your wife and
with David and with others, you've begun to see that the real bonds
of affection and friendship are stronger and more durable than the
artificial ties. Nevertheless, I think your recent more effective severance of synthetic ties to your cousins has made you feel that David
could do the same thing with you. You're afraid David's independence
will take him away from you because you have relied so much on these
artificial ties. You've lost sight of the existence of the genuine affectional bonds which made David *want* to be close to you."

The patient heaved a deep sigh of relief and said quietly, "That
fits completely."

In discussing the meaning of dreams it was said that a dream represents an attitude or practice of which the individual is unaware and
which he is reluctant or unwilling to acknowledge when awake. The
patient here very quickly stated in his interpretive remarks following
the presentation of the dream that he always thought he believed that
"kids should be encouraged to be independent." The attitude he was
reluctant (but not entirely unwilling) to acknowledge was that his concern was not for his son's welfare, but for his own.

In contrast, the patient had healthy attitudes as well toward his
son, and wished him to become independent. He had struggled hard
in analysis to identify and relinquish his enslaving tactics toward his
son. He had *unequivocally* encouraged overnight visits by the boy to
the homes of friends, and in other ways too had succeeded in the framework of healthier values—in spite of his anxiety about failure within
the framework of his pathological values (enslavement of others). By
my delineating for him the existence in him of healthy values, of feelings and behavior showing genuine love for his boy, he was relieved
and reassured. (This is an example of authentic reassurance.)

Six months before, at the time of the Spilling His Guts dream (the time of another assertion of independence from his cousins) the patient had reported saying to his closest friend, "I'm over forty and I'm not a man yet." Now, as he again made a maturing spurt, he again worried about his capacity to maintain firm relationships without the use of dependent techniques. The pathological sense of self that derived from functioning with enslaving techniques had been further threatened by his maturing relationship with his wife. In an affective sense, his own growth was echoed in his observation of his son David's "beginning to have an adolescent maturity." And so, during his later encouraging, independent business negotiations, "that frantic feeling—*David, David!* —has been persisting for the last two weeks." It was not that he needed to hold on to David to survive; it was that as new, healthier techniques of living developed, he had come closer than ever to completely abandoning his pathological-dependent-enslaving behavior, and he distortedly sensed this change as a weakening. Basically it was not David that he feared to lose, but his own personality as it was identified with a dependent way of living. This then is another example of the commonly occurring anxiety that develops in the context of evolving health.

Dream Index

NOTE: *Many of the dreams in this volume appear again and again, in different contexts. Sometimes they are referred to very briefly, at other times more extensively. The* **BOLD FACE TYPE** *indicates the pages on which the fullest presentation of the dream may be found.*

Analyst-Chauffeur, **123–124**, 127, 136, 169, 188, 259, 287, 294

Annoyed with Mother, 52, **113–114**, 127

Atomic Reactor, 164

Battle Tactics, 8–9, **186–187**, 200n

Bear Man, 4, 196, **197–198**

Bird of Prey, 4, 7, 31, **115–117**, 127

Bleeding Patient, 58

Blowing My Top, 6, 50, 51–52

Breech Presentation, 3–4, **5**

Burning Man, **56–57**, 61

Captain-Woman, 46, 184n, **254–257**, 282n, 292, 293, 294, 310

Child-Woman, **320–323**, 325

Chinese Laundry, 239, **240–241**, 242, 243, 244

Contemptible Passion, 7, 63, **120–121**, 127, 145, 216, 275n

Crazy Woman Nightmare, 51n, 53, **73–77**, 79, 83, 85, 86, 98, 99–100, 151–152, 162, 165, 170, 203, 234, 246, 275, 278, 298

Crude and Ugly Things, 194–195

Dancing Teacher, 209

Danny's Climb, 295–296

Death of Husband, 190n, **204–205**, 254n, 269n

Disturbingly Adequate Husband, **172–173**, 190n, 192n

Dog Eat Dog, **93–94**, 99

Dragging Feet, 51

Driver Does Not Stop, 195–196

Dying and Being Reborn, 296–297

Edging Sideways, 53–54

Egyptian King, 94

Elevator Nightmare, 3, 165, 200n, 202n, **218–226**, 230–231, 234, 246, 324n

Eliminator, **58–59**, 18on
Empty Suit, **117–119**, 127, 171, 190
Enjoying Her Frustration, **185–186**, 202–203
Escaping the Photographer, **185**, 186
Execution, **193–194**, 195

Faking It, **104**, 107, 110, 127, 298
Fight with an Antelope, 11n, 101, **104**, 105, 106, 107, 109, 110, 127, 228, 234, 298
Fruit Store Man, 63

Growth Pills, **187–188**, 308

He's Not So Bad, **279–280**
Holding Him Back, 7, 245, 279, **316**, 317, 324, 325n
Homosexual Incest, **150**, 278
Hot Dog, 8, 38, 39, 45, 63, **112–113**, 127
House Alterations, **5–6**

Incorrigible Wife, **317–318**, 324, 325
Independent Mistress, **146**, 171n, 178
Induced Labor, **31–32**, 130, 185, 203, 210n, 215, 216
Irrigation Deluge, 3, **46**

Japanese Battlefield, **196–197**, 217
Just Friends, **148–150**, 244

Keeping One Coin, 187
Kept Calling Up, **89–90**, 175
Kindly Senator, **275**, 278

Long Corridor, **141–142**
Lost Son, 31on, **327–329**

Madman, **288–290**
Making a Play for Her, 216

Mother Just Died, 266
Murder Trial, 159, **160–161**, 175, 178, 180

Night Club, 239, **241–242**, 244
No Destination, **311–312**, 313
No Intercourse Yet, 279
No Time for Cousins, 315
Not Listening, 51

Oil Well, **235–238**, 245, 246
Old Negro Prostitute, 7, **147**, 148
Old Woman Masturbating Him, **148**, 282–283

Parachute Nightmare, **275**, 276–277, 278
Pissing, 87, 166
Poisonous Dachshund, 8, **45**
Poor Guide, 56, 58
Poor Sprinkler, 54
Positive Throat Culture, 166
Principal's Office, **282–283**, 291, 292
Prodigy, **45–46**
Puppy-rat, 6

Rabbis' Curse, 19on, **293**, 294
Rat Eyes, **173–174**
Recurrent Dreams of Lionesses, 6, 41, **122–123**, 127
Restaurant, 239, **241**, 242, 244, 245
Rocking Chair, **54–55**, 58
Royalty Coming to an End, **285–286**

Sad Young Lady, 46
Scared Shitless, 50, 51, 52, **114–115**, 127, 203n, 230
Screwed Up, **190–192**, 231
Shark in Swimming Pool, 3, 8, 125, **126–127**, 158, 167, 168, 18on
Shit Piles Up, 51n, **78–80**, 86, 298
Shitty Behavior, 51

Sickle, 40

Sideways Approach, **146–147**, 171n, 178

Skating Rink, **125–126**, 127

Sledgehammer Attack, 146, **163**, 171n

Something to Tell, 51

Son Sucking Me Off, **133–138**, 178, 269

Special Gun, 287–288

Spilling His Guts, 4–5, 19, **299–302**, 308, 327, 330

Statuesque Masturbation, 50–51, 52–53, 130, **143–145**, 146, 147, 163, 171n, 178, 190n

Straight and Narrow, 4, **103–104**, 105, 107, 110, 127, 298

Supermarket Baby, 45

Three Bedraggled Cats, 8, **143**, 311–313, 314

Three Condoms, 67n, 91n, **153–154**, 173

Tiny Cobras, 94, **138–141**, 159, 175, 180, 231

Toaster, **106**, 110, 127

Token Kindness, **67**, 275n

Two Drunken Sailors, 231–233

Two or Three Cents' Worth, 32

Unkept Date, 311

Urinating in the Bottle, 55–56

Very Contented, But . . . , 25, 51, 190n, 245, **315**, 317, **320**, 323, 324, 325

Wading in Deeper, 56, **125–126**, 127, 168, 180n

Wand and the Apes, 41, **169**, 259

What Are You Doing Here? **315**, 324

Wheelbarrows, **189**, 190, 251, 259, 291n

Whirling Dervish, 164

White Hot Car, **59–60**, 163

Woman on Barren Beach, **121–122**, 127

Wooden Earth, 46

You Hold Me Close, 148, **275–278**, 279

General Index

All dreams are indexed separately in the Dream Index, which starts on page 331.

acceptance-out-of-existence, 201–202, 207n

action, as dream element, 24–39
  and episodic dreams, 239
  reflection of waking behavior, resistance, 198–199

Adler, Alfred, ix, x, xi

affection, for analyst, 148, 226–228, 290

aggression and sexuality, 131

ambivalence (*see also* the dreams Shit Piles Up; Death of Husband; Captain-Woman; Spilling His Guts):
  intensification of, near termination, 292
  between marital warmth and domination, 314
  and reassurance in depression, 306

analyst, activity of, *see* associative activity; collaborative process; interpretive activity; interpretive hypothesis

analytic "brinkmanship," 202–203

anger:
  as antidote for anxiety and other feelings, 213
  and anxiety, 159, 161, 162–164
  and bladder urgency, 163
  and depression, 59–60, 162–163
  and headache, 100, 138, 163
  and intestinal tensions, 138
  and resistance, 199, 210–211

animal as individual in dream, 6–7, 41, 78, 115–117, 122–123, 126

anxiety, 157–181 (*see also* functional effectiveness; self-concept; sense of self; unreality, feelings of; Elevator Nightmare)
  competitiveness a source of, 157
  defined, 157
  denial of emotion as source of, 162

anxiety *(cont'd)*
    evaluation of, associated with use
        of early dreams, 108
    as an experiential feeling in
        dreams, 51
    and guilt, 174–175
    intimacy as source of, 162
    with new emotions, 100
    and omitted dream data, 246
    in psychotherapist, 174
    pursuit of, in schizoid and other
        patients, 180
    rejection as source of, 175–176
    as result of failure to ward off in-
        terpersonal influences, 173
    and sex, 177–178
    tender emotions as source of, 165,
        178
    threat to manipulative techniques
        as source of, 170–174
associations of analyst, 15–16
associations, contextual, 11, 16 *(see
    also* personal glossary)
    occurring years later, 289, 294–
        295
    related to psychosomatic symp-
        toms, 101
    stimulated by a similar dream, 140
associations of patient *(see also* mo-
    ment of association):
    after the session, 104 *(see also* as-
        sociations, contextual; personal
        glossary)
    before dream report, 78
    during dream report, 104, 185–
        186, 317–318
    explanations and analogies, 98
    psychosomatic signals, 100–101
associative activity, 2, 10–19
    of analyst, 16–19
    of patient: following the session,
        107; practical suggestions to pa-

    tient, 98; process, 14–15; psy-
        chosomatic focal point, 101
attitude, relation to behavior, 121

bargaining with insights, 206n
Bartlett, Doris, xxiii, 264n
Bartlett, Francis, xxiii
beating analyst to interpretation,
    250–251
blurring in verbal communication,
    97–99, 217 *(see also* insulating
    terms; loose terminology)
Breuer, J., 13n
brief therapy, 21, 42

castration fear, xvii, 132
changing symbolism, 40, 45–46
childhood, demand for unrealized,
    183–184 *(see also* transference)
childhood memories, importance of,
    269
collaborative process, xvii, 19–22,
    26–27, 35, 47–48, 102–103,
    108, 110, 115, 117, 124–125,
    138, 146, 147, 171 *(see also*
    mutuality)
    avoided by interpretive filibuster,
        250
    basic feature of curative process,
        258
    beating analyst to interpretation,
        250–251
    as counter to anxiety in therapy,
        180–191
    criterion of strength, 214–215
    false cooperativeness, 188–189
    fullest expression in interpretive
        activity, 251–252
    increased with spouse, as termina-
        tion criterion, 288
    in joint decision to terminate, 296
    overcoming resistance, 183, 228

in pursuit of meaning through feeling, 235
rushing into new topic, 251
as subjugation, 25
undermined by false reassurance,
265
undermined by therapeutic "tricks,"
212
competitiveness, 86–95
defined, 87–88
in marriage, 313
between men and women, 92
pathological view of analytic dyad,
273–274
reinforced by cynicism, 86, 87, 95
and resistance, 182–183
sense of defeat with change, 292
and sex, 177
as source of anxiety, 157
techniques of, 86–87, 94
collective unconscious, 37
condensation, 38 (*see also* multiple
reference)
conflict, emotional, *see* ambivalence
consciousness, x–xi, xiv, xxi–xxii
change of, in analysis, 257–258,
263
cynical distortions of, 70
dream symbolism and waking consciousness, 233–234
evolution of, 53
healthy, 68–69, 170
and sexuality, 133
sleeping consciousness and resistance, 182
contradictory emotions, co-existence
of, 60–61, 67, 73, 75, 83
and health, 60
and therapeutic progress, 61
control over others:
and anxiety, 169–170
and depression, 308

countertransference, 17
and anxiety, 174
"culturalist" psychoanalytic approach,
viii, xi, xv–xvi, xxi–xxiii
culture, and dream symbolism, xv–
xvi, 32–33
cynicism, xii, xvii, 64–86, 170n
analysis of, 71–86
clinical illustration of, 275
as cultural influence, 64
defined, 65, 68
and depression, 70
evolution of, 68, 70
as reinforced by competitiveness,
95
and resistance, 25, 183
and the schizoid patient, 180
and trust, 274–275
and tricks of analyst, 212

Dement, William, 239n
dependency, 124, 259, 294
coercive dependency, 308
demand for an unrealized childhood, 183–184
helplessness, 215
near termination, 293–294
depression:
and anger, 162–163
and cynicism, 70
danger of false reassurance, 305
discouragement, contrasted with,
317
dreams of depressive patients, 51,
59–60, 117–118, 121–122, 153–
155, 163–164, 204–205, 219–
220, 298–300
and evolving health, 187–188, 324
and fear of future, 309
among friends, 94
of husbands, 92–93
as an interpersonal practice, 215

depression (*cont'd*)
  and rejection, 175–176
  as resistance, 138, 210–211, 215
  over responsibility for own happiness, 232
  and retaliation, 92
  and therapeutic goal, 177
discrepancy between emotion and concept of it, 60–64
  found through introductory dreams, 112–113
  in marriage, 63
  obscuring initial reactions, 99
  pathogenic effect of on children, 63
  relationship to behavioral discrepancy and self-concept, 157–158
dream, *defined*, 34, 120
dream, elements of, 2, 38
  and symbolism, 38
  traced through three episodes, 239–245
dream process, 44
dream symbols, 31–48 (*see also* changing symbolism; psychosomatic symbols)
  abstractions, 34
  and common cultural experience, 33
  emotional connotations of, 35
  origin of, 32–33
  personal glossary, 32–33, 40, 42, 245, 292, 294
  repetition of, 40–42
  semantic specificity, 31
  sexual, 40, 129–156 (*see also* homosexuality; phallic symbols)
dream wish, 37n
dream work, *defined*, 38
dynamic concept of the dream in the therapeutic situation, 1–29

Ehrenwald, Jan, xix
emotion (*see also* discrepancy; feeling; meaning):
  and competitive tactics, 86
  denial of, 53–59
  detection of, 94, 110
  disorientation by denial of, 278
  emergence of new, 77, 79, 100
  emotional control and anxiety, 164, 168
  initial reactions, 99–100
  and intellectual exchange in analysis, 258
  as measure of therapeutic commitment, 101
  synthetic exaggeration of, 203
  technical considerations and suggestions, 95–101
emotional similes, *see* similes, emotional
empathy, 97, 261
engagement, therapeutic, 22, 23, 24, 25, 59, 107–108, 147, 183, 192, 199, 200, 210–215, 222, 291
episodic dreams, 238–245, 315
equality:
  between patient and analyst, 111
  between the sexes, 92–93
  struggle against, in marriage, 190, 288–289, 313–327
euphemisms, 96, 171
evolving health (*see also* the dreams Crazy Woman; Death of Husband; Oil Well):
  emerging in context of pathology, 266
  feelings of unreality, 263–264
  growth without analysis, 263
  reflected in episodic dreams, 245
  sadness and uncertainty during, 265, 290–291
exhibitionism, therapeutic, 21

experiential feeling, *see* feeling, experiential

feeling, xv, 2, 9–10, 49–101 (*see also* emotion)
  experiential, 10, 38, 39, 50, 78
  symbolized, 10, 39, 52, 59, 67, 78
filibuster, interpretive, 27–28, 202, 250
"flight into health," 217
free association, 13, 102, 109 (*see also* associations; associative activity);
freedom, concepts of, xii–xiii
Freud, Sigmund, x, xii, 13n, 37n, 38, 40, 129–130, 132
  Culture, Sex and Anxiety, re-evaluation of, 178–180
frigidity, 91, 130, 313
Fromm, Erich, viii, x, xiv
Fromm-Reichmann, Frieda, 274n
functional effectiveness:
  and anxiety, 157–158
  and competitiveness, 157
  evolution of healthier, 258
  and materialism, 179–180
  and resistance, 182, 224
  and sense of self, 157–158

game of dreams (resistance), 205
glossary of symbols, *see* personal glossary
grandiosity, 126, 142–143
  recognition of, at termination, 286
  source of anxiety, 165–166
  symbolized, 144, 146
Green, M. R., ix, 274n
guilt, xvii, 97, 175

health, 253–266 (*see also* evolving health)
  and changing symbolism, 45

and contradictory emotions, 60–61
  detection of, 61
  early in therapy, 105, 106, 107, 117, 126
  environmental influences toward, 68–69
  evidence of, in depressed patient, 306
  and feeling in dreams, 49, 253–266
  healthy individual, description of, 170
  marital partner's health as source of anxiety, 171
  patient overcoming resistance, 209–210
  and realistic analyst in dreams, 278
  replaces anxiety, 181
Hoch, Paul H., 263n
homosexuality, and homoerotism, 39, 112–113, 135–138, 146, 150, 152
  and anxiety, 177
  characteristics of, 138–139
Horney, Karen, vii, x, xi, xiii, xxii
hostility, *see* anger
hypothesis, *see* interpretive hypothesis

inappropriate documentation (resistance), 200
individuals (a dream element), 2, 4–8
  analyst as individual, 7–8, 267–280
  animal individual, 41
  as attributes, 4
  as surroundings, 38–39
  various forms: animal, 6–7, 41, 78, 115–117, 122–123, 126; human, 4; of others, 7; of self, 256; inanimate, 5–6; multiple, 5
infantile sexuality, 132

initial (emotional) reactions, 99–100
insecurity, 90, 97
insight, 98, 257, 258–259, 262, 316
instinctual concepts, ix, 53, 132, 156
insulating terms, 27, 97, 217, 247–
    248
intellectual exchange, role of an anal-
    ysis, 258–259
interpretation, by analyst alone, 74,
    104–105
  vs. symbol-labeling, 108
interpretive activity, 136–137, 229–
    252, 304–330
  of analyst alone, 20–22, 22–23, 24,
    25, 124
  correlation with symbolism, 47–48
  heart of the curative process, 251
  of patient alone, 25–27, 28–29,
    251
interpretive hypothesis, 20–22, 102–
    103, 104–105, 107–108, 110–
    111, 112–113, 114, 116, 120
  introduction of, 118–119
  of patient and analyst, 122, 124,
    125, 136, 206, 250
  related to nondream data, 260–261
  as resistance, 250–251
intimacy, 70
  with analyst, 149, 228
  fear of, 310
  and interpretive activity, 251–252
  precluded by grandiosity, 145
  and sex, 180
  sexual metaphor for problems of,
    152
  as source of anxiety, 162, 275–278
  at termination, 290
introduction of associations, 140–141
    (*see also* associative activity)
introductory dreams, 102–128
  clinical examples, 10, 53–54, 103–
    111, 112–128

evaluation of associated anxiety,
    108
feelings, focus on, 102
significance of, 102–103

Jung, C. G., ix, x, 37

Kelman, Harold, x
Kleitman, Nathanial, 239n

Langer, Susanne K., 44n
loose terminology, 96–97
love:
  and blurred communication, 97
  children's, 64
  and competitive triumph, 64
  and contradictory emotions, 61
  cynical use of, 170n
  healthy, 69
  increased capacity for, as a crite-
    rion for termination, 281–282
  love for analyst, 226–228, 243,
    277–278, 290
  and moral blackmail, 65
  oversolicitous, 66
  prevented by competitiveness, 93
  schizophrenic distortions of, 64

Masserman, Jules, 92n, 159n, 176n
meaning, pursuit of, through feeling,
    83, 104, 235–238
metaphor, ix, 34, 132, 164
  sexual, 146, 152
moment of association, 11n, 73, 204,
    209n, 219, 231, 232, 235, 263
  clinical examples of, 313, 317,
    319n
  defined, 234–235
  failure to note, 234
  link to behavior and emotion, 234
multiple reference (condensation),
    38, 39

mutual enslavement, 307
mutuality, 251–252, 273–274

needs, 65, 146–147
  and anxiety, 176–177
  and therapeutic goal, 176
negation, of associations and insights,
  248–250, 325–326
negative therapeutic reaction, 190,
  214–215, 324
nonverbal communication, 96n

occurrence of analyst in dreams,
  267–280
  cynicism toward analyst reflected,
  274–275
  in introductory dreams, 102, 105,
  117–118, 120–121, 123–125
  outwitting analyst (resistance),
  185–187
  relation with analyst, symbolized
  sexually, 146–152
  transference, 268–269
Oedipus concept, xvii, 132, 155,
  179–180
"olive incident," 42–43, 44, 159–
  160, 175
overdetermination, 40

passivity of analyst, *see* collaborative
  process
pathological integrity, 187, 198, 199,
  256, 266, 296
penis envy, xvii, 37, 132, 179
personal glossary of symbols, 245,
  293, 294 (*see also* associations,
  contextual)
  defined, 32
  individual symbolism, other aspects of, 40
  and waking symbols, 42

personality, xxi–xxii, 157–158, 257–
  258 (*see also* consciousness)
phallic symbols, 36, 133, 141
physiological studies of dreaming
  and sleep, vii–viii, 239n
premature ejaculation, 91, 156
primal scene, 64, 179
priority of dream material, 246
processes, progression of in analysis,
  260
pseudo-conscientiousness (resistance),
  199–210, 250
psychosomatic clues to emotions,
  100–101
psychosomatic confusion, 14, 206,
  215, 325
psychosomatic symbols, 11, 47–48
psychotic processes, 159n (*see also*
  unreality, feelings of)

rapid-eye-movement technique, vii–
  viii, 239n
reassurance (false and authentic),
  264–265, 305–306, 329
  in depression, 305
rejection, 90, 97, 175–176
repetition, of unresolved problems
  in dreams, 40–41, 320n
repetitive dreams, 40–42, 122–123
repression, 53, 270n
resistance:
  analysts's contribution to, 271
  to analyst's interpretive activity,
  23–25
  antagonism and challenges, 210–
  215
  beating analyst to interpretation,
  250–251
  case study of, *see* Elevator Nightmare
  and commitment, *see* episodic
  dreams

resistance (*cont'd*)
defined, 182
demand for unrealized childhood, 183–184
in dreams, 182–228
escape into genesis, 201, 221
filibuster, interpretive, 27–28, 250
flight into health, 217
and genuine love for analyst, 226–228
"glorified self-confronter," 27, 246–247
helplessness and self-pity, 215
intense form of, 196–198
negating associations, 27, 249–250
outwitting analyst, 185–187
pseudo-conscientious forms of, 199–210, 250
rushing to new topic, 251
as sadness during emerging health, 265–266
through seduction, 216–218
slowing the pace, 187–188
at termination, 290–291
in waking life, tactics of, 198–199
thwarting spouse, aimed at, 190, 225
Rifkin, Alfred H., 17n
Robbins, Bernard S., x, xi–xii, xiii, xxii, 263n, 270n
rushing to new topic (resistance), 251

schizophrenic panic, 263–264
schizophrenogenic force, 64
security, 90, 176–177
seduction of analyst, 216–218
self-concept:
ability to function, related to, 167n
and anxiety, 159, 161, 162, 165
change in during analysis, 258, 263
defined, 158

of "goodness," 168–169
healthy, 170
manipulative ability as basis of, 169
rooted in emotional stoicism, 226
self-recrimination, 200
semantic specificity, 31
sense of self:
analysis as a threat to, 169, 256
and anxiety, 159–161, 162–163, 165, 168, 330
defined, 157–158
and functional effectiveness, 157
healthier, derivation of, 258
healthy evolution of, 170
healthy and pathological sources of, 168–169
manipulative functioning as source of, 169
pathological, near termination, 283–284, 296
sexual impotence, 91, 180 (*see also* premature ejaculation)
sexuality:
anxiety, interpersonal pathology, and sex, 177–178
in dreams, 40
Freudian view, differences from, 130–133
instincts, personality, and dreams, 156
nonsexual aspects of personality in sexual symbols, 153–155
and relationship with analyst, 146–152
sexual passion symbolizing all deep emotion, 145
similes, emotional, 13, 16, 98, 233
sleep, relationship of dreaming to, vii–viii
speculation (during evolving health), 82, 85, 262–263

Strachey, J., 38n, 132n

Sullivan, Harry Stack, viii, xiii

surrogate, xviii, 268, 319–320

surroundings (dream element), 2, 8–9, 39, 106, 112

symbolism, xiv, xviii, xix, xxi, 31–48 (*see also* changing symbolism; feeling, symbolized; personal glossary; psychosomatic symbols; semantic specificity; universal dream symbols; waking symbolism)

Tauber, E. S., ix, 274n

terminal dreams, 281–297

termination, 20n, 281
  anxiety, see Principal's Office and Madman dreams
  collaborative decision, 296
  criteria for, 284–285
  resistance to, 290–291

therapeutic exhibitionism, 21

therapeutic goal, 23, 25, 26, 28, 47, 176–177

therapeutic opportunism, 203

therapeutic process, viii

Thompson, Clara, 37

thought and feeling, interrelationship of, xv

transference, 268, 273 (*see also* occurrence of analyst in dreams; resistance)

traumatic neuroses, 41–42

"tricks" of analyst, 211–212, 215

Ullman, Montague, vii–xix, xxiii

unconscious, the, x–xi, xii, xiv, xvi, xxi

unexplored dream data, 245–246, 324–325

uniqueness, pathological criterion of

self, 167, 169–70, 188 (*see also* grandiosity)

universal dream symbols, 32–36, 133, 141, 142
  Freud on, 132
  vernacular, correlation with, 143

University of Chicago dream laboratory, vii

unreality, feelings of, 263–264

validation, 57, 106, 107, 115, 233
  as criterion for termination, 285
  definitions of, 29, 229–230
  documentation (an analytic process), 261–262
  replacing resistance, 327
  of interpretation of a depressive patient's dream, 306–307, 325n
  of a resistance dream, 191–192
  of a terminal dream, 283

Van Den Berg, J. H., xin

waking symbolism, 42–44
  "olive incident," 42–43, 44, 159–160, 170

western culture:
  and competitive pressures on parents, 65n
  competitiveness and cynicism in, xi, xvii, 87, 92–94, 157, 273
  denial of emotion in, 162, 165
  emotional pathology of, 53
  use of people to bolster self-concepts and functional effectiveness, 170n

writing of dreams, 99

young adults, resistance of, 190n

Zubin, Joseph, 263n

BABY GIRL

I was born in Baltimore twenty-seven years ago, and then I died—twice. I died both times because my mother was filled with drugs and so was I. Crack babies are messed-up babies, and, according to what the doctors were saying, I didn't have a prayer.

But they brought me back from death's door. Someone or something keeps bringing me back from death's door.

I don't understand it, but maybe writing this book will help me see who I was and who I became.

Sometimes I close my eyes, take a deep breath, and imagine myself back then:

A little-bitty baby small enough to fit into the palm of the doctor's hand, no bigger than a puppy or kitten; a baby who has to be fed with an eye dropper 'cause her mouth is too small for the nipple of a bottle; a baby born cross-eyed due to the drugs running through her system.

A baby born to die.

But that same doomed-to-die baby finds a way to live.

How?

Why?

Sure wasn't because of Mama. Mama was Loretta Chase. The woman may have wanted me—I can't know that for sure—but I do know that she couldn't care for me. Later I learned that Mother was the kind of lady that always kept a drug dealer around to fill her needs. She could do that because she had a pretty face, long wavy hair, and a fine figure. Men flocked to her. My daddy ran from her—or she chased him off. I never did get the story.

I didn't get a lot of the stories about my real parents. They're ghost figures in my childhood. I saw them in my dreams when I was a little girl. Sometimes they creep back into my dreams now that I'm a grown woman, but they're always covered in mystery.

The mystery was heavy because as soon as I was born I was put into a foster home owned by two people who had a row house in the toughest neighborhood in East Baltimore. Their names were Cora and Levi Pearson and their place was on East Oliver Street, three doors off the corner of North Montford. That's where I grew up. Oliver and Montford is where it all happened.

When I arrived the Pearsons were already in their early sixties. Sweet folk. They took care of me, but I still wanted my mama. And when I heard that Mama was calling for me, I got happy all over. I wanted to see her.

All little girls wanna see their mothers. All girls need their mothers. The earliest dreams I can remember are dreams of my mother. I'd see her standing there before me, holding out her arms, hugging me tight, putting me to bed and tucking me in.

"You're my precious baby," she'd say.

I'd smile at her, close my eyes, and fall asleep inside my dream.

THE CLOSET

My memories of Mama's visits are like dreams.

During the first two visits we were at the park. I remember clouds and rain, I remember a dark sky, wet grass, and plastic slides in the playground. I remember Mrs. Simms, the white social worker, who held my hand until, from behind a tree, a woman appeared. The woman was beautiful. She ran to me with her arms wide open. I didn't move. I didn't know what to do.

"It's your mother," said Mrs. Simms. "Go to your mother."

I let the woman embrace me. She smelled of cigarettes and perfume. Tears ran down her cheek. I didn't know why she was crying. She held me tight and said words I don't remember. I imagine that she said she loved me. We walked for a while. She, Mrs. Simms, and I went to a candy store where I got a soda and a little bag of M & M's.

"You and your mother look just alike," Mrs. Simms said.

I loved hearing those words because I knew my mother looked like a lady in a magazine.

The rain stopped—I can't remember if this was the first visit or the second—and children were in the park. My mother said something about my pigtails. As a little girl, my hair was done up in little pigtails.

"If you let your hair grow out," she said, "it'll look like mine."

She let me touch her wavy hair.

"Can I bring her to my house? Can I be alone with my daughter?" she asked Mrs. Simms.

Mrs. Simms said, "Maybe. Maybe next time."

Next time came soon. The night before I was too excited to sleep.

What would my mother's house look like? I was sure it'd be pretty because she was pretty. I was sure it'd be big. The house on Oliver Street had three floors and three bedrooms, but I knew my mother's house would be bigger. The house on Oliver Street had all sorts of people living there—grandchildren and cousins to Mr. and Mrs. Pearson. But I was my mother's only child. I wouldn't have to share the house with anyone but my mother. Maybe I could live with her forever.

I always hated dresses, but I wore one to visit my mother because I wanted to look pretty. I wanted to look like my mother. My dress, lavender and embroidered with white lace, was brand new. My foster mama had bought it for me to wear to church.

My excitement built as Mrs. Simms drove me to my

mother's. But when we arrived, I was sure she had made a mistake. It wasn't a house at all, but a tiny one-room apartment with a small kitchen, and a couch that opened up into a bed. The room was messy and didn't smell good. This couldn't be where my mom lived. But it was.

When Mrs. Simms left us, my mother sat down on the edge of the bed. Something was wrong. She was crying and shaking. I didn't know why. She didn't hug and kiss me like she had in the park. She didn't even look at me. I just stood there.

Then her mood changed. She got up from the bed and told me to take off my clothes. I didn't understand why. I wouldn't do it.

"Do it!" she cried.

She screamed at me until I did it. I took off all my clothes, dropping them on the floor.

"Now get in there," she ordered, pointing to the closet.

I tried to run but my mother caught me. She pushed me into the closet and locked the door behind me. I began wailing at the top on my lungs.

"Stop crying," she said. "I'll be back."

Then the sound of her leaving the apartment.

The darkness.

The fear of being locked in.

Naked fear.

Baby girl fear.

Pure terror.

I carried on. Kept crying. Kept screaming louder, but no

one heard. Cried so loud and long that I cried myself out. I finally fell to the floor and started kicking. I had to get out. Someone had to hear me.

I don't know how much time passed, but when I heard the voices of Mrs. Simms and my foster father, I screamed my head off. They broke open the door and set me free. I was hysterical.

"Imagine that," I heard Mrs. Simms tell my foster father, "selling her little girl's clothes to buy crack."

I was never allowed to be alone with my mother again.

Sometime in my childhood my mother reappeared at the house on Oliver Street.

Each time the visit was short, and with each visit she looked less beautiful. Her eyes were crazy. Sometimes her dress was dirty and worn. She'd come into the front room and just look at me. She'd try to smile, but the smile wouldn't come. She'd cry and leave.

Her visits became more infrequent. Finally they stopped.

That's when Mrs. Pearson became Mama and Mr. Pearson became Pop.

COLD-BLOODED KILLER

For the first eight years of my life, I was not only teased for being a foster child, I was teased for being cross-eyed. Mama told me I looked fine, and so did Pop, but I knew better. I knew because the kids on the block wouldn't leave me alone. They teased me something fierce. They called me weirdo. Called me ugly. "How many fingers am I holding up?" they'd ask. And they'd laugh and say I was blind as a bat.

At first I didn't fight them. I was too small. Their cruelty hurt my heart, but I didn't know what to do about it. Didn't cry. Didn't lash out. Just held it in and kept to myself. Became a loner.

"You ain't ugly," said a handsome man who came to visit one afternoon. "You as pretty as your mama."

He wasn't talking about Cora Pearson. He was talking about Loretta Chase, the woman who took off my clothes and locked me in the closet.

"This here is Bernard," Pop said to me as we sat in the front room. "This here is your real father."

Unlike light-skinned Loretta, this man was black as midnight. Like Loretta, though, he had his hair in waves. He brought me a little doll I didn't want. I didn't like dolls. As he sat there, I looked into his eyes and saw ice. I felt ice.

"You a good girl?" he said.

I looked down at the floor and didn't say nothing.

"You got all those pigtails," he said.

I still didn't say nothing.

He got up and put his hand on my cheek. His hand was cold.

"Be a good girl," he said.

He left without another word.

Later I heard Mama and Pop talking in the kitchen.

"He's a stick-up man," said Mama.

"Worse than that," added Pop. "Man's a cold-blooded killer."

Didn't take long to learn what that meant.

Killing was part of our neighborhood. Death lived on our block. Death was the business of Collins Funeral Home, just down the street. Seemed liked death rode down Oliver Street more often than the ice cream truck. Death was a regular. Even as a baby girl, death—up close and real as rain—was part of my life.

THE SMURFS

Death is a lot for a kid to contend with.

The Smurfs are the opposite of death. Smurfs never die. Smurfs live forever in a dreamland where I want to be.

First time I learn about Smurfs is over a friend's house. They're on TV.

"Who they?" I ask.

"They the Smurfs."

I fall in love with the Smurfs, so deep in love until Mama buys me Smurf sheets and Smurf pillowcases. I have Smurf pictures on the walls and Smurfs cartoons by my bed. I surround myself with Smurfs.

Man, I even have me some Smurf dreams.

In one dream I wake up and I'm not on Oliver Street no more. I'm in a mushroom house. That's right. A house cut out of a big-ass mushroom. Far as I'm concerned, it's a Smurf World. If you don't like it, you can go Smurf yourself.

Got me four fingers like a Smurf. Got me a little white

hat, puffy feet, and Smurfy eyes. I still got my braids. I'm Braidy Smurf.

Braidy Smurf is meeting Brainy Smurf. Here's Hefty Smurf who's got a tattoo on his arm and can kick plenty ass. Harmony Smurf is hanging with Handy Smurf.

I'm chilling with all the Smurfs. Even Smurfette. Especially Smurfette. She's wearing a dress and high heels. She's flirting with me just like she flirts with the boys. Invites me to her crib. I go in and get comfortable.

I'm sure-enough falling for Smurfette.

But if Smurfette is a girl, what does that make me?

In real life, I wasn't relating to girls. I was relating to boys.

In school, the uniform was skirts. But I was bony and didn't like showing my knees. I wanted to wear baggy jeans like the boys. Soon as I got home I got out of that skirt and put on jeans. Got out of that blouse and put on a boy's shirt.

"Put on that cheerleader skirt," Mama said.

"Don't want to."

"You need to, baby," she insisted. "You're going to make an adorable cheerleader. You're pretty as a picture and you're the best little athlete in that school. I want you to try out."

Loved Mama and wanted to make her happy, so I tried out. Went to the audition where they made you dance like Janet Jackson.

Don't get me wrong. I been in love with Janet my whole life. Loved her when she was Penny on *Good Times* with JJ and them. I watched those reruns till I had 'em memorized. When homegirl hit with "Control," I loved her even more. I love her today.

When "Control" dropped, we were all caught up in the videos. "Nasty," "What Have You Done for Me Lately"— those jams were poppin' everywhere I went. But when I went to the cheerleader audition and saw that they wanted me to do Janet's chair routine from "The Pleasure Principle" video, I said, "Thanks, but no thanks." Janet can do that stuff, but not Fefe.

Fefe was what they were calling me when my eyes were still crossed.

"Fefe's fucked up," said one of the boys who saw how I liked to wear jeans and shoot hoops. "Fefe's a straight-up bull dyke."

I didn't know what that meant, but I beat his little ass anyway.

"Fefe's a tomboy," said someone else.

I could deal with that word because it had "boy" in it.

The big change for Fefe came when Mama, bless her heart, paid for the operation to fix my eyes. By then I had taken her name, Pearson, and was officially Felicia Pearson. But it didn't take long for Fefe to turn into Snoop. Happened when I was eight. I'll get to that story in a minute.

KNIGHT RIDER

Mama went to a Holy Roller church where everyone was jumping for Jesus. I could feel it. You had to feel the spirit. The music was fresh, the Holy Ghost on the loose, and the people cool. Those big church ladies were out in the kitchen cooking up collard greens, neck bones, and pig's feet. Jesus was all right with me.

Pop was one of those Jehovah's Witnesses. I liked going to his prayer meetings 'cause there were all kinds of folk up in there—black, white, Latino—who thought my pigtails were cute. They were always dropping change in my purse.

But church went on for too long and got me restless. I was an outside kid. Inside bored me. Outside stimulated me. I loved the streets. Loved to sit on the stairs in front of Mama's house and just watch the world go by. Early on, Mama let me wander. She really had no choice 'cause I'd be wandering anyway. Wander down to the corner store where they sold meats and candies. Wander over to the beauty parlor where the women were deep in their dish. Wander to the liquor store where the old winos spun their stories about back in the day. Wander to Gibson's, the sub shop where they got a little arcade with Pac-Man. No one could beat me at Pac-Man.

Wander across the street to play with Curtis. Like me, Curtis followed *Knight Rider* on TV. I didn't know about *Sesame Street* or *Electric Company*, but I sure knew about *Knight Rider*, the show where the star was KITT, a black customized Pontiac Trans-Am. I wanted KITT because KITT could ride through fire. Nothing could stop KITT and nothing could destroy KITT. I had dreams about being in the world of the Knight Rider like I had dreams about being with the Smurfs. In my Knight Rider dreams, when I was commanding that car, nothing could stop me.

You can imagine how happy I was when I got me a toy version of the Knight Rider car.

"How come you don't play with dolls?" asked Curtis.

"How come *you* don't play with dolls?" I asked him.

"I'm a boy. My people say you a butch."

"What's a butch?" I wanted to know.

"That means you ain't right."

"But I got the right Knight Rider, don't I?" I said, holding the car up to the sun and watching the light bounce off it.

"Let me see that thing."

He grabbed the little car from me and let it fly down the street until it knocked into a light pole so hard that black paint chipped off the right door. That got me seeing red. I lost it. I took a swing at Curtis that caught him upside his head. I nearly took his head off. He came back at me, but I was too strong for me. I kept slamming him.

"You a butch," he kept screaming at me.

I slammed him so hard that people passing by had to break it up.

Curtis never fucked with me again.

Back in the crib, Mama used to scold me when she learned I was fighting. After my eye operation I wore glasses for two years. I broke many a pair due to squabbles. I knew Mama wanted me in dresses and ribbons, but Mama was also wise enough to know that wasn't me. Mama knew to accept people the way they are.

Pop got a kick out of having a tomboy. He was a handy-man who ran his own little business. He could fix anything mechanical and he liked teaching me. I'd go up on the roof where he taught me to lay tar. Taught me to fix the pipes. When I got a bike—a red-and-black boy's style with the bar under the seat—Pop taught me to take that sucker apart and put it together again. I'd put an empty juice carton on the spokes of the back tire to make that rat-rat-rat-rat noise. Me and the boys would call 'em our dirt bikes. At age eight, that's how we rolled.

Pop would watch me roll down Oliver on my Huffy and smile.

"Girl," he said, "you got an extra dose of get-up-and-go."

Pop had a good dose himself. He'd get up and go visit girl-friends behind Mama's back. Found this out the hard way:

One day we were in the pawnshop where he picked out a gold necklace. He wrote a little card and put it in a box. Because I was looking at all the pistols behind the counter, Pop didn't think I was noticing him. But I noticed everything.

Get home and get ready for dinner. Dinner's always an event at Mama's 'cause you never know who'll show up at the table. Fact is, you never know at any given moment who's living in the house. Mama's grandchildren are always around, not to mention cousins of all ages.

Tonight's macaroni and cheese. Mama puts a hurting on mac and cheese.

"Hey, Mama," I say. "Pop bought you a beautiful necklace."

Pop looks at me like he wants to kick me in the head.

"That's lovely," she says. "Let me see it, Levi."

Pop starts stuttering. "Not sure—not sure where I put it."

"You put it right in your pocket," I say, running over and digging it out for Mama to see.

"There's a card and everything," Mama says.

When she reads the card, though, her eyes turn red as fire. Just like that, she puts Pop's ass out the house. Poor Pop's in the doghouse for weeks. He finally pleads his way back in, but the beautiful thing about the man is that he's not mad at me.

"Give her a whupping for what she done to you," says a cousin of Pop's, a teenaged boy who likes to get high down in our basement where he lives for free. "Whup her bad."

But Pop ain't giving me no whupping.

Pop is saying, "That's my girl. She just told the truth, that's all she did. You can't go off on no one for telling the truth." And with that he'd pat me on the head and have me go with him down the street to fix someone's washing machine.

KEN AND BARBIE

Sheila was Barbie.

I was Ken. I was five, maybe six years old.

We were playing house.

Sheila had golden brown hair. Her body was developing faster than the other girls'. She already had a little booty.

"You the mommy," I said. "I'm the daddy. I just got home from work. How 'bout a kiss?"

Sheila kissed me on the cheek.

"You make dinner," I said. "I gotta go back to work."

"Where you work?" she asked.

"On the streets," I answered.

"What you do?"

"Woman," I said, acting like Pop, "I do what I need to do. I take care of you, that's what I do."

"Do you love me?" she asked.

"Sure," I said. "Ken loves Barbie and Barbie loves Ken. That's how it go."

"We gonna have babies?"

"You want babies?"

"Three," she said. "Two girls and one boy."

"Okay, we'll have babies."

"You know how to make babies?" Sheila wanted to know.

"Well," I hesitated. I really didn't know, but I said, "We just kinda rub together."

We kept our clothes on and just kinda rubbed together.

"Okay," I said, "you wait awhile and then the babies come."

That was our game, and we played it for months.

Sheila was my first girlfriend. Our song was LL Cool J's "I Need Love."

That song had me falling in love with slow jams. Funny to think of me as a little girl dreaming of being the man of the family.

But that's who I was.

Another girl, this one a little older, would sometimes have me sleep over at her house. She'd call it a pajama party. She also liked to play LL's "I Need Love." She also liked to play house.

When we got into bed, she played like she was asleep, and she let me do sneaky shit to her. But I knew she was awake and loving it. She just didn't want to admit it. That was my first experience being with a girl who liked to pretend she wasn't liking it. As time went on, I learned that she wasn't the only one.

I learned that lots of girls have different sexual feelings. The honest ones will admit to it. They'll even talk about it. Sometimes they like a boy. Sometimes they like a girl. Sometimes they like a girl who acts like a boy. I never had problems talking about those different feelings. I did what felt good and natural. Never had no guilt. Never felt like I was doing nothing wrong.

But I'd soon learn that not everyone has an easy attitude about sex. Sex gets people confused, guilty, and crazy. If you're open about your feelings, and those feelings are different from everyone else's, you might be laughed at or even beaten down. You might be secure about your sex life, but the more secure you are, the more insecure you'll make others—especially folks who hate the different sex feelings running through their heads and heating up their hearts.

They say your life is secure long as you got a roof over your head.

When I was eight, the roof blew off our house—just like that—and water started flooding in. We ran down to the basement. I thought we'd drown, but we made it through. In 1988, some kind of crazy storm hit Baltimore real hard and nearly did us in.

Next day, though, Pop was up there banging on a new roof.

"Anyone wanna help?" he asked everyone. Mama had some relatives living there that I didn't even know.

No one wanted to help—except me.

"She'll fall off," said a woman I called my aunt.

I paid her no mind, climbed up there and started hammering.

From the streets, a guy looked up and saw me.

"Hey, Levi," he yelled at Pop, "ain't that child labor?"

"This child," Pop yelled back down, "ain't no child. She's smart as a whip and twice as strong as any two boys on this block."

"Well, you keep her close to you, Levi, 'cause this block's getting worse every day. This here is the Wild West."

Pop knew the neighborhood well as anyone. He saw the dangers. He saw how the shit was turning worse before his very eyes. He'd tell me that back in the day it was a nice place to live and raise kids. He'd complain about the hoodlums.

Once I even saw Pop come face to face with a knucklehead trying to jack him up.

It was the end of the workday. I happened to look out a window and saw Pop walking down the street. That's when a gangsta jumped up outta nowhere and stuck a gun in Pop's back. Pop wheeled around and gave this boy such a heavy look—I mean fire was coming out Pop's eyes—the thug backed down. The gangsta melted into a punk. Never saw nothing like that before. But that was Pops.

He was strong. He worked hard, earned his money, provided for his family. Him and Mama both did things right. They were the right models for a young girl growing up.

So why didn't I grow up the way they wanted me to?

Why couldn't I follow their lead?

Why did I wind up doing the things I did?

The streets were screaming at me—that's for sure. But the streets were screaming at everyone. Some kids ignored those screams. I didn't. I had to see what the screaming was all about.

EVERYTHING MOVES OFF MONEY

If you studied the streets like me, the truth was up in your face: Money made it happen. Money made people jump, duck, hustle, and hide. Big money made *you* big. The lack of money made you little. Your money could be dirty or clean. Didn't matter. Your money could be soaked in fresh blood. That didn't matter either. What mattered was having it. What mattered was getting it. What mattered was keeping it.

To an eight- or nine-year-old child looking at life from the steps of East Oliver Street, it was crystal clear that everything moves off money.

Then when the boys from New York started opening up shop, it became even clearer. New money was taking over.

A shop is where a dealer sets up operation, gets him a couple of corner boys to organize the merchandise and look out for cops, plus a couple of runners who deal with the customers in the cars or the customers walking by.

If you're a kid with half a brain, you scope out the scene in no time.

To me it was interesting.

Being outside Mama's house was always more interesting than being inside.

Action was better than no action.

"You're restless like a little boy," one of Mama's friends told me.

I was already thinking of myself as a boy—so I took it as a compliment.

The girls were inside with their sewing kits and baby dolls.

The boys were outside looking for trouble.

Trouble didn't scare me none. I didn't think twice about it. I figured I could take care of myself.

Rico thought so, too.

Rico was the first dealer who brought me into the game—even though he didn't bring me very far.

Rico was an ultracool cat from New York, half black, half Puerto Rican. Short, handsome, super-smooth.

Loved me some Rico. Rico spotted me right off.

"You just sitting there playing like you don't know what's happening," Rico told me.

I didn't say a word.

"You talk?" he said.

"Sure."

"What do you got to say?"

"Nothing."

A car rolled by with 2 Live Crew screaming from the speakers, "We Want Some Pussy."

"You know what that song's about?" Rico asked.

I nodded.

"I bet you do."

He came closer to me and said, "I got something for you to hold. You cool with that?"

I nodded again.

He handed me a packet. I knew what was inside.

"You put this in your pocket for a minute or two. I'll be back later."

He was testing me.

When he got back in an hour, I was sitting in the same place.

"Got that packet?" he asked.

I handed it to him without saying a word. He handed me three ten-dollar bills.

That was the start.

That was also when the cops wouldn't think that a kid might be holding dope for a dealer. Back then you could get away with it.

Back then, before the New Yorkers like Rico came through, the dope scene was calmer. You'd see people get high, but Rico and his boys raised the stakes: The highs got higher 'cause the dope got stronger. Things got crazier.

The crackheads were really crazy. It was like watching cartoon characters on TV. They had different names—Superman, King Kong, Wacky. If Wacky found a hole—a shop where the

dope was really good—the other fiends would see him trip-
ping and start screaming, "Where the hole at, Wacky?" Wacky
would point to the hole and the crackheads would run over
there to cop. The hole was the spot, the shop where the shit
was sold.

After they got high, they acted all funny, shaking and
dancing and carrying on.

To get the fiends from coke to heroin, which earned
the dealers more money, Rico and his boys would pass out
what they called Ts. Ts were teasers, free samples to get you
started.

"I see you understand the game," Rico said to me.

I didn't even bother to nod. I didn't have to.

The game on the street was so different—more complicated,
more dangerous and deadly—than the games we played in
the schoolyard. The schoolyard games, volleyball and basketball, were great for me because I excelled at them.

I wasn't intimidated by the taller boys who were older
and stronger. I was quicker and more aggressive. I couldn't
be backed down. That attitude earned me a good reputation
in the schoolyard. And my high grades earned me respect in
the classroom. School was cool. School was guarded by security niggas with real guns. School was no joke.

But school was boring. School didn't excite my eyes or
my mind. School was routine. You could predict what would
happen from one day to the next.

On the streets, though, you couldn't predict shit. Might be quiet now, but a minute later, BANG! Something big comes down that changes up the game. The battles over territory, the fight for the best locations to set up shops, the new playas coming in and the old playas going out—the action never stops.

You have to be quick. And smart. If you react wrong, that might be it. If you react right, you can keep playing.

I kept playing.

UNCLE

I was eight years old when I fell in love with Pam Grier.

Mama's grandson was living in the basement where he played the tapes of her movies from the seventies. I was glued to the screen.

Pam Grier was Coffy, a chick with a giant Afro and a body from heaven. She works as a nurse during the day. At night she takes on the bad guys and blows them away, one by one. She's got her own private arsenal and her own style of killing. The poster hanging on the basement walls says, "She's the godmother of them all . . . the baddest one-chick hit squad that ever hit town."

In another movie, Pam is Foxy Brown. This time her hair is curly and her dresses even skimpier. Foxy Brown is so down she don't hesitate cutting off some guy's dick. You don't fuck with Foxy.

But Foxy is make-believe and the streets are real. I can't deal with make-believe for too long. I'm back on streets, just looking around, holding a packet or two, seeing what the day brings.

One day I was sitting on the steps when a man came by. He was in his twenties, good-looking, two golds in his mouth, happy attitude. I knew he was dealing.

"Hey, Snoop," he said, "what you doing?"

"Who's Snoop?" I asked.

"You."

"I ain't Snoop, I'm Fefe."

"No, you Snoop."

"If you say so."

"I say so."

He sat down on the steps next to me.

"You too young to be doing what you doing," he said.

"How you know what I'm doing?" I asked.

"I seen you, Snoop," he said. "I seen you watching this mess out here. You watch like a hawk. You don't miss nothing."

I didn't say nothing.

"You a girl who thinks you're a boy," he said. "But I think you're Snoop."

"Why Snoop?" I asked.

"Snoop out of Charlie Brown. Snoop's that puppy who's always saying cute things. He's sweet but he's sad."

"All right."

"Yeah, you Snoop all right. And I'm telling you you should be in school."

"I am in school. Today's a holiday."

"You do good in school?"

"Real good."

"What subject you like best?"

"Math."

"Figures," he said. "You gotta be good with numbers."

"I am."

"And you're real sure of yourself, ain't you?"

I just shrugged. Where this guy coming from? What did he want? Why was he so interested in me?

His two gold teeth sparkled off the sunshine. He had this big smile across his face. I didn't know what to think.

"What I think," he said, "is that you're smarter than the other kids playing out here. You're one step ahead of them."

I stayed silent.

"Well, in this game it's good to stay one step ahead, but it's even better to stay out completely."

"You out?" I asked him.

"I'm in," he said. "Deep in."

———

That's the first time I met the man who named me. His name was Arnold Lonly. When I tried calling him Mr. Arnold, like my mama taught me to address my elders, he say, "Just call me Uncle."

And that was that.

Uncle didn't live in the neighborhood but he knew the neighborhood. He worked it. He set up shop and had him a thriving business. From Jump Street, he always had an eye for me. Didn't take long to learn that he really didn't want anything from me. He was just wanted me to stay clear of trouble. He saw something good in me. And I felt his love. He tried to steer me right, but I was gonna do what I was gonna do.

NINE-MILLIMETER

Death lived on our street.

Me and my boy D used to play in front of the Collins Funeral Home, one block down East Oliver, where we'd watch them bring in the bodies. Mr. Collins was a twisted dude.

One day he said he'd pay us to clean out his basement. We backed off, but the promise of money lured us down there. Next thing we knew, old man Collins locked us in.

The room was filled with corpses. One casket was open. A man was in there, and he was still alive. I know because I saw him stretch out his arm and I heard him take his last breath. Frightened to death, we ran up the basement stairs, banging on the door until our hands turned bloody. But old man Collins wouldn't let us out. We finally broke a window and crawled out. I felt like I had escaped death.

Few months later death returned. This time death got all over me.

When it happened, D and I were playing in the alley. By then I was in the sixth grade and running wild—going to every house party I could find and holding packs for the most vicious dealers in the game. Mama and Pop were nice folks, but they couldn't control me. Besides, they had no idea what I was doing.

Me and D weren't doing much that day when two niggas came running down the alley, one chasing the other. The nigga being chased didn't see our bike and tripped over it, falling right in front of us. The nigga chasing him had a gun. Just like that, he pumped four shots into the dude's head.

I watched blood gush out of his skull; I saw his brains splatter out on the concrete.

Never had seen a murder before.

Never had seen anyone shot up right in front of my eyes, inches from where I was standing.

How did I feel?

I can't remember feeling. Just remember looking.

How did I react?

Can't remember reacting. Just remember standing there.

Inside my head I was saying, *Oh, shit, that nigga just got his brains blown out.*

But on the outside I wasn't crying or screaming. I wasn't moving. I was cool as a fuckin' cucumber.

Just stood there.

The killer looked at me, and I looked back at him.

I didn't know what he was going to do, but I wasn't moving.

I wasn't scared 'cause he didn't look like he wanted to shoot me. He already did what he had to do. I think he also saw that, though I was an eyewitness, I was cool. I didn't look like no snitch. I wasn't interested in getting my brains blown out.

So just like that, he tossed the gun at me—a heavy-ass nine-millimeter.

He nodded at me, like it was okay. It was a gift. The gun was mine. I nodded back.

I picked up the joint and put it in the pocket of my baggy jeans.

And that's when everything kicked off.

BOW AND ARROW

In the world of nine-millimeter handguns and semi-automatic weapons, you don't think about bows and arrows murdering someone. Bows and arrows are off some old Robin Hood movie. Who knows anything about bows and arrows?

"Miss M was killed by a bow and arrow," D told me.

"What!" I said. "What you talking about? Miss M is nine months pregnant and about to have her baby."

"Bow and arrow went right through her stomach and into her baby. Killed 'em both."

"That's crazy. Why's anyone shooting an arrow at Miss M?"

"They say it was an accident."

Miss M was the mother of a close friend of mine from school.

I didn't want to believe it. I knew it couldn't have happened. Some fucked-up rumor.

But the rumor wasn't a rumor. The rumor was real.

I went with my friend to the funeral home where her

mother was laid with her little infant. They were both wearing white. They'd taken the child from the womb and placed it next to her mama.

Never seen nothing like that before in my life.

People were screaming with grief, moaning and shouting, "Lord, have mercy!"

I got up and walked by the casket. They were so still.

Mother and child.

Dead.

Silent.

Frozen.

By then I was ten, and I'd seen boys killed. I'd seen men shot down in cold blood. But this here was different. This was a mommy and a baby. This was the saddest sight I'd ever laid eyes on.

My heart was so heavy it was hard to get up when the service was over. I didn't want to leave them alone in that casket. I felt empty. I felt like nothing really mattered if a bow and arrow can go through a mother's tummy and kill both her and the innocent little thing growing inside her.

What kind of world is this?

I didn't have no answers. I didn't want no answers. I didn't want to cry. I could usually keep myself from crying. But not this time. This time I broke down along with everyone else.

This time was the worst.

"YOU BAD"

Boys start humping on girls at a young age. That's just how it is. I started seeing it when I was ten or eleven.

But when they tried humping on me, I fought 'em off. After I beat the shit out of a couple, they left me alone. The boys who understood me became my best friends and running buddies. They looked at me like I was no different than them. In my mind, I wasn't.

Once I had that gun, I was on my way. I hid it under Mama's summer kitchen, a porch in the back of the house where I could crawl under the foundation.

Life went on.

Me and D played basketball with hoops made out of crates. D had game and so did I. He was also tenderhearted, thin-skinned, and hated being teased. When kids at school ganged up on him and started calling him names, he ran to me and said, "Get the joint."

"We don't need to be fooling with no gun," I said.

"I don't wanna shoot 'em, I just wanna whip it out and scare those niggas real bad. Go get it."

I got it. Gave it to D. And the two of us went looking for the boys who'd been ragging on D.

We found them. All ten of them. They saw we were looking for trouble, and they were ready. They had baseball bats and knives, but they weren't ready for a nine-millimeter.

Neither was D. He didn't know how to use it. He didn't distance himself to get good range. He got too far up in their faces. Had no leverage.

"Yo, D," I said, "back up."

But by then he was whipping out the gun. One of the niggas saw what D was doing and knocked the joint out of his hand. Gun fell on the ground. Before anyone could react, I grabbed it. I aimed at the nigga who had plucked it and shot the boy through the leg.

For the first time in my life, I'd fired a gun. The guys backed off. The fight was over before it started. D was all smiles.

"You bad," he said to me. "You ain't scared of nothing."

I got this reputation. And I got this attitude. If anyone questioned what I was doing, I'd say, "What the fuck do you care?"

You feel what I'm saying?

I'm saying that no one cared about me. Mama and Pop were cool, but they were off in their own little cocoon. They couldn't relate to me. They couldn't control me.

I remember looking at Mama while she read her Bible and listened to her gospel music. She'd be smiling and nodding her head to the good grooves. The Word was making her happy. She was a woman who lived the Word. She tried her hardest to put it on me.

"God loves you," she said. "Don't you know that?"

I said I did, but I really didn't. Didn't know who God was.

"God is Jesus," she explains. "He died so you can live."

"I *am* living, Mama."

"He died so you can live forever."

"No one lives forever."

"That where you're wrong, child. Heaven is forever."

"I don't know nothing 'bout no heaven," I said.

Mama smiled and started quoting scripture. The words sounded pretty, but the words didn't mean much to me. I imagined heaven as some make-believe place folks invented to make themselves feel better about living down here in hell.

Pop was the same.

He liked to talk about how Jesus would come down at the end of the world and swoop up all the true believers.

"When is the end coming?" I asked.

"Soon, baby," he said. "Real soon."

"How soon?"

"Could be tomorrow. Could be tonight. That's why we gotta get ready and stay ready."

I loved me some Pop, but I couldn't buy that line. Tonight the sun would set. Tomorrow it would rise. Tuesday would follow Monday and Thursday would follow Wednesday. Same old shit, day in and day out. Far as I could see, no magic Jesus would be dropping out of the sky any time soon.

I couldn't fault Mama and Pop for believing in the magic,

though. The meaning behind the magic was beautiful. But the magic did something to Mama and Pop that removed them from the world—at least the way I looked at the world. They were characters in some goody-goody movie where there's always a happy ending. I liked looking at the movie, but I knew it wasn't for real. I couldn't live in that movie. I was living in another movie—a shoot-'em-up.

Mama and Pop were super-sweet folk, and I know that sweetness must have rubbed off a little on me. But I saw them as two people with their heads in the clouds. They didn't see what was really happening in my world. My world was ruled by street smarts.

If you have them, you survive; if you don't, you die.

That was an exciting idea.

But the idea that Jesus was coming back to get the good guys and punish the bad didn't mean anything. I didn't believe that shit for a minute.

AIN'T NO AVERAGE DAYS

Every day can be a little scary. Or a lot scary.

When I was coming up, fear came early and quick, but I think I musta blocked it or forgotten it.

Some scary shit, though, I ain't ever forgetting.

Ain't ever forgetting the day I was just standing up in the kitchen washing dishes. Mama had just come back from a little vacation. She was upstairs taking a nap. I'd just gotten home from school.

Just your average day.

Until I hear a knock on the door.

"Your cousin home?" asks this nigga standing there. Nigga looks all jittery.

"Who you?" I ask.

"T."

"I'll go see."

I go look for my cousin, who's a man about twenty-one. He's back in the bathroom.

"T is up in here looking for you," I say.

"Tell him I'm in the bathroom."

I tell T.

T says he'll wait.

Meanwhile, I hear my cousin slipping out the back door.

When I look up, T is gone.

I go back to washing a plate.

Then *Pop! Pop! Pop! Pop!*

I drop the plate.

Somone's shooting.

Someone's shot.

Someone's screaming, "Your cousin's down."

Look up the street by Collins Funeral Home. My cousin is laid out on the sidewalk, blood all over him. Homeboys are going through his pockets, stealing his drugs and his money.

Cop sirens are screaming.

Helicopter whirling overhead.

Cousin ain't dead, but he's paralyzed.

It was T who shot him. Later I learned that my cousin had fucked up T the week before, and this was payback.

This was life on East Oliver.

Cousin was running down Oliver to get his piece that he had stashed in another crib. T caught him before he got there.

I think to myself—T could have started shooting back at the house, could have shot me, or Mama, or all of us.

This is how it goes.

Cousin shot. Cousin I loved. Same cousin who always brought me Chinese food. Cousin who liked to get high on weed and laugh with me for hours.

One day Cousin is running around.

Next day Cousin is paralyzed.

Ain't no average days.

"SHE MY DAUGHTER."

When folks asked Mama about me, she'd always say, "She's a good girl. She's a good daughter."

That was Mama. Mama saw the good in everyone.

Truth is, I *was* a good daughter—or least tried to be. Wouldn't ever let anyone say a bad word about Mama or Pop. Anything they asked of me, I did. Willingly.

I worked. Scrubbed floors, washed dishes, did laundry. I liked being Pop's little helper. Liked being Mama's right arm. Liked when Mama told her friends how much energy I had. She was proud of me and I was proud to be called her daughter.

At the same time, you could say I was the daughter of the streets. That was the Snoop Mama and Pop didn't really know. Maybe if they had looked, they would have seen that side of me. But they didn't wanna look. They didn't wanna know. And that was cool with me.

Pops had his cronies who dropped by on some Saturday

nights to drink their beers or sip their whiskey. When I ran through the room where they'd be sitting, Pop would stop me and say, "This here's a fine young girl who's growing up to be a fine young woman."

"Sure-enough," the cronies would say. "You doing a fine job with that child."

All this praise was falling on my head. All this praise was feeling good, except I knew that Mama and Pop had their heads in the clouds.

They missed what was really happening.

For instance . . .

One day Mama says we're low on some grocery items. Would I pick them up for her?

"No problem, Mama. I'm on it."

I skip down to the corner store. I got a list and it's taking me a minute or two to tell the man what I need.

Nigga waiting on line behind me says. "Move your li'l ass out the way."

I ignore him, but he leans on me harder.

"Yo bitch, or butch, or boy, or whoever the fuck you are, get moving," he says.

I say, "I'm almost through."

He says, "Butch, you through now."

Then out of nowhere this grown man comes up to the nigga. The man is dark-skinned and tall. He's got on a green leather suit and alligator shoes.

"You best apologize to the young lady," he tells the nigga.

"I ain't apologizing to no fuckin' butch kid," says the nigga.

"I do believe you are," says the man, who pulls out a gun and sticks it in the nigga's ear.

Nigga says, "I do believe I am. I'm apologizing."

"You better show her some respect," says the man. "She my daughter."

That's how I met the man I wound up referring to as Father. He wasn't my real father—I hadn't seen that man since I was three or four—but this nigga was better than my real father. My real father was small-time. My new father was big-time.

Like Uncle, Father was a dealer, but not your average dealer. Father controlled all of East Baltimore. Uncle was in the game. Father *was* the game. Father was King.

Father took a liking to me. I can't tell you why.

Once he gave me fifteen hundred dollars for school supplies.

Another time he took me out to see his mansion that sat way beyond the county line. Looked like something out of *MTV Cribs.* Marble and gold and red silk curtains. Pool tables and Jacuzzis and stained-glass windows.

Father was fast-talking and super-smart. He was nice as he could be to me, and didn't want nothing back. But I heard some niggas say that if you got on the wrong side of Father he'd kill you and your whole family.

Father liked having me around 'cause I stayed quiet and just observed. He knew I was thinking.

"I can hear you thinking," he'd say. "You're thinking one day you'd like having all this shit up in here." He pointed to the circular staircase in the entryway to his house.

I didn't say nothing, but Father was right.

GODMOTHER

"You don't need no gangster godfather," she said. "You need a good godmother. I'm your godmother."

The woman talking was Denise Robbins. She lived right down the street. I was coming out of the sub shop when she was going in. She stopped me to say we needed to talk. I'd known Denise most of my life.

"You know I love my godmother," I told Denise with a smile on my face.

"But you love running these streets more," she snapped back. "Look here, baby, I understand what's happening with you. I see it."

"What do you see?"

"These fools out here, these drug dealers and drug lords, these gangsta godfathers look at you like a mascot. They see you like a pet. To them you're a puppy or a kitten. You think they're protecting you. Ain't that right?"

I just shrug.

"Well, I got news for you, babygirl. Those godfathers only care about one thing—and that's cash money. Maybe they'll reach down and pet their cute lil' puppy from time to time, but they ain't real family. They're hoodlum family. Real family's based on love and caring. Hoodlum family's based on crime and killing. Girl, you better learn the difference before it's too late."

"I know the difference, Denise," I said.

"You say you do, but you sure don't act that way. You're an agitator. You're looking to agitate whenever you can. You thinking agitating is cool. Well, it's not."

"I got people who got my back," I said.

"I know those people," said Denise. "I've known them a helluva lot longer than you. And the gospel truth is that they don't got nothing. They don't have no decency. They don't have no basic respect for human life. They ain't God-fearing and they ain't God-loving. They worship the golden calf. They about money and power. They live by the gun and die by the gun. Is that what you want?"

"I ain't dying any time soon."

"I'm not saying you are, baby. But I am saying that the people you're following will lead you to an early grave. What's the point of that?"

"What's the point of anything?"

"God. God's the point of everything. Comes down to one simple thing—we're here to love each other, not kill each other. In this here neighborhood, you're doing one or the other. I'm saying this not to preach to you, sugar, but just to let you know I love you."

"I love you too, Denise."

"Then I wanna see you change your ways—and change them now. Can I have a promise? Can I have commitment?"

"My sub's getting soggy," I said.

Denise shook her head.

"I want you to think about what I said," she practically begged me. "At least tell me you'll do that."

"I will."

But I didn't.

HE'S THINKING, *SHE TURNED YOU OFF.* I'M THINKING, *SHE TURNED ME OUT.*

Father looked after me from afar.

Uncle looked after me from up close.

Because he was the King, Father was ruling an entire kingdom. Uncle was a Prince with a smaller territory. The King spent a lot of time holed up in his castle, but the Prince was always around.

Uncle had always been convinced I really wasn't gay. He'd been watching me grow up for a few years now and didn't like how I dressed.

"You dress like a boy," he said, "and you act like a boy because the boys are getting all the action. You want some of that action. I understand where you coming from. But if you ever had any real-life sex with a grown woman, you'd get straightened out in a hurry."

I didn't say nothing.

"You don't believe me?" he asked.

I still didn't say nothing.

"All right," Uncle said. "I'll prove it to your stubborn ass. I'll set you up with a horny bitch and see how gay you are after she gets hold of you."

I looked at him, expressionless.

"You think you man enough to handle that?" he asked sarcastically.

I offered up a little smile.

About a week passed.

"I found her," said Uncle when I saw him on the corner.

"Found who?"

"The bitch."

"Oh."

"Here's her address. Go by there tonight."

I went by.

By then I must have been twelve. I'm guessing the woman was nineteen or twenty. She was fine as she could be. I just called her Miss Fine.

"What you know about chopping?" she said to me.

Chopping meant fucking.

"Not too much," I said.

"Ever do it?" she asked.

"Well, not really."

"Maybe you not ready for that. Maybe you ready for this."

For a long while she gave me oral sex. I mean, *a long while*.

Next time I seen Uncle, he was real curious.

He's thinking, *She turned you off.*

I'm thinking, *She turned me out.*

"What did you think of it?" he asked me.

"Well," I said. "It was different."

"I knew you wouldn't like it."

"I didn't say that."

"So what are you saying?"

"I'm saying I think you set me up with a good experiment. And I wouldn't mind experimenting a little more."

Uncle cracked up. "Girl," he said, "you are crazy."

Crazy or not, I went back for more. This time Miss Fine gave me some instructions on the fine art of chopping. She taught me how to strap it on. And it's been on ever since.

Where I grew up, the boys started chopping young. They'd find some wild girls and get them a cheap motel room. The boys would take me along. I was one of them. I was accepted, even in the motel room.

When it was time to chop, I'd strap on but never take off my boxers or undershirt. I didn't have to be butt naked. I didn't want to be butt naked. I could take part and slam as hard as any other boy. And of course I'd last as long as was needed. That was a real advantage.

Another advantage was that Uncle and I never had a falling out, even after he saw that his attempt to change me up sexually wasn't working. He resigned himself to the fact that I was who I was. He never judged me or tried to change me.

I'll always love him for that.

Despite his love and watchful eye, though, there was no slowing me down.

I'm not sure why, but I was hell-bent on working the wild side of the street. The wilder the better.

By the time I hit twelve, I was straight-up out of control.

That's when things went nuts.

DEATH UP CLOSE

I seen death up close when that boy got his brains blown out right in front of me. I seen other niggas get blown away on the streets. When it happens, you stop and look. You stop and think. A life's been snuffed out. That's it. Cat's gone. Ain't never coming back.

Maybe 'cause it happened so much I didn't let myself feel what most people would feel—fear or horror or confusion. I didn't wanna feel too much 'cause if I felt too much I might go crazy living where I lived. So the easiest thing was just to watch in wonder and say to myself, "That's how it go sometime."

I thought I could deal with death. Shit, I *knew* I could deal with death. Death didn't flip me out and death didn't make me scared of the streets. I did all that in spite of the death around me.

But then this one death worked on me a whole different way.

Pop.

One day something needed fixing on the roof and Pop said to me, "Hey, girl, would you mind going up there to fix it."

Didn't mind at all, but Pop always liked going up on the roof. I knew something was wrong.

"You feeling okay?" I asked him.

"A little tired, that's all."

I saw that in his eyes and later asked Mama about it.

"He got a bad report from the doctor" was all she said.

I wanted to ask more about it, but something told me not to.

As weeks went by, he lost weight. Slowed down. Slept during the day. Well, Pop *never* slept during the day. The man was a worker.

Finally Mama said the word.

"Cancer."

Cancer was eating him up, and it was happening fast. So fast that from one day to another you'd see him getting smaller and thinner. Soon he was at the point where he couldn't work at all.

Doctors said he should be in the hospital, but Mama said no. By then she knew he was not getting better. She also knew that he didn't wanna go to no hospital. He wanted to be in his bed at home.

Every night after I came in from running the streets, I'd go in and check on him. He'd be in bed next to Mama. I'd kiss him on his nose. That always made him smile. He'd open his eyes, look at me, and just nod. He was too weak too speak.

Then one of those nights Mama came to wake me up. Had to be around 2:00 or 3:00 A.M.

"Come with me, child," she said.

I followed her into the bedroom. I knew. I felt it. I kissed Pop on the nose, only this time he didn't smile.

His eyes were still open but he wasn't breathing. I took my fingers and gently closed his eyes.

"When the sun comes up," said Mama, "go tell the family. Go tell them in person."

I did like Mama asked me to do. I told everyone that needed telling.

I can't remember crying. Can't remember mourning the man. I knew I loved him and I knew he'd loved me. I was his helper on the roof and in the workshop. He never got mad at me for being a tomboy and never thought I was strange. He took me the way I was.

His being taken away might have gotten me mad. Can't say for sure.

Lots of things got me mad.

Back then, though, I wasn't thinking about how I was feeling.

I was just doing.

"YOU A BOY"

I was doing all I could.

I was running with different crews.

My first crew was all girls. Must have been twenty of them. If I was twelve years old, they were sixteen. All big girls. Big-boned, tall, and strong. I was the shrimp. They let me hang with them 'cause I was nervy. I'd do anything they'd do—and then some.

They weren't lesbians. They had boyfriends. But in most cases they could kick their boyfriend's ass if the nigga got out of line. We called ourselves LMP after three streets in our hood.

We'd go to the movies together and talk to the screen. We tripped on a picture called *Juice* with a rapper who just came out with his first record. He went by 2Pac then and he was something different. He had these eyes and he had this attitude. He had his own flow and burned up the movie screen. Nigga was on fire. *Menace II Society* was another story that spoke our language. Probably the freshest was *New Jack City*. We saw that one until we knew every line. Wesley Snipes chewed that up, Ice T was cold, and Chris Rock had us believing he was a fucked-up crackhead. We were seeing our lives up there.

Day by day, week by week, LMP's little shit got bigger. We got bolder. We started out by mouthing off when other girls came through our territory. Then we got meaner. If a girl we didn't know glanced in our direction, we'd say, "Who you staring at?" Then if she mouthed off, one of my girls would encourage me by saying, "Pop that bitch, Snoop. Pop her hard." I'd smack her in the face or punch her in the jaw. My girls liked to see me fight 'cause I didn't have any quit in me.

What did I have in me?

What the hell was I was so angry about?

I couldn't tell you.

We'd go to a house party and see another girl crew, this one from the west side. They'd get to dancing. LL Cool J had "Mama Said Knock You Out." Dre was rocking *The Chronic*. Or maybe the girls from across town were grinding with our boys to Janet's "That's the Way Loves Goes." Everyone was grinding to that jam. But if the grinding got too sweaty, we'd jump in there and straight-up start throwing the west side bitches out on the street. There were some serious fights, and I don't remember losing any of them.

Because I looked like a little nigga, not a girl, I was a novelty. Sometimes I felt like a mascot. And because I was the youngest and the smallest, I felt privileged to hang with the big girls. But I was always on the outside of the group. My size kept me on the outside, and so did my age, the way I dressed, even the way I walked.

"You a boy," the girls liked to say, "who got born a girl by mistake."

I didn't mind hearing that, but it made me think I really do belong with the boys. So I went back and forth. I ran with both crowds. Both crowds accepted me but both crowds really didn't.

I was in and I was out. I was here and I was there.

Whatever I was, I was hitting the streets hard because nothing was too crazy for me. I could handle it all.

At least I thought I could.

"YOU A GIRL"

Maybe I was always trying to prove what I wasn't—maybe that was it.

Nigga come up to me and say, "You a girl."

I wouldn't say anything back.

He'd shove me real hard.

"You a girl who thinks she's a goddamn boy, ain't you?"

Then he'd shove me harder.

Still don't say nothing.

"If you were really a boy, you wouldn't take this shit off me."

Then he shoved me so hard I nearly went down.

But I didn't. I found my balance and coldcocked the motherfucker.

I heard that question many times—"You think you a boy?"—but never again from him.

Right around then—must have been twelve or thirteen—I got the news from some relative.

"Your mama's dead," she said.

I knew she was talking about my real mother, not the mama who cared for me. I wasn't surprised because I'd seen it coming. Every time my real mother had come by, her eyes were already dead. I could see the life draining out of her. And there wasn't a damn thing anybody could do about it. She was cracked out. It's amazing she lived as long as she did. Finally, her body just couldn't take no more. A kidney disease killed her.

I didn't know how to mourn. Truth be told, I didn't even know how to feel about it. So I didn't feel nothing.

Sure, certain memories of her floated through my mind—the times I met her in the park, the time she locked me in the closet. I thought about her beauty. And how she died the death I'd seen my whole life on the street. Her highs took her to an early grave. I didn't even go to her grave. I don't know where it is.

You'd think her death would have scared me or set me straight. But hell, I wasn't no junkie. I wasn't about to blow coke up my nose and shoot dope in my veins. I wasn't interested in the crack pipe. That shit was for fools.

What interested me was danger.

Going to the edge.

And then over the edge.

I can't tell you why, but at a time when other thirteen-year-olds were buying frilly dresses and training bras, I was buying guns.

I was leaving the LMP crew to hang more and more with the boys.

I was running wild.

Mama saw what was happening. She saw me skipping school for days at a time and coming home late or not at all.

One morning I got home just as Mama was making breakfast. She stopped cooking her oatmeal and gave me a look. Wasn't a hard look and it wasn't a mean look. Mama don't got no mean in her. It was a look that said, *Girl, you breaking my heart.*

"Can we talk, child?" she asked me.

"Sure, Mama."

"You been out there on those streets," she said.

"I'm okay," I assured her. "I know what I'm doing."

"I'm afraid for you, baby."

"Mama," I said, "you don't gotta be afraid."

"I'm afraid I'm losing you."

"That ain't ever gonna happen," I told her.

"I pray for you every night, Felicia. When you ain't home, I pray that angels be watching over you. I pray for your protection, honey."

"I know you do," I said, "and I love you for it."

"I fear those people out there, baby. I fear they turning you the wrong way."

I hated when Mama talked this way 'cause I had no answers. She was right. I *was* being turned the wrong way. I saw it, but I wasn't about to stop it. Something like a fever had come over me. But it wasn't no twenty-four-hour fever. The fever felt permanent. The fever provided chills and thrills. Even when Mama was talking good sense to me, I felt the fever. The fever had more power over me than Mama's warnings.

"When you gonna stop this nonsense, Felicia?" she asked.

"Soon, Mama," I lied. "Real soon."

BONKERS

Mama wasn't the only one who warned me.

Uncle did the same. Fact is, Uncle was always preaching to me.

I remember one afternoon when the streets were slick with rain. We were riding in his Cadillac, going from one of his shops to another. He was making sure his business was straight.

"You gotta get out of this business," he said. "You gotta just think about school."

"I'm thinking about school," I said. "I'm doing good in school."

"You doing good in this business," he said. "See, that's the problem, Snoop. You do good at something you got no business doing."

"Same as you."

"No, ain't the same as me. I'm a man and I know what I'm doing. I got kids. I got money to make. You don't gotta do nothing but study."

"I am studying," I said.

"You ain't studying nothing but these here streets."

He wasn't wrong. And he wasn't convincing. Neither was Father. Fact is, my street shit was getting bigger. I was doing more than just working the corners. I was doing little jobs for operators who needed someone they could count on.

For example, nigga came up to and said, "See that bitch over there, she stole my dope. I want you to beat her ass."

"I ain't killing no one," I said.

"Don't want her killed, Snoop. Just hurt real bad."

"How much?" I asked.

"Fifty now. Fifty when it's done."

I waited a day, followed her down the street, and pulled her in the alley. Pistol-whipped her hard, then beat her with a table leg. Broke her leg and shoulder.

"Satisfied?" I asked the nigga.

He handed me the other fifty, no questions asked.

I was in the back of a stolen car. We pulled up to a gas station. My partner, the driver, started pumping gas. Cops pulled up next to us. The driver got scared and started looking all paranoid. When we saw the cops running our plates, we jumped out of there, tires screeching, cops chasing, chasing us through downtown, chasing us past the fancy houses in Fell's Point, running red lights, jumping curbs, speeding the wrong way down one-way streets, sirens screaming. We dumped the car in a deserted lot and ran like hell. Found an open cellar door, ran down the steps, and kept the rats company for a couple of hours.

Cops never did find us.

Me and my niggas were hired by a dealer to go after some deadbeats. The guys thought they gave us the slip. They went to the mall. They figured with all those shoppers around, the mall had to be safe. They figured wrong.

We followed them past Shoe City. One of them turned and gave us a look that said, "What y'all going to do? Pop us in the mall?"

We popped 'em in the mall.

My little man K did the shooting.

Then there was shooting on the corner of Biddle and Marfat.

I'm walking down the street with my nigga. Just chillin'. Here comes a U-Haul truck. Me and my boy look at each other like this ain't right. The U-Haul truck is going real slow. You don't see slow-moving U-Haul trucks on this street every day. And the driver's looking nervous. I catch his eyes and see something I don't like.

We step back.

U-Haul pulls to the curb.

Back of the truck slowly rolls open.

And suddenly the spraying starts.

Niggas from the west side with nothing better to do than to come east and start spraying.

Fuck those motherfuckers.

Me and my boy duck behind some garbage cans. I pull out my nine-millimeter and blast back. The fools in the U-Haul are sitting targets.

Two of them go down.

They don't touch us.

They run outta there with us still shooting at their asses.

Then there's the graveyard. Seems like we always go to the graveyard. The funeral home and the graveyard.

The graveyard is all foggy this afternoon. It rained in the morning and now a thick fog has moved in. We're there 'cause our friend J was killed by mistake. They killed J thinking he was B. J was a sweetheart. J was our homeboy. B is an asshole. The sweetheart got shot and the asshole is still walking around. B is up there with us telling J good-bye.

We walking toward the grave to bury J when, behind us, we see this guy approaching. We don't know who the fuck he is.

The eyes. The eyes always give it away.

This stranger's eyes are showing nervousness. And before we know it, he starts shooting at B. Shooter was sent to J's funeral to get B, the nigga they wanted dead to begin with.

We say, "Oh, no. Not up in here. You can't disrespect J by turning his funeral into a fuckin' shooting gallery."

My man hits the shooter with a silencer. He goes down slowly, slumped over someone's grave.

We leave him there and go bury J.

A few days later someone catches up with B and shoots him dead.

Wu-Tang Clan is out with "Protect Ya Neck." Later they screaming about "C.R.E.A.M. . . . cash rules everything around me."

Word.

LEAD BAT

Who did I think I was?

Why was I doing what I was doing?

I look back and wonder why.

I look back and ask myself questions that are hard, maybe even impossible, to answer.

But at the time questions weren't part of my life. Questions weren't part of my thinking.

I didn't ask.

I just did.

"What the fuck you doing?" Uncle would ask. "Word out there is that you crazy and getting crazier every day. You got to slow down, Snoop."

"What for?"

"To keep your little ass alive—that's what for."

I knew Uncle loved me. I knew he cared. But Uncle wasn't stopping me.

Neither was Father. I'd see Father roll by in his hundred-thousand-dollar ride. He'd pull over and say, "You staying outta trouble, Snoop?"

"No way," I'd answer honestly.

He'd laugh and lay a hundred on me.

"This is for schoolbooks," he'd say, "and nothing else."

I'd take the money and buy another joint.

Seeing what I saw, being who I was, I knew it was my balls and my nine-millimeters that was keeping me alive.

I wasn't backing down from no one. I wasn't backing down from life.

Life was the streets and the streets didn't scare me none.

Then these dreams. The details were fuzzy but the dreams kept coming back to me. They'd change up, but one thing was always there:

In the dream I'd be driving a car when a lead baseball bat would fly through the window, right at me. I'd wake up in a sweat.

In another dream I'd be walking through downtown Baltimore, kicking it with my niggas, when I'd look up at a lead baseball bat about to crack my head open. I'd wake up drenched in sweat.

There was a dream when I'm in a roller coaster and I look down and see some crazy man beating the controls with a lead baseball bat until the roller coaster starts collapsing and I start plunging to my death. Wake up in more sweat.

I don't understand dreams—then or now. There's nothing you can do about what you dream. But I have to say that in this case those dreams saw something I didn't—until I saw it in the flesh.

———

This shit was strange.

This was what happened in sure-enough life. This was no dream.

Can't remember the day of the week when it came down. Can't remember the weather. Might have been cloudy. Might have been clear. Don't know what jams were banging back then. Maybe MC Lyte and "Ruffneck." Maybe Da Brat getting "Funkdafied."

I remember that rumors were floating around how Tupac had shot two cops in Atlanta. Tupac might have been on my mind 'cause Pac had just come through our neighborhood.

He knew a lot of the niggas on our block. Couple of weeks before the day that changed my life, I was on the corner when I heard everyone saying, "Pac's around. Pac's down on the Boulevard, Pac's chilling with the niggas." I went down there to see for myself. And there he was.

Beautiful cat. Eyes all bright and lit up with love. Lit up with intelligence. No security either 'cause he knew he was safe with us. We loved Pac. He was short, compact, killer good-looking, and had huge feet. All the big-time dealers came out to see him, protect him, and welcome him.

I got to say, "Whassup, Pac," and see him smile right at me.

His smile was real sincere and his attitude real cool. Seemed like he had time for everyone. I was wishing I could hang with him, but so many people were wanting that same thing. Figured I better leave him alone. Wish him well. Go on my way.

It's something when you see a real star.

On the day when my dream came to life, I wasn't looking for no stars. Wasn't looking for a damn thing. Fact is, I was minding my business, walking my usual walk.

Father once told me, "You don't walk, Snoop. You stalk. You walk like you don't want no one to fuck with you."

"I don't," I said.

So I was stalking through the neighborhood. Forgot where I was going or what I had to do. Doesn't matter 'cause I looked across the street and saw a fight about to come down.

Didn't know the people. Didn't know why they was fighting. Didn't know nothing except fights always drew me. Something about the energy of a fight. The excitement. The danger. I wanted to get close and see what was happening.

So I crossed the street.

I fuckin' crossed the street.

Had I gone straight or turned the corner away from the fight, my whole life would be different.

Funny how so much hinges on five or six little steps.

I took those steps across the street and saw that tempers were boiling over. People calling each other motherfuckers and dirty bitches. Fists were flying.

Then it happened.

The bat.

The lead baseball bat.

A girl looked at me with murder in her eyes. I didn't know her. Never had seen her before. Don't know why she came at me. Made no sense. I wasn't cussing her. I wasn't threatening her. I was just walking by, watching this fighting, when she picked a slugger lead baseball bat—the same bat that had been coming at me in my dreams—and started swinging it at my head. If she caught me, I'd be dead.

I screamed for her to stop, but she wasn't interested in stopping. She wanted to take my head off.

I tried to get away but by then the crowd was too thick. I couldn't move. I was hemmed in by people while this crazy lady was lunging at me with a lead bat.

There was only way to stop her.

I took out my shit. I figured once she saw it, she'd back off. But she wasn't backing off. Even the gun couldn't stop her.

Only one thing could.

Shooting the gun.

Before she got to me, I got to her.

I shot her clean.

My lead stopped her lead.

She fell to the ground.

Dead.

I ran.

MURDER WAS THE CASE

Snoop Dogg said it. Snoop Pearson lived it.

Snoop kept running until she got to one of her niggas' house.

She stayed there for a night. That night she dreamed. Baseball bats were still flying at her head.

In the morning, there was a knock on the door. She peeped through the blinds. Uncle was standing there.

He hugged her. She expected him to cuss her out but he didn't.

"I know what happened," Uncle said. "I done heard all about it."

"The bitch was coming after me with a goddamn bat," Snoop explained. "What was I gonna do?"

"You did what you did," said Uncle. "But now you can't stay here. This neighborhood's too hot."

"Where am I gonna go?" asked Snoop.

"My crib," said Uncle.

Uncle's crib was way 'cross town. Uncle put Snoop in the back room and told her, "You lay low."

Laying low was hard for Snoop. Snoop had to hit the streets. Snoop hated being cooped up anywhere for long.

"If you don't lay low you gonna be cooped up for a lot longer than you can imagine," said Uncle.

"How long I gotta stay here?" asked Snoop.

"Long as I say," Uncle made clear. "Lot of people saw what you did."

"What I did was done in self-defense."

"Whatever you did, the heat's on. Don't move from here."

Snoop had a hard time not moving.

On the television she'd watch *The Cosby Show*. She loved *The Cosby Show*. She pretended like her daddy was a doctor and her mama was a lawyer. Her daddy would say funny things and act the fool, but he'd always be there for her. Her mother was young and beautiful. She'd have all these sisters and brothers, one cleaner than the next. They'd have their little dumb-ass problems like the new dress is too long or the curtains in the bedroom are the wrong color. Snoop would imagine being surrounded by all these people night and day. Nothing could happen to her. Nothing could go wrong.

"Nothing will go wrong long as you keep your ass right where it is," Uncle would tell Snoop soon as he came home from supervising his shops.

"Can't even go out to buy some chips?" Snoop asked.

"We got chips up here in the crib. Stay put."

Staying put meant watching more television.

Reruns of *Mama's Family*. Snoop loved *Mama's Family*. Loved laughing at those crazy white people. Loved how Mama would shoot her mouth off any damn way she pleased.

But how many hours can you watch TV without going nuts?

Snoop would peep out the window. Car rolling by. Snoop Dogg spittin' 'bout "Murder Was the Case That They Gave Me."

Biggie blowing up with "Ready to Die." "Big Poppa" and "Juicy" all over the streets.

The streets were calling.

"Stay inside," Uncle kept saying.

"Just wanna see what's happening," Snoop kept saying.

"I'll tell you what's happening," said Uncle. "They after you."

Snoop stayed in. Four days, five days. Then a whole week. More *Cosby*. More *Mama's Family*.

More dreams.

More nightmares.

Then came the rain, thunder and lightning. Rained like holy hell for days on end.

Cooped inside. Going crazy. Going stir crazy. Rain pounding against the roof. Pounding and pounding and pounding.

Then silence. Sweet silence.

Snoop woke up. It was morning. House was empty. Went to the window. Peeped through the curtains.

Sunshine!

Blue sky!

No clouds! No rain!

Beautiful, beautiful day!

Had to get out.

Just for a minute.

Just for a quick walk to the corner store to buy a little candy bar.

Wouldn't take more than a minute.

Once I was out, I was gone. I was feeling bold. Feeling like they'll never find me. They'll never catch me. I'll duck in this alley. I'll hide behind this van. I'll keep moving so fast, changing up routes and crisscrossing the city, that no one will trace my path.

I had all the moves.

I had all the confidence in the world.

I was so confident, in fact, that I even went back to East Oliver. Stopped by to give Mama a quick kiss. Mama didn't know that I was on the run. She didn't have to know.

"Go by and see your godsister, Monique," said Mama. "She been asking for you."

Monique lived just two doors down on Oliver. I ran by and found her in the kitchen making greens.

She gave me a taste. I love greens.

"Haven't seen you in a while," she said. "Where you been, girl?"

"Here and there," I told her.

I heard the front door open.

"You expecting someone?" I asked.

"Nope."

When I turned, I saw a policeman standing there.

Just like that, I started out the back door. But a policeman was standing there as well.

Nowhere to run, nowhere to hide.

Cop in the kitchen said, "We just wanna question you."

I didn't say nothing.

He approached me with cuffs.

"You gotta cuff me to question me?" I asked.

"'Fraid so," he said.

By then the kitchen was filled with cops. Must have been six of them.

They escorted me out the front door. Now the whole neighborhood was out there. Everyone was looking to see what was happening. There was a whole squadron of police cars.

I could see Mama coming out her front door. She caught a glimpse of me. I saw the hurt in her eyes.

There was nothing I could say, nothing I could do.

MORE THAN
A MINUTE

The Snoop that shot a woman before the woman bashed her head in with a bat, the Snoop that ran and hid, the Snoop that was stupid enough to go out the house, only to be seen and caught—that Snoop was me.

Hard to believe the things I did when I was barely a teenager, but I did them. I watched myself get into this mess, figuring my protectors would get me out.

Mama didn't have no money for lawyers, but Uncle did. Uncle and Father both told me to stay cool, they'd find me the best criminal defense attorney in the city.

I tried to stay cool, but how cool can you stay in the city jail waiting for your case? That shit takes forever.

"How long?" I asked Uncle when he first started explaining about the criminal justice system.

"More than a minute," he said. "There were a bunch of witnesses who saw you shoot."

"Well, I did shoot," I said, "but only to save myself."

"The witnesses might not have seen it that way," Uncle explained. "They might have heard the gunfire and then seen you holding the gun."

"Who knows what the fuck they saw?"

"That's my point, Snoop. I gotta talk to those witnesses."

"How you gonna find them?" I asked.

"I'll find them," said Uncle.

"How long do you think that'll take?"

"I keep telling you, Snoop—more than a minute."

23/1

They had raided Mama's house and taken away pictures of me. They put me on wanted lists and were hunting me down from different directions. I should have known better than to step out like that.

I stepped out and got snagged.

And that was that.

I'd been arrested before, but it was all petty stuff. In and out after an hour or two.

Now my ass was in city jail for God knows how long.

I can't say I was all that scared 'cause most of the niggas in there were boys I knew. Half of them was from around my way. It was like homecoming week.

"Whassup, Snoop," they said. "We glad you gonna kick it with us in here."

I wasn't glad, but I sure as shit wasn't lonely.

Uncle came by. Father too. Both said, "Look here, baby-girl. This here lawyer's coming through to help you. And besides that, we talked to the witnesses and none of them saw you shooting no one. Cops got a weak case."

Whether the case was weak or strong, the case took forever to get going. There were all sorts of delays.

"Delays," said the lawyer, "work in your favor."

Maybe so, but because the judge didn't trust me with no bail, I had to sit in city jail while the wheels of justice turned awfully fuckin' slow.

City jail was boring and bad. Same old damn thing day after day. Go to school in a trailer. Boys on one side, girls on the other. Of course I wanted to sit with the boys, but that was prohibited. The teaching was lame. The teacher was half asleep. The TV at night only got two channels.

I studied my lessons—always did good in school—but that didn't make the boredom go away.

There was no sex, at least none on my part. I didn't know any of the girls well enough to get that close to them. I was getting my survival shit together, and sex was the last thing on my mind.

One thing that was on my mind was escaping. Wasn't my idea, but a girl in my cell called N. Actually, N got the idea from watching *MacGyver*, the TV show about a secret agent.

In one episode, some dude escapes jail through a ceiling. Then he sprinkles pepper behind him so the dogs can't pick up his trail.

"We can do that," said N. "Look up in that ceiling. We

can push back that tile and crawl out to the street, pepper it up and be outta here."

I was skeptical, but what else did I have to do? N convinced me and also convinced S, the other girl in our cell.

N had me to steal some pepper from the kitchen. Then we got us extra blankets and towels we'd use to climb up to the ceiling.

N thought she had her little operation together.

But then S freaked out.

"I ain't doing it!" she screamed. "We'll get caught and get shot."

"Shut the fuck up," I told her.

She wouldn't shut up so I stomped her a few times until she did.

"You don't gotta go with us," I said, "but if you say a word I'll bust you up so bad you won't be able to open your mouth ever again."

I thought that settled that, but I was wrong.

S kept freaking out and a week later wound up telling the CO—the correctional officer—about our escape plan.

CO came by, saw our stash of pepper and stack of blankets and started laughing.

"You fools," she said.

We didn't say nothing.

CO got a stool and pushed back the tile where we'd hope to escape.

"Come on up here," she told me and N. "Look at your escape route."

"I don't need to look," I said. "I know what's up there."

"What?" asked the CO.

"A brick wall thick enough to keep a tank from breaking through," I said.

"If you knew that, why in hell were you looking to climb up there?" she asked.

"I wasn't. We dropped that idea soon as I saw the wall. We innocent."

"Well, you'll have time to think about your innocence when I put you both on administrative lock 23/1," said the CO.

That meant holed up for twenty-three hours with one hour for fresh air.

"But we didn't do shit," I said.

"But you *were* going to do shit," she snapped.

I started to argue, but why?

THE STRIP

I'd never been more than a few miles outside Baltimore.

Probably Father's house beyond the county line was the farthest I'd even been.

Never been to L.A. Never seen Hollywood. Other than what I'd seen on TV or in the movies, didn't know nothing about Las Vegas.

So why am I dreaming about that big Strip with all those fancy hotels and their huge neon signs flashing Stardust, Caesar's Palace, the Mirage, and Treasure Island?

Why am I seeing myself in Vegas, shooting craps at the table and playing the roulette wheels?

In this dream, I'm riding around in limos and sipping fancy drinks in the VIP sections of the nightclubs where the rap stars go to chill. I'm sitting in the front row of a heavyweight fight and I'm betting heavy. My man is winning and the crowd is cheering, the money's rolling in, the chips are red and green and yellow and blue, the blue lights of the after-party are low and I see the faces of all the stars. Mary J. is there.

"That's my wife," I declare. Biggie's there. Faith. Dre. Coolio. Da Brat. Latifah. Nas. Fugees. The party's on and poppin'.

But moving around the room, I feel something's wrong. I don't know what, but my stomach ain't right. My head ain't right. My head is starting to spin. My stomach is starting to ache. I'm feeling sick. Did I eat something rotten or drink some poison?

For all the bad feeling, I keep looking for someone. Don't know who it is, but I gotta find this person because this person is in deep trouble. I leave the party room and run through the casino, run outside on the Strip, run down the Strip, the neon lights racing over my eyes, my eyes searching every which way to find—who?

Everything goes blurry. Everything gets scary. Now there are niggas with knives and guns chasing me and I'm sweating and screaming, "Don't! Don't! Don't!"

"Wake up, girl," says N, who's standing over me.

"Man, this dream freaked me out," I say.

"The way you shaking, looks like a nightmare."

I look at my hands. They are shaking. I don't understand why. A dream has never before made my hands shake.

I try to forget it.

And I do.

Can't tell you how much time passed—maybe a few weeks, maybe a few months. But when the news came, I remembered every detail of that crazy dream.

"TUPAC SHAKUR SHOT IN LAS VEGAS."

That's what the news said on September 7, 1996.

For those of us sitting around city jail, it was like the president was shot. Only worse. We couldn't relate to the president. But all of us sure as hell could relate to Pac.

Now I understood my dream. It was so clear. And so goddamn scary.

He was shot in a drive-by and was laid up in some Vegas hospital. Pac was fighting for his life.

The crowd down at city jail wasn't a praying group, but we had us some prayer meetings. We prayed that Pac's life be spared.

We talked about when he was a young kid backup dancer for Digital Underground. We talked about his first record, *2Pacalypse Now*, and his last record, *All Eyez on Me*, and his new joint as Makaveli, *The Don Killuminati: The 7 Day Theory*. We talked about his genius.

We heard his lines in our head: "No matter what you think about, I'm still your child."

"What you feed us as seeds grows and then blows up in your face—that's thug life."

We waited for his change to come. We wanted him to live so bad. We wanted more Pac joints, more Pac movies. We knew he'd blow up to be bigger than anyone in the history of the game.

We wanted him to stay alive.

And then on the sixth day after the shooting, he died. Respiratory failure. Cardiac arrest.

I didn't wanna talk about it. Didn't wanna think about it. Still don't.

Uncle came by.

"We gotta talk about your case," he said.

"You were gonna make the case go away," I said. "You said the witnesses didn't really see nothing."

"Well," said Uncle, "almost all of them told us that."

"What you mean, 'almost'?" I asked.

"One witness can't be turned around," he said.

"Man or woman?"

"Woman," said Uncle.

"What's she saying?"

"That she saw you shoot her."

"What does my lawyer say?"

"Your lawyer wants to talk to you."

"Does the lawyer know what he's doing?"

"He's the best. He'll get you the best deal."

THE BEST DEAL

I was up in the gym. I was playing point guard, and I was making all the moves. I'd always been good at hoops, but on this particular afternoon I had a hot hand. Everything was falling.

Game over. I headed back to my cell. Note said my lawyer was there to see me. Cool.

Lawyer was smiling when I came in the room.

"No witnesses will testify against you," he said.

"Word."

"Of course the trial will go on. There's no way we can stop that, but it's pretty clear that their case is weak."

"So you think I'll walk?" I asked.

"I can't guarantee anything," the lawyer said. "But it's looking better than it ever has. Now it all rests on the trial."

I thought about the word "trial."

There's a trial down in the courtroom. Those kinds of trials happen all the time.

Then there's what Mama likes to call the trials and tribulations of life. That kind of trial was already happening with me being locked up in city jail. City jail smelled bad, looked bad, was bad. City jail was a trial of my patience. I saw some niggas lose their cool in city jail and straight-up flip out. They couldn't stop either crying or shaking or screaming shit no one could understand.

City jail was a trial.

The trial in the courthouse came up two years after I'd been sitting in city jail. I thought it'd go great.

It didn't.

First day we got there I saw this woman walk in the courtroom with the prosecutors.

"Who's she?" I asked.

"She's the one who said she didn't really see what happened," he said.

"So what's she doing with the prosecutors?"

My lawyer didn't have an answer.

I did.

They'd done flipped her. She was getting ready to testify against me. I could see it in her eyes. I could feel it in her walk. Bitch was ready to do me in.

As the days of pretrial proceedings went by, she walked in the courtroom every day.

I'd seen enough.

"See what kind of deal they'll give me," I told the lawyer.

"You're sure you want to deal?" he asked.

"Sure as shit."

That witness looked clean as a whistle. The jury was going to love her. I didn't stand a chance.

"Cut me a deal," I told my man.

He did.

"This is the best deal they'll give you," he said.

I looked it over and didn't hesitate.

"Take it," I said.

The sentence was reduced down to second-degree murder. They also reduced my jail term down from ten years to eight for the time I'd been sitting in city jail.

Of those eight years, the first five were without parole. That meant that I could be a perfect angel but my ass wasn't going nowhere for five years.

After five there was a possibility of parole.

I was fifteen. Maybe I could get out by the time I was twenty.

Looking at the big picture I felt like I could deal with that.

Five years was a long time, but five years was no lifetime.

I'd adjusted to shit before. I'd adjust to this shit now.

Besides, the move out of city jail was a good thing. I hated that fuckin' place. And from what everyone told me, the joint where I was headed—Maryland Correctional Institution for Women in Jessup—was an upgrade.

They said Jessup was a cleaner, bigger, more modern facility where they tried to actually rehabilitate bitches.

I didn't care about the rehabilitation. I didn't believe in it. I just wanted something better than that stinking sickening city jail.

Jessup was okay with me.

I was eager to get up to the place called the Cut.

A DIFFERENT WORLD

A Different World was a spinoff from *The Cosby Show*. Denise Huxtable goes off to college. That's the "different world."

Denise's world was filled with clean-cut college boys and cute little college girls.

I loved the show.

But watching the show from the Cut—which was another world—was a trip.

The inmates had another term for the Cut. They also called it Grandma's House

The Cut sounded hard. And Grandma's House sounded soft.

The Cut was hard.

Like *A Different World,* the Cut had a campus. Only don't look for no wholesome college kids.

Sinbad the comic was in *A Different World*. He was always cracking jokes and making everyone feel okay. We didn't have Sinbad at Grandma's House. We didn't have any happy-go-lucky comics brightening our day with sunshine and laughter. No, sir.

At the same time, the Cut was cool compared to city jail. The Cut had better food—thank you, Jesus—and the Cut had more activities.

Even though I wasn't free, being able to walk from building to building gave me more of a sense of freedom than I felt during those long months I was sitting in city jail.

Also there was a window in my cell. That window was real important. The window overlooked the fields beyond the prison yard and let me watch day turn to night and night turn to day. The window let me study the seasons. It let me see the world, a piece of sky, the foggy mornings, the rain in spring, and the snow in winter. That window opened my eyes to the grass that started growing and the leaves that started falling, the new flowers being born and the old flowers dying, the trees swaying in the storms, the branches broken off by the lightning, the thunder booming in the dead of night with dark clouds racing past the yellow moon.

The window was a beautiful thing.

You might think that sex in a women's prison would be a beautiful thing, too. All those girls cooped up together. They've made movies about that shit. You'd think that me, a sixteen-year-old lesbian, would have the time of my life. Well, you'd be wrong.

In the five years I spent in Grandma's House, I had sex once. Here's why: I value my health. I value my fuckin' survival. The Cut was full of straight-up crazy ladies, fucked-up crackheads, women who had cut off their boyfriends' balls. For real.

I love sex as much as anyone, but I love living more. Early on I saw how romantic relationships in Grandma's House got out of hand. You'd be loving on some woman, then come to learn she belonged to another bitch and wind up with a scissors in your throat. No, thank you.

For romance, I turned to *Guiding Light*. That was my joint, every day at three. I was hooked on that soap and couldn't wait to see what would happen next. It was like *A Different World*. I knew it was fake and had nothing to do with real life. But that only made those shows better. They let you escape from a place where no one was escaping.

I also liked watching Jerry Springer 'cause that motherfucker is crazy. He'll have men on that show who are fucking their mother-in-laws. Then he'll have the daughters breaking chairs over their mothers' heads. All kinds of shit.

So you get in the Cut and you find your place. My place was to fly under the radar. I didn't want to be no star in Grandma's House. I'd rather not be noticed. Why attract attention, especially from the crackheads who were out of their minds and might do anything to you? I stayed to myself.

I played volleyball and was damn good. I overcame the disadvantage of being short by jumping high and spiking hard. We even had a coach from the outside come in and train us. We had big tournaments in the Cut and my team won the trophy.

After I was in there for a month or so, Uncle came to visit.

"You all right?" he asked.

I nodded yes.

"You ain't getting rough with these girls, are you?"

I shook my head no.

"Didn't think so," said Uncle. "You know better than that."

"Sure as hell do."

"What about the schooling in here?" he wanted to know.

"They got a GED program."

"You going for it, Snoop?"

"I think I should," I said.

"I know you should."

He took my hand and patted it.

"Mama been down here to see you?" he asked.

"No, and she's not coming down. I don't want her here. Don't want her to see me in a place like this. It'll break her heart."

"Well, that schooling thing is great," Uncle said. "You'll probably do better in here than you'd do out there. Less distractions."

"Oh, I seen some distractions."

"Well, avoid them," Uncle warned.

"For sure."

For the most part, I did avoid those distractions. Eventually, though, some of those distractions caught up with me.

They had to. No matter how good your intentions, you just can't sit in jail, year after year, and not get your ass in a little trouble. Least I couldn't.

Meanwhile, though, the best entertainment—and the scariest—wasn't the nightmare Freddy Krueger movies they had on VHS. The best entertainment was the stories that women inside the Cut told about themselves. That's some shit I'll never forget.

"I COULDN'T HELP IT. THE MAN JUST HATED KIDS."

You'd hear these stories.

You'd be eating dinner. Or out in the yard. You'd be up in the gym or down in the laundry. The stories you'd hear would burn your ears. You had to listen. You wanted to listen. The stories on TV and the movies were okay. Getting off on *A Different World* or that fool Jerry Springer was one thing; that shit was mildly entertaining. But the real stories told by the real-life women at Grandma's House would blow your goddamn mind.

Of course in jail you had a long time to twist your story any way you wanted. You never knew how true someone else's story might be. But it didn't matter. You sat there and you listened and, after hearing how some lady wound up in the Cut, you just said to yourself, "Lord, have mercy, this bitch is crazy."

No matter how crazy she might be, you sat there and listened. That was the way you passed the time at Grandma's House.

I remember one inmate I'll call L. L was a light-skinned bitch who reminded me of my real mom. She was fine. She had these green eyes that looked like marbles and she had a refined way to talking. When she started into her story, she began telling it like a lady. Like she'd been to college or even law school. She talked like she had no ghetto in her.

"My mother was a schoolteacher," she said. "My grandmother had been a schoolteacher too. My father was a salesman who did very well and I always had lovely clothes. I sang in the choir in the Methodist church and I won all the spelling bees. Even today, I'm a superb speller. My older brother went on to college to become an engineer and I was supposed to go to a fancy college but I began dancing when I was very young. You've probably seen me in the videos. That's how I got out to California—video directors were hiring me. Practically every week I was dancing in a different video. I had an agent, a very important agent, and a famous lawyer who would go over my contracts before I signed anything. I was in demand.

"And I was in love. I don't want to name him, but a famous movie star fell in love with me. He was married at the time, but his wife wasn't interested in lovemaking. She was a social climber and just using him to get to all the parties you read about in the magazines. She didn't love him. I thought I did. I thought he'd build his world around me. That's what he said. That's what the man promised. He took me to Hawaii, to a luxurious resort right there on a private beach. Every day at sunset, the hotel would move the massage tables out by the water and I'd have my massage out there in the open with the breezes from the ocean and that Hawaiian music floating in the air. It was quite something. That's where I learned about skin care products.

"The movie star set me up in business. I was doing extremely well—it was a mail order business—and then I became pregnant. When my first baby came, the movie star left his wife for me. Yes, he did. We moved to a different part of Los Angeles, a very exclusive part, and I became pregnant again. That's when I knew he was cheating on me. But it didn't matter all that much because I'd known for a while that he wasn't the man I'd met in the beginning. He was addicted to gambling, he started getting fat, and his career was going downhill fast. He gave me a settlement for the kids. Big settlement. By then I was fed up with Hollywood. Hollywood is so phony. I wanted to come back to the East Coast where people are more educated and not as crude.

"When I moved back, I had many opportunities to marry. Men have never been a problem for me. There was a banker who wanted to marry me, and there was also a gentleman who owned a chain of fine clothing stores. He bought me a full-length mink coat. I have pictures of me in that coat. I went to New York many times and stayed at the Waldorf, the best hotel in the city, and ate in restaurants that overlooked the river and the bridges. There were very wealthy stockbrokers who wanted to marry me and a man from Egypt who owned factories all over the world. But these men meant nothing to me.

"Then Prince Charming came along. I call him Prince Charming because he was Prince Charming. Tall as a prince. Handsome as a prince. Dark eyes that melted you the minute he looked your way. Big hands and beautiful teeth. Size thirteen shoes. Low, sexy voice like Barry White. He had houses all over the state. A Bentley, a Ferrari, two motorcycles—one white, one black. He had white blood in him, maybe more white than black, because his skin was lighter than mine. He said he had a gold mine in South Africa. He showed me the pictures. He was going to take me there. He said he'd been looking for me his whole life and now that he'd found me, he could never let me go. He was the one.

"We'd talk for hours on end and never got bored. We'd talk all night. We'd love all night. He was one of those men who could control his body. He'd say, 'I'm not coming until you come at least five times.' The lovemaking was like nothing I had ever known. Even now, talking about him gets me wet. He was a man among men.

"He was writing a book about his life and told me, 'Now I have the final chapter. You are the final chapter.' Different businessmen from foreign countries would come to his house for dinner and he'd introduce me as a queen. He gave me a diamond necklace worth eighty thousand dollars. He gave me a gold diamond watch worth fifty thousand dollars. He took me to Florida where a designer custom-made all my outfits and modeled a line after me. The line became famous. The designer wanted to photograph me for his ads, but Prince Charming wouldn't allow it. 'She's mine and mine alone,' he said.

"So my life was perfect. Absolutely perfect. He wanted me to go with him to France for the summer. Of course I loved the idea. But then this one little problem kept coming up: my children. He hated children. He said I couldn't take the children to France. By then, though, Mom had died and all my aunts had moved away.

"'We'll hire a nanny,' I told him.

"'I don't want a nanny,' he said. 'I don't want kids. Kids ruin everything.'

"'I have my kids, though,' I told him.

"'Long as you have your kids, you don't have me,' he said.

"I tried to reason with the man, but he wasn't reasonable that way. He had his attitude. He also had his choice of any woman in the world. I knew that. I saw them coming and going. But I also saw that he was ready to make me his queen. How many women get a chance to be a queen? So I did what I had to do."

L stopped talking. Her green eyes were cold as ice. I didn't want to ask her, but I had to.

"What did you do?" I pried.

"I burned down the house," she said matter-of-factly.

"But it was okay. The children were asleep. It happened so fast they couldn't feel anything."

Wait a second, I was thinking to myself, *this crazy bitch done burned her house with her kids inside? And she's sitting here saying it like it was no worse than overcooking the hamburgers. This is one wack job I'm avoiding for as long as I'm staying at Grandma's House.*

One of the bitches who'd been listening to her along with me couldn't contain herself.

"That's some horrible shit," she said.

"I couldn't help it," said L. "The man just hated kids."

"THAT'S WHY THEY CALL IT GRANDMA'S HOUSE."

I heard a lot of stories about why the Cut started being called Grandma's House. The one that gave me the most chills, though, came down through a woman I'll call Z. I didn't know whether to believe her, but I had a couple of nightmares over her story.

She was in her forties, maybe even older. Had scars all over her face. She'd been cut up and burned something awful. She was ugly to begin with—maybe that's why she was so pissed off at everyone. If you got close to her she'd hiss at you like a cornered cat, so you sure-enough left her alone. No one wanted to fuck with her. There were dozens of rumors about her case but she never talked to anyone. Then she started playing basketball with us. She was over six feet so we put her at center. Even though she was older, she could keep up with the young girls. With the passes I'd feed her, she scored like crazy. That got her to like me.

One day we won a big game because of her inside moves. That put her in a great mood, and she started talking to me. She had a low voice that was scratchy. Even her lips were scarred something awful.

"I know no one likes looking at me," she said, "and I don't give two shits. Fuck 'em."

I didn't say nothing.

"Everyone wants to know what happened to me," she went on. "You wanna know too, don't you?"

Still didn't say nothing.

"Everyone wants to ask me but they too scared. You scared too, ain't you?"

"Hell, yes, I'm scared," I said.

That made her laugh. Made her like me even more.

"Happened when I young. When I was young. My grandma listened to this song that said, 'When I was nothing but a child, all you boys tried to drive me wild.' You ever hear that song?"

"No."

"Old fucked-up blues song. I don't know nothing about those old blues. Grandma would drive me crazy with those old blues. Sounded like shit to me. I don't even like music. Music gives me a fuckin' headache. You like music?"

"I like Pac."

"Oh yeah, Pac. Well, that ain't music. That's poetry, ain't it?"

"Yeah."

"Grandma played her blues music night and day. I hated that shit until I busted up a few of her records. She'd just go out and buy more. She did it to drive me crazy. You know how bitches will drive you crazy."

"Yeah."

"You have a grandmother?"

"Well, I have a foster mother who's like a grandmother," I said. "I call her Mama but she's old enough to be my grandmother."

"You like her?"

"Yeah. She raised me. She didn't have to, but she did."

"My grandmother raised me too," said Z. "My mother up and left after I was born. Just left. How 'bout your mom?"

"Crackhead. She dead."

"Shit," said Z. "That's the stuff that done me in. You ever deal with the pipe?"

"No."

"The pipe is deep. The pipe is so deep until you ain't ever the same again. That's where all these scars come from. You wanna know about the scars?"

"If you feel like talking, I'm listening."

"I'd pick me the meanest motherfuckers to get high with. Don't know why. But every last one would be lowdown and nasty. When we run out of shit, they'd make me chase after more. I'm the kind of bitch who'd say, 'Fuck you. *You* chase after the shit.' They'd cut me. I'd cut 'em back. They'd cut me again. And that's how it go. Went that way for years. But the thing about the pipe is that the pipe takes you all the way down to places you didn't know were there. You been to the crack house?"

"I've been by to take a look."

"So you know what's happening in there."

"I have some idea," I said.

"Well, if you hanging in the crack house, you okay. That's the nice part of it. That means you getting loaded and you cool. It's when you don't even have enough money to buy nothing in the crack house—that's when you fucked up. That's when you out on the street doing stick-ups and shit. Doing anything to get you some money to buy some crack. You feel me?"

"Oh yeah," I said. "I seen that my whole life."

"Well, you ain't seen nothing like what happened to me. I done so many stick-ups in my neighborhood there was no one left to stick up. So I started robbing my grandmother. Ain't that something?"

"You ain't the only one," I said.

"But I'm the only one who took it as far I took it."

For a couple of seconds, Z fell silent.

"How far is that?" I asked her.

Z took a deep breath and went on. "She and her three friends play poker every Friday. Penny poker. Her three friends, they grandmas too. Old bitches. They be sitting in there listening to those blues records and playing their little card game. One of those Fridays I came into the house looking for Grandma's purse. I find it in the bedroom and start snatching out her money. One of the old bitches sees me and starts yelling. Grandma gets up and tries to stop me. I ain't in my right mind. I'm in my crack mind. Grandma starts smacking at me. I smack her down. Knock her down. The other bitches start screaming."

Z stopped again. Her eyes got funny. She took all these deep breaths.

I didn't say a word. Nothing I could say.

"I cut her throat," she finally said.

I just nodded.

"Killed my own fuckin' grandma."

"That's really something."

"That's why they named this here joint after me. That's why they call it Grandma's House."

GG

Called her GG because she wore everything Gucci. Gucci belt, Gucci shoes, Gucci sunglasses. For all we knew, she wiped her ass with Gucci toilet paper.

In real life GG had been a Gucci whore pimped by a cat she called Valentino. Valentino was notorious for training his girls to rob their johns. This here was the story GG told me:

"Valentino was known as the man who couldn't come. That's why he was so beloved by his women. They'd be popping off like firecrackers and Valentino, well, he'd be as fresh as when he started. A half hour, an hour, I've seen him go ninety minutes on three different bitches. Didn't make no difference to Valentino. The porn people were all after him, but he said, 'Fuck y'all. Y'all can't match the money I'm making out here running my girls.'

"See, to be a Valentino girl was a way to get famous. He didn't choose just anyone. You had to have class to start with. The right look, right goods, right everything. Once you got the nod, though, that was just the beginning. Then my boy would school you. School you hard but school you right. He'd tell you about johns. When they bumpin' you, some of 'em wanna last. Some of 'em don't. Here's how to make 'em last. Here's how to pop 'em right quick. Valentino would school you on psychology. The man's a genius. See, psychology is what it's all about. Getting inside a motherfucker's head. If the john want Mama, give him Mama. He want a schoolgirl, you be a schoolgirl. He dreaming of Halle, start purring like Halle. Valentino had this saying, 'Know your john, double your earnings.' Valentino was right.

"Problem was, Valentino had him some expensive taste. Loved the big cars and the big cribs and even got him a big boat somewhere out there on the bay. The boat had a captain and a cook. I know 'cause I was about the only working bitch who done seen that boat. Boat was seriously tricked out. Looked like a church with all the marble and gold on the walls. But paying for that marble and gold became a problem for Valentino. He got himself squeezed between two hard-nosed money men. He needed serious cash.

"That's when Valentino changed up his game. Game used to be, 'Some guy fucks you and you get paid.' Now the game was, 'Some guy fucks you, and while he's fucking you, Valentino has a dude sneak in the room to take his money.' So my job is to scream so loud during the fucking until the john can hear nothing but my fuckin' screaming. That's kinda fun. But when the john sees what's happening in the middle of the fuck and jumps off me, I'm supposed to knock him over the head with a chair. I'm no good at that. I don't like it. 'Tough shit,' Valentino says, 'You'll do it.' Did it for a while. More I did it, though, more I hated it. Some guy wanna fuck me, cool. But I don't wanna fuck him up. See, I'm one of those nonviolent people like Dr. King was talking about. I'm tired of smacking motherfuckers upside the head. I refuse. 'Fine, bitch, then I'll smack *you* upside *your* head. How you like that?' I don't like it. Don't like it one bit, but Valentino's getting rougher and I'm getting sorer and the shit's getting crazier until one night I got a rich john up in there and I ain't screaming loud enough to drown out the noise of the man robbing the john. The john sees what's happening and jumps off me right quick. That's when I'm supposed to crack him over the head, but I ain't playing. He and Valentino's man get into it. Valentino's man ain't fucking around. He up and shoots the john through the heart. Just like that, we got us a dead body on our hands.

"Valentino's all pissed. Makes me help bury the john out in the country somewhere. That gets me pissed. Cops come round looking for the dead guy. They start pointing at me. But I ain't pointing at no one. I ain't saying nothing. But then they start getting serious with first-degree murder charges and I start pointing to the place where we buried the man. I get accessory to murder. That's a helluva lot better than first degree. I get to come to Grandma's House and chill for a minute."

"How 'bout Valentino?" I want to know.

"Money men who was squeezing him dealt with him."

"And did what?"

"What do you think? Squeezed the fuckin' life out of him."

DILDOS FOR SALE

Doing business at Grandma's House is a different deal. It ain't like setting up a Starbucks in the mall.

The girls have different needs and, if you're interested in making cash, you will find a way to supply those needs.

What does everybody need at Grandma's House? What does everyone want?

Sex.

So I started thinking about sex—not for myself, but for my business. I was still too cautious to get crazy with sex in the Cut. But sex was happening all around me and, as someone used to hustling one kind of merchandise or another, I was trying to figure out how to combine commerce and sex.

What kind of merchandise did the girls need most?

Dildos.

Whether bi, straight, or straight-up gay, women want it; or they want to give it. Anyway you look at it, they need it.

And since the Cut didn't exactly have a gift shop that sold

sex toys, I figured I'd set up my own. I also figured that I'd keep it simple. One product and one product only. The essential product. The ever-popular dildo, the product that never goes out of style and is always in demand.

Problem is, where do you get them? Who do you order them from? Who's your supplier?

I saw that I had to be my own supplier. And with that in mind, I'd find my way into the medical supply room to get some Ace bandages. Ace bandages are the building blocks to a good sturdy dildo. If the supply room was closed off, I'd fake an ankle injury and get me some bandages through the nurses.

I took orders.

I crafted them in four sizes—small, medium, large, and extra large. Made them as real-life as possible. Took me a few hours to make a real good one. I knew my workmanship had to be solid or I'd get complaints. Not to brag, but all the time I was in business, never had one complaint. Word went out— "If you need a do-right dildo, see Snoop."

Payment would come in different forms. Sometimes cans of soup. Sometimes packs of cookies. Sometimes candy. You couldn't get rich in the Cut, but you could keep yourself busy.

My dildo business was a good thing.

One girl loved her fake dick so much she gave me a gift. A fat joint. I'm no pothead, but it's easy to get bored at Grandma's House. I looked at the joint and said, "Hell, why not?"

THE TRIP

Just one joint—one little innocent joint. A simple commonplace cigarette stuffed with commonplace marijuana.

Or so I thought.

I didn't have a lab to analyze the shit. Maybe it was something more than pot. Or maybe a strain of pot grown to fuck you up for good. Who knows.

But there I was, sitting out in the yard after having done my clean-up duty early. I had about a half hour to kill. The afternoon was windy. Some of the girls were playing basketball, but I was feeling tired. And the joint this bitch had slipped me was looking pretty good.

Why not?

Off in the corner of the yard, no one was looking my way. Besides, I wasn't known as a troublemaker. None of the guards gave me attitude.

Lit it.

Sucked up the smoke.

Kicked back and watched the clouds roll by.

Cool.

Clouds are cool.

Weird, but one of those clouds looked like an angry old man. I could see his eyes and his mouth. His motherfuckin' mouth was moving. I seen it moving. There was some thunder, but, wait—wasn't thunder. He was talking. Saying something. But what? Holy shit, I could make out his words. His words were, "Snoop, you getting high. Snoop getting fucked up." The thunder was talking. Thunder can't talk, but I'd be goddamned if I didn't hear it again.

Then I seen the girls playing basketball look at me. They heard the thunder. They knew I was high.

Better take another hit.

Took another hit.

Deeper hit.

Kept that shit inside. Held it. Let it swim up through my brain so it could straighten out my thoughts. But my thoughts were getting more crooked with every puff. My thoughts were saying, "The sky is screaming your name. Get your ass inside."

So I finished off the joint and went inside. Went to my cell and sat there, eyes closed, trying to see pretty pictures and hear pretty music. Instead I heard this chanting. Sounded like all the bitches in the Cut were chanting my name, saying, "Snoop's high. Snoop's high. Snoop's high." When the guarded passed by my cell, she looked at me like she knew.

Everyone knew.

I'd been high before, so I realized paranoia is part of being high. But for some reason I couldn't call this paranoia. I had to call it the truth. This was real. The chanting was real. I heard it distinctly. Came right at me.

I put my hands to my ears but the chanting got louder. When I tried to lie down on my bunk, my skin felt all bumpy. I was getting bumps. I'd study one bump and it looked like it was getting bigger. Bumps all over me. Bumps and that fuckin' chanting. I started itching. Started scratching. Bumps started blowing up. Looked in a mirror and saw my eyes bulging out. Felt like my goddamn eyes were about to pop out of my face.

Now I was getting scared.

Now I wanted the high to stop.

But I was still going up, not down, and the chant had turned into screams—bitches screaming my name—and the screaming wouldn't stop and I went to the bunk and curled myself up like a baby and started crying to myself, crying 'cause I was scared I wouldn't come down from this fucked-up high, crying to myself 'cause I was scared to cry out loud 'cause I was ashamed of crying and ashamed that a lousy joint had wacked me out.

I was crying when a CO came in the cell and saw me there.

"You okay, baby?"

I looked up at her. She was pretty. Her eyes were soft.

I sucked in my breath and tried to act strong, but she saw me falling apart. She put her hand on my forehead.

"You gonna be all right," she said. "Sometimes it just gets that way in here. But it'll pass, sugar. You'll be fine."

I let her touch me. I liked her touching me. I liked when she held my hand. Didn't want to tell her that I was high on some crazy weed, but I figured she already guessed that. She didn't care. But she did care about me. She sat with me for a long spell. When I started shaking, she held me.

"I'd take you to the clinic," she said, "but you're better off here. They'll give you blood tests in the clinic. You don't want no blood tests."

The CO was a sweetheart.

That night she became my sweetheart.

That night she got me through the worst trip of my life.

CO became my first and only love in the Cut.

CO
_____

Falling in love in Grandma's House is a different kind of falling in love. You're not in the world. You're in jail.

You ain't going to the movies and ice-skating or taking a walk in the park. You'd like to snuggle by the fireplace or book a room at the Hotsheet Hotel. But there's no fireplace and not much time to snuggle. You got to sneak, and sneaking ain't easy in the Cut.

Truth is, me and CO never did make love. We made out. We kissed in the dark corners and found some time for hugging, but straight-up screwing never happened. Neither of us wanted her to get fired. That would be the end of our relationship and the end of the only romance I was having.

CO did me favors. One big favor was getting me a bunch of colognes and perfumes from the outside so I could sell 'em on the inside. Had me a good little business going.

Bitches all over Grandma's House came to know me as the perfume lady. Had me a bunch of different brands—one for every taste.

CO was a lady. Naturally I was the man in the relationship. I would have loved to have been fucking CO, but just the idea that another woman was caring about me and loving on me made a difference. She'd slip me little notes that told me to meet her here or meet her there. Then she started writing letters about her life on the outside. How she was lonely. How she'd never met anyone like me. How, once I got out, she could see us hooking up forever.

"You mean it?" I said.

"With all my heart."

But hearts are changed by the Cut. Once inside, you don't have the same heart you had on the outside. Least I didn't.

At age eighteen, my heart had hardened.

It was hard to begin with, but seeing what I saw and hearing what I heard, my outlook on life got even more basic: Life was shit. So fuck it. Get what you can.

I know that folk talk about rehabilitation in jail, and for a while I thought maybe I'd become a different person. But forget about it.

Maybe if I had had a good teacher to inspire me—maybe that would have made a difference. But the truth is that I had this one teacher who made my life miserable. She had the opposite temperament of CO.

She had it out for me. She called me all kinds of things.

But I had only word for her . . .

BITCH

Bitch look at me and say, "You got your homework?"

"Yeah, I got my homework."

"Read it."

I read a little essay I wrote about basketball players.

Bitch say, "I didn't tell you to write about basketball."

"You said to write about what I like on television."

"Television *shows*," Bitch says, "not television sports."

"Well, a game is a show."

"Tear up your essay."

"What!"

"You heard me—tear it up."

"But I wrote it real carefully."

"You wrote it real sloppy."

"How you know that?"

Bitch say, "'Cause everything you do is sloppy. Now write a new essay and present it in class tomorrow."

I look at the bitch like she's crazy.

Problem is, I believe she's crazy in love with me. I truly believe she likes girls, and she has the hots for me in particular. But because she don't like liking what she likes, she takes it out on me. She knows I ain't ashamed of being gay. I like it. I'm proud of who I am. Meanwhile, this bitch is scared of who she is. So she makes life in Grandma's House miserable for as many girls as she can.

Next day I come into class with something I wrote about *The Fresh Prince of Bel-Air*.

I say something about how Will Smith has a funny point of view that makes everyone laugh, regardless of whether they're rich or poor. He's a homeboy that everyone loves.

Bitch says, "You missed the point."

"So what *is* the point?" I ask.

"The point is the contrast between life in the affluent suburbs of Los Angeles and the ghetto attitude of a boy from Philadelphia."

"Isn't the point that Will's funny as hell?" I ask.

"But what's underneath the humor?" Bitch asks.

"What's underneath your piss-ass mood?" I ask.

"I'm going to have to cite your negative behavior," she says.

I say, "I'm going to have to cite your lousy sense of humor."

"You're making it worse for yourself."

"You ain't helping none, bitch."

Bitch say, "That does it."

I say, "I hope so. You kicking me out of here?"

Bitch say, "No, you're not getting out of the final exam."

I took her fuckin' final exam and got all the answers right. Except she changed my answers around and failed me. She rigged it to make it look like I didn't know anything.

On top of that, she reports me to the supervising administrator.

"Your teacher feels that you're uncooperative and disruptive," says the supervisor. "Plus, you failed the exam."

I say, "Fuck that bitch. She switched my answers to *make* me fail. She's a dyke who don't know it. That ain't my fault."

Supervisor tells me I have to change my attitude or I'll never get my GED.

"Fuck that too," I say.

And with that, I go back to my cell.

That damn teacher sets off a bad period for me. For weeks afterward, I skip my classes. That teacher turns me against book-learning.

I go through this heavy-duty anger period.

I see anger all around me.

Old woman inmate who been living in the Cut for years gets angry at her cellmate. Cellmate won't stop talking shit. Cellmate badmouths this old woman night and day.

Then one day in the rec room, the old woman throws a pot of boiling water at her cellmate and disfigures her face for life. That stops the bitch from talking shit.

I get angry at my own cellmates.

One of my cellmates says I gotta cut her hair. I don't wanna bother with her hair.

"You got to," she keeps saying. "I seen how you cut that other bitch's hair and I liked how it looked. Now cut mine."

I can't get her to shut up, so I figure it's easier cut her goddamn hair than listen to her yap.

I do it. I design a little style for her.

But she hates it.

"You got me looking like Mr. T," she says.

"I like the way it looks," I tell her.

"You did it to spite me," she says.

"Fuck you. You were the one who kept after me till I did it. Well, I've done it. This ain't no beauty salon up in here."

"Fix it!" she starts screaming. "You gotta fix it!"

"I don't gotta fix shit."

"I ain't going out there looking like Mr. T."

"Exactly where you going?" I ask. "You in prison, bitch. Ain't nowhere *to* go."

"I'm telling you to give me a different cut," she keeps saying.

I'm through arguing. I start walking away. She grabs my arm.

"Let go," I say.

She won't let go. I pull away.

Then she makes a mistake. Big mistake.

She slaps me.

I see red. I go off. I take the clippers and go across her face. She starts shrieking. Blood everywhere.

She never asks me to cut her hair again.

Supervisor calls me in again.

"You're going to have to do something about your behavior."

"What?" I ask.

"You tell me."

"I don't know," I say.

"You mess up in school. You cutting up your cellmates."

"That one cellmate was fucking with me. That's the only reason I cut her."

"You're headed for more time not less. Is that what you want?"

"I just wanna be left alone," I say.

"And I want you to correct your conduct."

I roll my eyes up and study the ceiling.

"Look," says the supervisor, "is there someone from the outside you'd listen to? Your mother, for example."

"She dead."'

"Your stepmother."

"I don't want her here. I don't want her to see me in this mess."

"Anyone else?" she asks.

I think for a while.

"Call Uncle. He can talk to me. Uncle can talk to me any time he wants to."

BRAIN DEAD

Sitting there across the table from me, he looked beautiful. He put a smile on my face.

"Girl," he said, "looks like you haven't smiled in a while. Looks like they done turned you mean in here."

"Why you say that?" I asked.

"That's what they told me."

"Who told you what?" I wanted to know.

"The supervisor said you turned against your classes and turned against your teachers."

"One teacher," I said. "One bitch that has it in for me."

"Why's that?" Uncle asked.

"Closet case. She hates that I'm out and she's in."

"Sounds like you've been taking psychology classes," Uncle said.

"I don't need no psychology to see what she's about."

"Whatever she's about has nothing to do with what you're about."

"That's what I'm saying," I said.

"That's what you're saying but it ain't what you're doing," Uncle explained. "What you're doing is fucking up your education over one teacher. That don't make good sense, does it?"

"I don't need to kiss anyone's ass."

"I ain't telling you to kiss ass, Snoop. I'm telling you that you've been in this place two, three years already. You're eighteen years old. You'll walk out of here in another couple years. You'll walk out educated or you'll walk out brain dead. That's what it comes down to."

"The Cut will kill off your brain cells no matter what."

"Not if you change your attitude it won't," said Uncle. "Right now you're all negative up in here. You done made that choice. No one made it for you."

"Except the bitch," I said.

"The bitch is a bitch. That ain't gonna change. But how you react to the bitch is up to you. You can let her throw you off or you can go your own way."

"What way is that?" I asked.

"Well," said Uncle, looking at me square in the eyes, "there's only two ways. Up or down."

"And you saying I'm going down?" I ask.

"I know it. I see it. You got to check yourself, girl, or you don't got a prayer. You'll get more bitter by the day, and by the time you look around you'll be nothing but a crazy angry bitch yourself."

I started to answer back, but Uncle stopped me. He said, "Just think about what I'm saying."

I thought about that expression "brain dead."

Who the fuck wants to be brain dead?

"You serious about this brain dead shit, ain't you?" I said to Uncle.

"Serious as a heart attack, baby. You got to take advantage of what this place got to offer. If you can get your GED inside here, grab it. You'd be a fool not to."

We spent another half hour or so talking 'bout what was happening back on the block.

"You all right?" I asked uncle. "The shops in good shape?"

"The shit is always crazy," he said, "but you don't gotta worry about that. You just gotta worry about keeping yourself in good shape. You a jewel, Snoop. You a valuable jewel. When you get outta this joint, you gonna shine."

I had to hug the man for saying that.

I had to hug the man for coming down to the Cut to set me straight.

No one else could do that except Uncle.

LOOKING UP

Uncle was right.

Up's better than down.

Looking down you see nothing but concrete.

Looking up I see that window.

I look out that window.

Little buds are popping out all over the branches of the trees.

Soon the buds will burst open into leaves.

Soon spring will be warming us up.

Flowers will start blooming and things will smell sweeter.

Longer days, brighter light, more time to play in the yard.

In the Cut, winter's a motherfucker. Spring's a breath of fresh air.

Winter can make you crazy. Spring can make you hopeful.

After Uncle's visit, I was ready to get hopeful.

I needed that turnaround. I needed to put myself on a

sensible course of learning something besides making dildos in three different sizes.

I needed Uncle's energy and the knowledge that he really cared for me, no matter what kind of mess I got myself into.

I needed all the help I could get. Some of that help came from another piece of good news. This one was a surprise. I learned that my godmother, Denise Robbins, another big supporter of mine, had trained to be a correctional officer and was coming to work at the Cut. Denise was family and having family inside Grandma's House couldn't help but keep my spirits high.

She couldn't do me any special favors, but just seeing her from time to time did me a world of good.

Denise was another reason I started to turn the corner from negative to positive.

Around this time, a negative came up.

Word came down that the mother of the girl who had gone after me with a bat—the girl I killed—was being sent down to the Cut. Word came down that the woman would be looking for me.

I wasn't worried. I knew at Grandma's House they put people like that in protective custody—and that's just what they did with her. The woman had a lot of emotional problems. From time to time, I'd see her pass by, but she was always with an officer. She never said shit to me, and I never said shit to her.

Did I feel bad about what I'd done to her daughter?

Of course I did. I felt horrible about it. I felt deeply remorseful. If there had been some way to undo it, I would have. But in my heart I knew that what I'd done was done out of self-preservation. It was kill or be killed. There was only way to save myself—and that's what I did.

The women in the Cut knew what was happening. They kept the girl's mother away from me and, for the most part, out of my sight.

So I went my way without fear.

I kept my head up, my eyes open.

I went back into the classroom, where the teacher no longer bothered me. She tried her best—she was still a bitch—but, after Uncle's visit, I was a different person. I wasn't taking none of the bitch's attitude personally. She could dog me all she wanted. I didn't care. I was reading deep into the books. I was learning my lessons. I had the answers before anyone else. History class. English class. Math. You name it. Snoop was on the case.

When I met CO in a secret alleyway where no one could find us, when I held her in my arms and gave her a kiss, when she told me that she loved me and was proud of the progress I was making, I said, "Baby, everything's changing now. Everything's changing for the better. This here is the best day of my life."

THE WORST DAY
OF MY LIFE

When my dreams start getting crazy, I start to worry.

I'm not saying I can see the future. I can't. But I pick up vibes and those vibes creep into my sleep.

For weeks my sleep was disturbed. I was dreaming of bad shit. Can't remember it all, but it had something to do with knifings and shootings. Crews were being ambushed and sprayed. Then there were storms, hurricanes, tidal waves, and tornadoes blowing through the neighborhood and wiping out everything in their path.

I'd wake up sweating. Wake up wondering. Wake up with this bad feeling in the pit of my stomach.

Oh, well. There was work to do. I was on the cleanup patrol in the yard. I had my books to read and my lessons to learn. I had to keep my nose clean and stay outta trouble. I couldn't think of the other twenty or twenty-four months

I had to go, just sitting in Grandma's House. I had to get up and do things to make the time pass. I had to live the life of the Cut.

And I did.

I'd see bitches about to get in a fight, and I'd avoid them.

Bitches might threaten me. I'd ignore them too. I couldn't be provoked into a fight. Had no reason to fight. Had every reason to keep moving up.

So where were these dreams coming from?

In one, I'm walking through an open field and bombs are dropping on my head.

In another, a pack of wolves are chasing me down.

I'm drowning in the ocean and I'm being pushed out of a skyscraper.

I wake up with a headache, every single day.

The headaches get worse. Aspirin don't help. Advil don't help. The Cut has a pretty good doctor, but she says there ain't nothing wrong with me. She says everyone in jail gets headaches.

Then one day I'm looking out that little window in my cell and see dark clouds coming over the horizon. They coming fast. It's a storm from hell. Before I know it, day's turned to night, pitch-black night, and the thunder's booming and the lightning crackling and it sounds like God is dumping his anger down on Grandma's House. Feels like the ceiling's about to collapse and the walls above to cave in.

I'm walking down the hallways, on my way to the rec room, with the shit just getting louder and louder, when I see a girl on the phone. I know her from the neighborhood.

She puts down the phone and says to me, "Snoop, I just heard about Uncle. I suppose you know already."

"Know what?"

"He dead."

"What you mean dead?"

"What part of 'dead' don't you understand? The mother-fucker ain't breathing no more."

"He ain't dead," I say. "He was just here visiting me."

"He dead all right. Drug deal went bad. The word is that he went to drop off two bricks and some nigga turned on him. Shot him up real bad."

I look this bitch in her eyes. I see she ain't lying. But I also know that I can't deal with the truth.

I go through something strange.

I tell myself this ain't happening.

I haven't walked down the hallway.

I haven't seen homegirl talking on the phone.

She didn't look at me.

I didn't look at her.

She didn't open her mouth.

She didn't tell me nothing.

She didn't say Uncle's dead.

Uncle's not dead.

Uncle's alive.

None of this happening.

Uncle was just here visiting me. Uncle gave me good encouragement. Uncle gave me the word I needed.

He'll be back to visit. Maybe next week. Maybe the week after.

Everything's cool.

When I get out of here, first thing I'll do is run over to Uncle's crib. He'll be there with his wife and kids. He'll greet me with that big smile of his. We'll hug. We'll sit down to lunch and he'll tell me how proud he is of me.

It'll be beautiful.

Uncle's beautiful.

Uncle's not dead.

He can't be.

It didn't happen.

LOSING IT

It did happen.

It took me a few minutes, and I was back to reality. Homegirl had told me that Uncle was dead. Her words were true, and just like that, I snapped.

I ripped the pay phone from the wall and threw it on the cement floor. Then I threw myself on the floor and started screaming.

Never in my life had I ever gone into this kind of rage: hitting my head on the floor, hitting again and again until I passed out.

Later they told me that the Turtles—the armed guards who worked at Grandma's House—had to haul me off. It took four of them to contain me. When I woke up, I was in the mental ward. The way I was acting, they were scared I'd kill myself. And they weren't wrong to be scared.

If it weren't for the good-hearted guards that stayed by my side and saw me through, I might have done just that.

But those guards were like the doctors who saved me when I was a cross-eyed crack baby. They got me through some of the worst days and nights of my life.

I can't remember everything that was going through my mind during those long hours. I know it was despair, and depression, and anger, and confusion, and heartbreak, and fear. I was afraid that I couldn't make it without Uncle. Uncle had been the rock. Uncle had been my biggest believer.

Despair said that nothing was right in this world. Depression said that nothing would ever get better. Anger said that the world was fucked. Anger cursed a world that would kill Uncle in cold blood. Confusion said nothing made sense. Heartbreak said something sweet and good was gone and would never be back. Fear said that what happened to Uncle could happen to me. *Would* happen to me.

CO tried to comfort me. She came to the mental ward and, when no one was looking, she held me. CO told me I'd get through it. CO was cool.

I was anything *but* cool. I was sweating at night and freezing in the morning. I had the chills. The killer headaches came back. The nightmares got worse. I kept thinking—*If Uncle's dead, why should I be alive?*

You can only stay in the mental ward so long. You can only take sleeping pills and tranquilizers for so long. After a while, the pills turn on you and the tranquilizers get you crazier than you were before. So you have to make up your mind. As Uncle put it, ain't but two ways—up and down.

I was going down.

When I got out of the mental ward, I felt myself going down. In my cell, I looked out the window. When the sun was shining I hated the sun because it made things look good when things were bad. When the sun went away it reminded me that there was no sunshine in my heart. When I looked out the window at night I couldn't see stars, only darkness.

I went about doing what I had to do, lining up, mopping up, eating a little bit of this and a little bit of that. I lost weight. Refused to play basketball. Barely knew where I was or what I was doing.

Went through the paces.

Didn't see no light, no hope, no nothing.

DOUBLE WHAMMY

Couldn't do the usual things that got me going.

Couldn't watch TV.

Couldn't read a book. Or a magazine. Or even the sports page in the newspaper.

Couldn't talk to anyone.

Couldn't listen to anyone.

Could hardly look at anyone.

Kept my eyes glued to the floor.

Kept my mind glued to Uncle.

Him getting shot. Him being dead. Him never coming back.

My mind was fucking me, getting me to remember the good times when Uncle first became my friend. When he'd give me all that good advice. When he'd stop by the corner to make sure his Snoop was all right.

Mind was messing with me night and day until I was dying to find a way to shut down my mind completely. Just close my eyes and concentrate on something other than Uncle. Something other than this fuckin' penitentiary. Something like good food. Or good pussy. Anything to get my mind off death and dying and doom and gloom.

I was eating alone, thinking those kinds of thoughts, when this girl who knew I came from East Baltimore came up to me.

"You know that nigga you call Father?" she asked.

I didn't answer. I didn't wanna hear nothing about Father. Didn't wanna hear that he was dead. But she kept talking.

"He just got life."

"For what?"

"For everything. They came down on him hard. Got him on every last thing you can imagine. And they made the shit stick. He gonna be gone forever and a day."

They got Uncle.

Now they got Father.

Ain't gonna see Father again no more. He ain't dead, but he might as well be dead. Motherfucker's now a lifer.

These were my guys, my lifelines. How did my lifelines become my deathlines. How did all this happen?

News of Father coming after news of Uncle deepened the hole I was sliding down. Blues got bluer. Funk got funkier. Everything got uglier.

If someone had said, "Take this here pill. Won't hurt you none and you'll be dead in ten seconds," I might have swallowed it. Anything to get out of a world that was going against me.

I slept.

I sulked.

I let the darkness surround me until everyone was saying, "Snoop, you look half dead."

I was half dead and knew it wouldn't be long before the other half would crumble.

From one of the other cells I heard someone playing a song called "Sugar on the Floor."

That's what I felt like. All the sugar had spilled out of me and was on the floor. Nothing sweet was left. Hope was gone. Wasn't any way in the world for this condition to lift. It was heavier than anything I'd ever felt before. It was permanent. No doubt, it was taking me down.

And then one night when my eyes were half closed I looked through the window and saw a half moon. That's when it happened. Still don't understand it. All I can tell you is that it happened.

GRACE AFTER MIDNIGHT

I've never had a vision. Ain't never seen no angel. Never heard the voice of God say, "Hey, Snoop, do this or do that." Never heard the voice of God say nothing.

Back when I was a kid, Mama took me to her Holy Ghost Baptist Church. Pop had me over to where the Jehovah's Witnesses praised God. Far as I was concerned, it was all good. Wasn't like I got caught up in that shit, but I didn't see it doing no harm.

As time went on, and I hit the corners, Mama would try to get me back me in church, but I wasn't having it. Church didn't mean nothing to me then. Didn't have the time. Didn't have the interest.

Then when I got stuck in the city jail and later sent down to the Cut, I seen ladies who couldn't stop jumping for Jesus. They looked as crazy as the girls who were in there for murdering their boyfriends. Lots of time they *were* the girls who'd murdered their boyfriends. I stayed clear of them bitches.

Someone's always trying to convert your ass in jail. Someone's always throwing a Bible at you and getting you to see the light. Well, the only light I saw was the light coming out of that little window in my cell. I didn't see no magical light.

But something amazing did happen to me a month after Uncle got hit. I'm gonna try to describe it best as I can, but it ain't gonna be perfect. It can't be, 'cause I don't understand it.

I was sleeping. I was dreaming. I don't even remember the dream, but I do remember when I opened my eyes I thought I was still dreaming. I actually pinched myself real hard to make sure I wasn't dreaming. I wasn't.

I felt something. I felt a presence. Something was in that cell. Something was surrounding me. I felt like it was coming in me; and I felt like it was coming out of me. It was a sweet warm energy flowing all around me. It had me smiling. I had no reason to be smiling, but I was. I don't smile all that much, so for me to be smiling in the middle of the night for no goddamn reason is crazy. But this was crazy. This was more than a good feeling. This was something moving me and changing me and causing me to smile. This was saying to me, "It's all right. It's okay. Everything's cool. Everything's right." It wasn't saying that in words, but that was the feeling.

Then I felt Uncle's presence.

I ain't saying he came back from the grave. I didn't see nothing. But he was there with me. I know how it felt when Uncle came round, and, believe me, in the dead of night he had come round. Motherfucker was there.

He was there and carrying love with him. He was saying—least the feeling was saying—that love is something that's always there. It comes to you. You accept or you reject it. You accept it and it's yours. Reject it and it's gone. That's it.

You go up or you go down.

This middle-of-the-night feeling had me up. More up than I'd ever been in my life.

I was rejoicing for the feeling. I wanted to wake up every last bitch asleep at Grandma's House and tell 'em the good news.

Love's all around.

Love's come to town.

Love's in the Cut.

And that love wasn't nothing we had to buy or work for.

Was just there.

Free.

Beautiful.

Next morning I saw my godmother, Denise. I had to tell her about it. Denise is church people, and I knew she'd understand.

"That's grace," she said.

"What's grace?" I asked her.

"God's free love. It's yours. You get it 'cause he's giving it. He done paid the price for you."

"Grace," I repeated.

"Amazing grace," she added.

"It came after midnight," I said. "Grace after midnight."

HOME STRETCH

This business of counting days will drive you crazy.

I was still eighteen. My new good behavior was being noticed, but I knew I couldn't risk another negative move.

Now that I saw the light, I wanted to move into the light.

The light from that little window in my cell was shining brighter every day. Even if the day was gray, I'd see light inside the gray. The sky might be coal black, but I'd see light in a distant star.

If you look for light, you find it.

If you pray for hope, you get it.

I found light and I found hope.

When CO and I could manage our secret little meetings, she'd say, "Snoop, you a whole different person. I see you smiling."

"Uncle put that smile on my face," I said. "The only way I could have learned that lesson was through the fucked-up pain of his death. I saw what happened to him, my favorite guy in the world. Exact same thing was gonna happen to me if I didn't turn this shit around. I'd get out of here and start acting the fool all over again. Those negative vibes were all over me. You saw that."

"I've always seen something better than that in you," said CO. "I seen someone decent and good."

We'd hug, we'd kiss, and that'd be it. Better to live with sexual frustration than to get caught screwing a CO in the Cut.

Caution was the word.

I read me some good books, about Malcolm X, Dr. King, Muhammad Ali, and other black leaders.

I listened to some good music.

When I heard my girl Janet singing 'bout "I Get Lonely," I was wishing I could keep her company.

When Busta Rhymes was spittin' 'bout "Put Your Hands Where My Eyes Could See," I kept looking out that window in my cell and hoping the seasons would change faster.

Lil' Kim was blowin' up big. MC Lyte had out this jam called "Cold Rock a Party." Missy Elliott was rocking "The Rain." Juvenile, Jay Z, J-Lo, Ja Rule, JT Money, Ol' Dirty Bastard, Monifah and Monica and all kinds of shit was coming into the Cut. These sounds made me wanna get out of the Cut. But believe me, I wasn't planning no escape.

I believed in the grace business.

I knew I was blessed.

And knowing that gave me patience. Gave me fortitude. Gave me the wherewithal to grind it out, hour after hour, day after day.

I got me that GED.

Thank you, Jesus.

Got me those good behavior reports.

Thank you, Lord.

Got along with every bitch that came my way, even the ones looking to claw out my eyes.

Found a way to chill 'em out.

I'd explain it clearly. "Look here, bitch," I'd say, "I ain't looking to fuck up anyone and I ain't looking to get fucked up. So you best be moving on. You feeling me?"

They felt me. By then they knew I had a reputation that said, "Snoop is cool, but don't get on her wrong side."

My reputation for violence kept me peaceful.

"I'm changing my ways," I told CO.

Told my godmother, Denise, the same thing.

"No more temper tantrums," I said. "No more bullshit. I'm headed outta here and nothing can get in my way. Nothing except my own stupidity."

"You got that right," Denise agreed.

"I got lots of blessings," I said.

"You got God to thank," she told me.

"And I thank him," I assured her. "I thank him every goddamn day."

THE DAY OF DAYS

It'll happen. Time will pass.

You can look at your watch ten hours a day. You can watch the second hand go round and round until your eyes cross and you can't see straight no more. You can feel like time's slowing down. You can even feel like time's stopped, but, no, sir, it hasn't. It keeps moving.

An hour.

An afternoon.

An evening.

A day.

A week.

A month.

A year.

And then two years.

The routine's kicked in:

You sleeping all right. You eating all right. You getting in the rec room and shooting hoops all right. You squeezing in a little hidden time with your girlfriend. You studying up those books real good. Passing those tests. Being nice as you can be to the officers and the supervisors and the guards.

You getting by.

You letting that time pass and, believe it or not, you being cool about it all.

And then one day, you look up at the calendar and see that you're there. The day of days has arrived.

You getting your ass outta Grandma's House.

You kissing this fuckin' Cut good-bye.

Like the old folk say, "Free at last. Great God almighty, we're free at last!"

The day wasn't sunny. The day wasn't warm. There wasn't no rainbow in the sky and the birds weren't singing. Fact is, the weather was rainy and the sky was dark.

But I didn't give a shit.

A hurricane could be blowing on the outside, but I'd walk into it with a big ol' smile. To get outside the walls of the Cut, to step out of that joint into the cold air of freedom was all that mattered.

I had my little suitcase in my hand and was feeling lighter than air.

July 7, 2000.

Felicia Snoop Pearson, age twenty, was stepping out.

Felicia Snoop Pearson, former prisoner, was getting out early 'cause of good behavior and the work time she'd put together.

Felicia Snoop Pearson, former corner boy, former drug runner, former friend of every bad-ass nigga in East Baltimore, was taking her first breath of free air.

No bars in front of her; no bars behind her; no lockup at night; no checkup every hour; no one breathing down her neck.

The rain fell on my forehead. The rain felt great. There, by the curb, was Uncle's wife, waiting for me.

"He'd want me to do this," she said. "He'd be proud of you. Wherever you wanna go, Snoop, I'm happy to drive you."

"Take me to Mama's, please."

Mama was the first person I wanted to see. Hadn't seen the lady for six years, since I first went into city jail. Hadn't wanted her to see me locked up. Hadn't told her when I was getting out. Wanted to surprise her.

That drive to Baltimore was the best trip of my life. Everything looked beautiful. The passing cars. The billboards. The telephone poles. The Burger Kings. The motels. Even the white lines dividing the highway.

I kept closing my eyes and imagining I was still in the Cut. Then I opened them and smiled. I wasn't in the Cut. I was passing by a gas station, a school, a factory, a car wash, a playground.

On the radio Da Brat and Tyrese were singing "What 'Chu Like." I liked everything, everything I saw, everything I felt. I liked Destiny's Child. I liked DMX talkin' 'bout his "Party Up in Here."

At the same time, I wasn't looking for no party. Didn't

wanna drink and sure as shit didn't wanna drug. I was looking for Mama.

"Child," she said, as soon as I ran up the stairs, opened
the door, and fell in her arms, "I sure wasn't looking for you.
But now that I found you, I gotta praise the Lord. Gotta say,
'Thank you, Jesus.'"

She started crying, and I started crying along with her.

"Thank you, Lord," she kept whispering. "Thank you,
sweet Lord."

She fixed me a big meal and called the relatives over to
greet me. Everyone was cool. No one said a nasty word about
where I'd been.

"We just happy to have you back" was the only word I
heard.

Everyone congregated around the kitchen table while I
devoured the best meal of my natural life. Baked chicken.
Macaroni and cheese. Greens. Corn. Hot apple pie.

You couldn't tell me that life wasn't sweet.

One cousin said, "Tell us the worst thing that happened
to you in there."

"Not being here" is all I said.

"She's prettier than ever," one of the aunts told Mama,
nodding in my direction.

"Pretty on the outside and inside too," Mama said. "Minute I laid eyes on my baby, I saw the Lord had been dealing with her. She changed. God done put her in there for a
reason."

I didn't disagree with Mama. On that day, I didn't disagree with anyone or anything. My mind was smiling as much as my mouth. I'd look out the front window of Mama's place, the windows where you see East Oliver, and remember the tiny window in my jail. How many times had I looked out the window?

Ten thousand? Ten million? Who knew?

When I looked out Mama's windows, I saw cars riding up and down the street. Kids playing. Dogs running. A taxicab. An ice cream truck.

I could just step out the house and buy an ice cream cone. No one would stop me. No one would look twice.

I did it. I bought the ice cream. Ate it. Sat on the stoop—that same stoop where I had first looked at the world, trying to understand the game—and just listened to the sound of my breathing.

Evening fell. The rain stopped. The city smelled fresh. I continued taking in the sights and sounds all around me. Sirens. Buses. Mothers calling in their children. The world going on. The world doing its thing.

I was back in the world.

I was going on.

But this time my thing would be different.

This time everything would be different.

LOVE, INSIDE AND OUT

There's inside love and outside love.

Love inside the Cut is strange love because you're locked up and nothing's normal. Your life ain't normal, your thoughts ain't normal, your dreams ain't normal. Your brain's scrambled by all the bricks and bars and the cold fact that you can't get out until they let you out. You're also surrounded by a whole lot of bitches who ain't never getting out. Their attitude about love will fuck you up.

You want love. You always want love, no matter where you at. At Grandma's House, when you find someone who seems sweet and nice, you grab on to her. Least I did. That was CO.

Inside the Cut, CO and I met in the secret corners to steal a kiss. That always felt good. She was cool. She talked about the day I'd be out of there, the day when we could be a couple, sleep in a bed together, and have us some real sex.

That day came soon after I got released. The sex was real. I liked all that. I thought CO and I had it going on.

We went to the movies like a regular couple. We saw silly movies like *Big Momma's House* and laughed our asses off. We saw scary movies like *Scream 3* and action movies like *Mission: Impossible II*. Having a date, ordering a Coke and a box of buttered popcorn, holding hands, and sleeping all night with a lady I loved—these were good things.

But I soon learned that love outside the Cut is different than love inside the joint.

"Where were you yesterday?" CO asked.

"Talking to my parole officer," I said.

"What about?"

"About getting me a job. You know, they got that re-entry program. I been trained real good to fill out applications. They taught me how to make a good impression during interviews."

"Is your parole officer that tall woman with the big tits?" CO asked.

"I'm an ass man," I reminded her.

"She likes girls, don't she?"

"She married with two kids."

"What difference does that make?"

"I'm just another case to her," I said.

"I thought you said she likes you."

"She does. But not the way you worried about."

"I ain't worried," said CO.

"You sounding worried."

"I just don't see how it could take all day to meet with your parole officer."

"Didn't say it took all day."

"Then what'd you do the rest of the day?" CO wanted to know.

"Helped Mama in the kitchen."

"You didn't go out?" she asked.

"I did go out."

"Where to?"

"The store."

"And then what'd you do?"

"Picked up a bitch with a big butt and fucked her brains out all afternoon."

"You don't need to be sarcastic," said CO.

"But that's what you worried about, ain't it? You think I'm fucking someone behind your back. Well, I ain't. I'm the loyal type."

"I still wanna know where—"

"I ain't answering no more questions," I snapped. "You can believe whatever you wanna believe."

Next day CO called and apologized. "There's a movie that's supposed to be funny," she said, "called *Miss Congeniality*. Let's go see it."

I said fine.

We went to a gay bar afterward. CO was anything but Miss Congeniality.

"I don't like the way that bitch over there is looking at you," she said.

I said, "Ain't shit I can do about it."

"You don't got to look back at her."

"I wasn't looking till you mentioned her."

"Let's get out of here," said CO.

"We just got here."

"If you stay, you're staying alone."

"I'm staying," I said.

"'Cause you wanna pick up on that bitch, right?"

"'Cause I wanna finish my drink."

"I got drinks at my place."

"Then why the hell did we come to a bar?"

"It was your idea," she said. "You wanted to check out the merchandise."

"Fuck you," I said.

"You chasing me off. Is that it?"

"I'm telling your bossy ass that I'm gonna sit here and finish my drink—that's what I'm doing."

"And I'm telling you it's time we got outta here."

That's when I turned my back on CO.

"If I walk out that door now," she threatened, "you're never seeing me again."

I didn't say nothing.

"All those years you were in Grandma's House," she went on, "all that time we spent together—you willing to throw it away?"

Still didn't say nothing.

"I'm telling you, Snoop, I'm demanding you leave with me right now."

She put her hand on my shoulder.

I knocked her hand away.

No overbearing bitch was gonna put me in prison. I'd just got outta prison. That prison was made of concrete. CO's prison was made of jealousy. Both prisons would make me miserable.

It was a tough lesson, but at least I was learning it early on: Love inside the Cut one's thing; outside it's another.

BOYS DON'T CRY

Breaking up with CO didn't put me in a bad mood. Being free to walk the streets and look for a job—man, that was enough to keep me happy 24/7.

I was gung-ho to follow up on this re-entry program and do myself proud. Living back at Mama's house, I was doing everything right.

I'd turned over a new leaf and wanted to stay on the straight and narrow.

I felt the blessing. I felt the grace.

And even though I was sorry the thing between me and CO didn't work out, I stayed away because I wasn't interested in hooking up with someone ruled by jealousy. Life is too short for that shit.

I didn't go running into another relationship. That ain't me. I've never been promiscuous. Never been known to run around with two different girls at once. Truth is, I've had only a couple of serious relationships. I don't need to be with a woman on a date to have a good time.

Lots of time I go out by myself. I like seeing movies alone.

Not long after I got out of the Cut, I went to see Hillary Swank in *Boys Don't Cry*. I'd heard it was about a girl who pretended to be a boy. People said it was a great movie. I wanted to check it out.

I sat in that dark theater, and I couldn't believe my eyes. Couldn't believe how much I loved the story and loved the movie.

I identified with the girl called Brandon who wanted to be a boy.

I felt that her pain was my pain, her dilemma my dilemma, her heart my heart. She was sweet and she was good. Wasn't looking to hurt no one. She was just being who she was. She was good people. I was rooting for her to get by.

I was deep into the love story. I knew that a girl who feels like a boy can fall in love with a girl. And I know that a girl can love a girl who dresses and acts like a boy. I been there. I done that. That shit's real.

The whole movie was real. Hillary Swank chewed it up. As an actress, she had balls, just like the Brandon girl she was playing had balls. That whole movie had balls to show what it was showing. It had balls 'cause it made you love the Brandon girl. Didn't judge her. Didn't make it like she was sick or wrong. The movie understood. The movie loved her. And you had to love the movie.

Well, I did. I was rooting for Brandon. I forgot, at least for a minute, that it was a real story that had a real ending. I was rooting for a happy ending. Come on, Brandon. You can do it. You can act like a boy, love on a girl, and have a happy life. You can get by. You can survive all the ignorance and hate that the world puts on gays. You get what you want and come out a winner. In the end, good triumphs over bad. Love wins all. Brandon's gonna get through this thing. Brandon's gonna survive. Gotta survive 'cause her heart is right and she ain't hurt a fly and there's no reason to hurt her.

And then it happens.

They rape her. And then they came in there with all the guns and stuff. And they murder her.

Boys don't cry, but I was crying. If you had a goddamn heart, you had to be crying. And then I got mad. Real fuckin' mad. And then I got to thinking:

If a big boy tried to rape me like that, I wouldn't fight back because, one by one, a big boy will beat up a smaller female. Ain't shit you can do. But afterward I'd come back. I'd come back when he thought everything was good. I'd come when he was sleeping. I'd come back and cut off his balls with a knife, slice off his dick, shove it up his butt and blow his fuckin' brains out with a gun.

That's what I'd do to the motherfucker who messed up Brandon.

That's what I'd like to do all the motherfuckers who make fun of gay people by scaring 'em and hurting 'em and torturing 'em and humiliating 'em and treating 'em like we dirt.

Boys Don't Cry broke my heart and enraged my mind that there's still all these assholes out there who got nothing better to do than mess up people different from them. Why? What's the point? What they trying to prove?

Ain't we all supposed to be children of God?

Ain't he supposed to love us the way we are?

Ain't this grace business about not having to do nothing to get God's love? He already loves you. He can't do nothing *but* love you.

He don't love just white or black or gay or straight. He don't say this church is wrong and that church is right.

He's just loving.

The guys who killed Brandon were a long way from feeling that love.

All they was feeling was blind hate.

Like Uncle say, you go up or you go down.

UP

Got that *Boys Don't Cry* movie outta my head. Got CO
outta my head, too. I got plans to make, a job to get, a life
to live.

I'm gonna jump into this re-entry program my parole
officer's been helping me with. Re-enter the city. Re-enter
society. Re-enter the workforce. Become a useful citizen. Use
the skills I learned in the Cut. Go straight. Stay straight. Stay
connected to hardworking people doing good. Avoid the assholes and hang with the achievers.

Got me a plan.

Got me new energy.

Good energy.

Clear-eyed clearheaded energy.

Got me this training that says, "When you fill out an
application, and if it asks whether you've been to jail, leave
it blank. Then during the interview, when and if the question comes up, explain how you did your time, earned your

GED, and are 100 percent rehabilitated. That way you have a chance to get a job. But if you indicate on that application that you've been to jail, that might prevent you from getting the interview."

I was ready, set, go.

The training had me thinking positive. I was clean. I was smiling. I was talking correctly and displaying good manners. When I went to the employment agency, I was on my Sunday best behavior.

Man looked at me and said, "You look like a strong girl."

"I am, sir."

"Looks like you wouldn't mind manual labor."

"Not at all, sir."

"Working in a factory bother you?"

"Working in a factory sounds good."

"You sure got a positive attitude."

"Gotta be positive, sir. Positive is what gets us through."

"Well, you're getting through to me," he said. "I see an opening at a car plant. They need a worker on the line where they make those bumpers. You interested?"

"Very interested, sir."

"When you can start?"

"The second I leave here."

He laughed. "You're not making bumpers in those nice clothes, are you?"

"I'll pick me up some overalls on the way, sir."

"You can show up tomorrow morning. I'll call the foreman now. He'll be happy to have someone this eager to work."

"And I'll be happy to help him any way I can, sir."

That was it!

I walked out of that agency smiling from ear to ear. First interview, and *swish! I score!* Nothing but net.

I had a job. I was on my way.

Went home and told Mama, who, of course, gave the glory to God. That was okay with me. Maybe it was God. Maybe it's always God.

Well, with God's light finally shining down on me, I walked past the corner where the boys were dealing dope and didn't give those niggas a second glance. My pay might be meager and my hours long, but the work was legit and the job was real. You had to be responsible to work this gig. And the company had to have some faith in me to put me in the factory.

I had followed the training course, and the training course was working. I didn't indicate I'd been to jail on the application, and, to my happy surprise, the guy never brought it up. If he had, I was ready with an answer—I'd paid my debt to society, I'd done my time and come out a better person. But the question never came up. He was a good guy. He saw that I was all about wanting a good job, and he gave me a break.

That night I sat in the bathtub listening to my Mary J. jams. I wanted to relax before the big day. I didn't want to go out and celebrate. Didn't wanna party because I was seeing that work would be my party. Work would be where I could find the real joy in my life. Work—honest work—is what I'd always missed. Having a boss. Being responsible to the boss. Learning quickly and getting ahead. I'd always bucked the system, but now I wanted the system. Wanted it to work for me. Would *make it* work for me.

Slept a dreamless sleep.

Got up early.

Felt refreshed.

Mama made oatmeal, fresh-squeezed orange juice, toast, and jam.

Put on a clean new pair of overalls. Fixed myself a couple of sandwiches for lunch.

Joined the other workers of the world as we waited at the bus stop.

I felt regular.

Felt good.

Caught the bus.

Got off at the plant.

Went through doors, walking proud, looking for my foreman.

"Hello, new world," I said to myself. "I'm ready."

THE LINE

I'd been in police lineups, but I'd never worked an assembly line.

Tell you the truth, I liked the assembly line. Had a rhythm, a definite groove. I liked the movement, liked seeing those auto parts dancing down the belt. It was sort of exciting.

I thought of Pop, the man who had me working next to him all during my childhood. Pop had taught me the value of hard work. He had shown me that I have a knack for making things and fixing things. Pop had given me the confidence that I was showing my foreman.

Foreman was impressed. He saw I was willing and capable of doing anything the men could do. He respected me.

I caught on quick. I could handle the speed of the assembly line in no time. I could handle placing the right parts in the right places. I could handle some of the guys looking at me like they wanted to say, "What's this bitch doing here?"

After a day or two, I even made friends with some of the guys. Once they saw I could stand with them toe to toe, they gave me props.

I got to work early. Worked my ass off. Sometimes I didn't even bother taking the breaks so I could get more work done.

I was on fire.

I wanted to shine.

I wanted to show everyone that I could hack it, I could do whatever they gave me to do.

At night, I went home tired, but it was a good tired. I'd go to sleep early and wake up at the crack of dawn, ready to go again.

"You sure are the eager beaver," said Mama.

"I'm working on a promotion," I said after I'd been there a short while. "Foreman says if I keep going the way I'm going, he could bump me up to an assembly line that pays a little more."

"Just keep at it, baby," Mama encouraged me. "I sure am proud of you."

I was proud of myself.

The shit had sure-enough turned around.

The way a good rap has a good flow, well, my work life had a flow. I was making bumpers and I was making friends. I was seeing how the straight life was the good life. When you get off from eight hours of solid manual labor, when you don't try to cut corners and give it your best, you feel good about yourself.

I was feeling great about myself.

"Snoop," said the foreman one afternoon, "would you step into my office for a minute."

"Yes, sir," I said.

Here's that promotion, I thought.

"Snoop," he said, "I gotta let you go."

"What!"

"Got no choice."

"I thought I was working out."

"You were working out great."

"Then what's wrong?"

"Your jail record. They told me you served long time down in the pen."

"I did," I said, "but I never said I didn't. It never came up in the interviews."

"Well, it's come up now."

"And you can't say nothing for me?"

"I said a lot of things for you, Snoop, but my boss over-ruled. He said you're dealing with sharp metal down here, and with your record, that's dangerous."

"That's bullshit. I ain't hurting nobody. I ain't even arguing with nobody. You seen me arguing?"

"Not once, but, like I said, Snoop, I don't got the final say."

"There ain't no way to appeal this?"

"'Fraid not. They say you gotta clear outta here."

"Today?"

"You'll get paid for today, but I've been told to escort you out."

"Like I'm a criminal," I said, "like I done something terrible here on the job."

"I don't like it any more than you do, but that's the way it is. All I can do is wish you luck."

"I'll need it."

IF AT FIRST YOU DON'T SUCCEED . . .

. . . try and try again.

That's what Pop always said when we were making stuff together.

If I hammered a nail crooked or patched the roof wrong, Pop would say, "Getting it right takes time."

Mama reminded me of that when I got home from being fired.

"Sure, you're discouraged," she said. "You can't help but be. But hang in there. You did good at that job. You'll do better on the next."

Gotta confess that it took me a week or so to get my spirits back up. I had a big resentment to shake off. Back in the Cut, they had told me if I followed this program and took their advice, I'd work.

Well, I took their advice and got canned.

Getting fired makes you feel like shit. And especially after you break your ass to do a good job. Getting fired unfairly makes you mad.

But what could I do with my anger?

Wasn't no one's fault. If the assholes who run this car plant wouldn't give me a break, I'd find someone who could. I'd keep my attitude positive. I'd think about the things that Uncle told me. I'd think about all the prayers that Mama and my godmother Denise said for me.

I'd go back out there and find another job.

"Glad you're not discouraged," the guy at the employment agency said to me.

"Not discouraged," I told him, "just determined. Determined to get something and keep it."

At first he didn't have anything, but I kept going back.

A week passed. Then two.

Finally, when I went the third time, he was smiling.

"Found something for you, Snoop," he said.

"I knew you would," I said. "I'm about to luck up."

LUCKED UP OR FUCKED UP?

Back at Grandma's House, they called it Job Readiness. They made a big deal of it. I took the shit seriously and wound up working at the car plant. After I got jacked up at the car plant, it took a little minute to clean up my attitude.

But I did.

I was back on the positive tip. I was ready to take this job the employment agency was offering at some book warehouse.

"What do I have to do?" I asked the guy.

"Haul boxes. Heavy ones. That bother you?"

"Fuck no."

First day of the gig, Mama fixed me another big breakfast. She prayed on me. She said, "Lord, thank you for blessing this child with your grace. Thank you for touching her heart with your love."

I caught the bus. I was back in the workforce. I'd gotten out of the Cut in July. Now it was September. The weather was still warm, the world still looking good to me. I couldn't help but remember back to how it was inside Grandma's House. Those bars, those bricks, those endless days, endless weeks, endless months and years.

Hell, I was grateful to be sitting on a bus, a free woman with a new job.

Foreman was a white cat. Nice enough. He presumed I was strong or I wouldn't be there—and he was right. I lifted the heaviest boxes they had. I hauled the shit all day long until one guy looked at me and said, "Girl, you stronger than two of us." I just nodded.

I got through the first day fine.

That night I went out to Buns, a club up on Lexington and Green. It was a mixed club, gay men and women, and since I got out of jail I had noticed how many more gay women were out of the closet. I had had me a couple of little romances, but nothing permanent. I wasn't interested in permanent. I was interested in celebrating the fact that I got another job. I was sipping on wine when a gal came up to me, real aggressivelike, and started talking. I don't like aggressive. I ignored her, but she got loud and testy. I could see she might be trouble. When she started cussing me, I ignored her. I'd learned my lesson about getting into it with crazy bitches. I moved on. Went home and went to sleep. Tomorrow's another day.

Tomorrow brought another challenge. Cat at work came up to me and said, "What's a skanky bull dyke doing working at a place like this?"

I just looked at the motherfucker. My eyes said, *Fuck with me and I'll cut your nuts off,* but my mouth didn't say shit. I kept doing what I was doing.

That didn't satisfy him.

"I hate dykes," he said. "Women ain't got no business eating pussy."

I kept on loading.

He kept on provoking, saying all sorts of raunchy shit.

I wanted to go upside his side so bad I could hardly contain myself. But I did. I pretended the asshole wasn't even there.

Finally, when he shoved me real hard, I was about to lose it and knee him in the balls. That's when God or good luck stepped in. The foreman was walking by, heard what the guy was saying, and fired his ass, right then and there.

Things were changing for me. The timing was good.

The job was good. I liked working in the warehouse more than the factory. Wasn't as loud. No sharp parts to cut your hands. Plus, other than the asshole who'd been dogging me, nicer people. Even made a couple of friends.

Life was finally taking a good turn. The days were going by. The nights were calm. The weekends could be fun, especially if I got lucky on Saturday—all girls' night—at Buns. I was staying out of trouble. And even saving some money.

Was completing my second month at the warehouse. Feeling confident. Finally settling into a routine that seemed to make sense. The guys were always complaining about sore backs and sore arms from all that lifting, but I was fine. I could do this thing.

Arrived on a Monday morning.

As usual, I was the first one there. Eager to get started. Went to the little locker where I stashed my lunch, opened it, and saw an envelope. Inside was a slip that said my services were no longer required.

Took the slip and went to the foreman.

"Why?" I asked.

"Your jail record."

I said what I said to the last foreman. I hadn't been asked about jail. If I had been, I would have told the truth, but it never came up.

This cat was cold.

"Tough shit," he said. "You're out."

I kept trying to explain.

He cut me off and said, "We don't want ex-cons here."

This was the same guy who'd been telling how well I'd been working out, the same guy who saw I could outlift almost every fuckin' man in the warehouse. I hadn't missed a day, hadn't gotten into a single argument, much less a fight. I was the model goddamn worker.

"Can I just say—" I began to argue.

"You can't say shit."

I thought about ending this job by slugging the foreman. I came awfully close, but I didn't.

What was the point?

Here all this time I thought I had lucked up, but I was really fucked up.

In my head, I was fucked up bad.

CAR WASH

There's a funny movie they made way back in the day called *Car Wash*. I watched it on TV a couple of times. Richard Pryor plays a hustling preacher. The jams are poppin' and the story's real good.

My story at the car wash ain't real good.

I took the gig to get my parole office off my back. After the first two fuckups, I was bummed out. I did what I was told to do and wound up getting screwed. I not only worked, I worked my ass off. I worked until I was sore from my head to my toe. Every muscle ached. Every good feeling I'd had went bad. Positive turned to negative. Sunshine turned to shit. All my eagerness, all my go-for-it energy, all my it's-gonna-turn-out-good energy turned rotten. I was sugar on the floor.

But I also figured I needed to do what I needed to do. Was a car wash any worse than slapping bumpers on cars or lugging around boxes of books? Besides, everyone in the movie *Car Wash* seemed to be having fun.

It was the end of summer. The last blast of heat was pushing through Baltimore. The radio was blasting Jay Z "Big Pimpin'."

The line never stopped. Motors kept churning. Engines kept burning. Put me on the wash line. Slap on the soap. Soap up the windows. Soap up the hood. Soap up the doors and the fenders. Soap up the Corvette, soap up the Jag and the Lexus. Listen to the rich bitch scream that we ain't using enough soap. Think about soaping up her big mouth. Think about the lunch break. Hear the bossman screaming, "Wash cars, hurry up, wash those fuckin' cars."

Do it all day Monday. Do it Tuesday and Wednesday and Thursday and Friday. Work a ten-hour shift on Saturday. Sleep late Sunday and when you wake up remember that all your fuckin' dreams were about washing cars. You can't stop washing cars.

I wanna stop washing cars. I wanna do something better with my life. I take off a day to go out on other interviews—office jobs, factory jobs, jobs at the mall, jobs in hotels. But every interview comes down to asking me about my past. In every interview I tell the truth. And in every interview I'm told they ain't interested. See ya later. Don't slam the door behind you. Have a nice day.

So it's back to soaping up cars. The tricked-out pickup trucks. The big-ass Escalades. The Ferraris that cost more than twice as much as my mama's house. Sometimes I think of getting behind the wheel of one of those motherfuckers and driving off. Up to D.C., up to New York City, up to Canada until no one can find me and the goddamn car is mine. Stupid fantasies. Just soap up the cars. Soap up my life. Soap up my brain. Wash the bad thoughts away. Thoughts of going back to the block. Thoughts of doing what it seems I'm supposed to do—work the corners.

You don't need no interview to work the corners. No one asks you questions and looks into your past. You don't gotta worry about being accepted. You don't gotta negotiate no salary. It's every nigga for himself. It's survival of the fuckin' fittest. That's what I'm fit for. That's what I'm born for. That's who I am.

But I think of Uncle, and I think of Mama, I think of Denise and all the good people in my life and I go back to soaping up the cars. It's ten in the morning. It's two in the afternoon. It's almost time to get off.

I smell of soap.

"You ain't soaping like you mean it," says the bossman as I walk out the door.

"Excuse me?" I say. *What the fuck does that mean?*

"You doing a lame-ass job."

"This *is* a lame-ass job," I tell him.

"You missing spots."

"Bullshit," I say.

"And the guys don't like working with no bull dyke."

I snap. "You know what? You and the other guys can go fuck yourselves in the ass. Fuck you, fuck the other guys, fuck this car wash, and fuck every motherfuckin' car-drivin' asshole who comes in here. I'm out."

LIFE AIN'T NO MOVIE

Life ain't no comedy. Ain't no folks singing songs on the car wash line. Ain't no cute jokes and ain't no happy ending.

That's how I was thinking when I told the car wash cat to fuck himself. I was fed up. Fed up with knocking my head against the wall. Fed up with niggas' fucked-up attitudes. Fed up with name-calling. This so-called straight world out here was no world I could relate to. It was a world I had to leave. I'd tried it and I'd fuckin' failed. So it was good-bye to bad garbage. I was going back to the only world where I'd ever done any good, the world where bad was good and where I was super-bad.

My rep was already established on the street. My shit was already standing. My shit was marked in stone.

I paid my dues. I had sat my little ass down in the Cut for a minute.

Now the minute was up.

Now I said, "Fuck everything else."

I was tired of struggling.

I could have talked to Mama, but I didn't.

I could have talked to my godmother, Denise, but I didn't.

Could have found a cool counselor or some righteous preacher, but fuck the counselor and fuck the preacher. I was tired of this fucked-up do-goody attitude. I was tired of being someone I would never be.

Back to the dog-eat-dog world.

Back to get it when you can.

Back to the goddamn block.

Ain't gonna fight with no one. Just bust a move and jump outta sight. Move outta Mama's house. Move in with a girl-friend. She's pretty cool. She lets me runs things. She knows I'm the man in the relationship. She don't bug me about where I'm going and how I'm making a dollar.

I got me five hundred dollars saved.

Take that five hundred, buy me a half ounce of coke, and work off that.

That's it.

That's the start.

Put that Mickey Mouse go-straight shit out of my head.

Think like I used to think.

Think ahead.

Start dealing with this coke and move up to heroin. More money in heroin.

Got one thought and one thought only:

Start slow, stay cool, but wind up the biggest drug dealer in East Baltimore.

This time fuckin' go for it.

I know the game.

Now I'm playing to win.

DICKHEAD

I called him a dickhead 'cause he *was* a dickhead. I called him a fuckin' prick cause he hated my ass so bad he bent the rules. He wanted the satisfaction of locking me up—and he did.

I was out there on the corner. Since the car wash bust, I had only been out there for a hot second. Got my shit together. Got me a couple of corner boys to watch for the cops. And got me a couple of hitters who would run the drugs to the customers in the cars. I knew what I was doing.

But this particular cop had attitude flying out his ass. Every time I was ready to open shop in the morning, he'd cruise by and talk much shit.

"Gonna get your ass, nigga," he'd sneer.

I wouldn't say nothing back. Wouldn't even look at the motherfucker. Naturally that made him angrier. He wanted some kind of reaction. I just turned my back. When he was gone, I went about doing my business.

It was like that for a while.

Then one morning he came by all worked up.

"This is it," he said. "Your time's up."

I just smiled, shrugged, and walked on.

Half hour later the dickhead's back. He runs his car up on the curb and pins me against the building, charges out, and cuffs me. Meanwhile, his partner comes out the alley with ten pills of ready-rock.

"These yours?" asks Dickhead.

"Hell, no," I say.

"I'm sayin' they are."

"I'm sayin' you're full of shit. You just puttin' this shit on me."

He smiled and said, "I told you I'd get you."

We go downtown. I know this is a setup. I know I'm getting out of this.

I'm feeling okay until the judge looks at my record, sighs, then closes his eyes, and then slaps on a seventy-five-thousand-dollar bail.

That means to stay free I gotta cough up three stacks (three thousand dollars) for the bail.

Here comes the lawyer talkin' 'bout another two and a half stacks.

Here comes all that pretrial stuff.

Here comes all the accusations, all the phony charges.

Here comes the pressure.

Here comes the knowledge that if this shit goes against me, my ass is back in the Cut for fifteen years.

Here comes the report saying I had drugs stashed in the alley.

But here comes my lawyer showing that if I was selling drugs I wouldn't stash them that far away. That's not how we do. He makes this logical and beautiful argument about how the case makes no sense. He chews up their shit and spits it back in their face.

Case dismissed.

I'm off. I'm out.

But, in addition to the five and a half stacks I had to pay for bail and lawyers, I'm out another fifteen stacks because my stash got hit while all this legal crap was coming down.

Dickhead costs me over twenty stacks.

But I'm cool.

Or am I?

"I'LL BUST YOU WITH THIS BRICK!"

That's what I'm screaming at the bitch. And I mean it. I'm ready to go upside her head.

She's a relative of Mama's. I call her Aunt, but right now I'm calling her evil 'cause she's calling me a "little dyke-ass bitch." She's saying, "Mama ain't even your real mama. You don't deserve no real mama. You born in garbage and you *is* garbage."

I'm walking down the street, on my way pick up Chinese food for Mama, while she's slinging these insults at me. She's screaming 'cause I put her out of Mama's house. I put her out the house 'cause she's high all the time. High as a mother-fucker and making Mama crazy. I put her out the house to protect Mama.

Now she's coming after me. And she done brought the police with her. She lied and told the police that Mama's house is *her* house. Well, it ain't. She don't got no house, which is why she's living off Mama.

She keeps yelling at me. I'm trying to walk away but the words keep flying and the cop wants to talk to me.

She prods the cops. She tells them, "Ask this dyke bull how many other dyke bulls she fucked down in prison. They let her out by mistake. She should be back there with all them other bull dykes."

The cop starts asking me questions, but this evil bitch keeps on screaming until I pick up the cinder block and say, "I'm gonna kill this bitch! Gonna kill her right now."

"You ain't killing no one," says the cop.

That's when they straight lock me up and hustle me downtown.

Just what I need.

Another charge against me. Another night in jail. Another reason for the judge to send me back to the Cut.

Another long hard night. Another jail cell with another window with another full moon reminding me of all the moons I saw from the little window at Grandma's House.

In the morning I'm scheduled to go before the judge where charges will be pressed.

I got a lot on my mind.

Takes a long time to fall asleep.

When I do, I dream of my dead mother. She's alive in the dream and we're back together. We're walking down the street, about to go in a pawn shop where she's going to buy me a nine-millimeter to protect myself, when someone comes up from behind her and shoots her dead in the head. I wake up and remember I'm back in jail.

God knows what'll happen to me.

Does God even care?

Do I even care?

It'll be what it'll be.

But true to form, this bitch is too high to show up in court. There's no one to press charges.

I'm free.

Another chance.

I dodge another bullet.

I could see this is as an opportunity to mend my ways and go straight. But I've been through that straight shit before.

It don't work.

Besides, my business is going good. My shops are thriving.

My corner is hot.

COP SAYS, "CRACK YOUR ASS CHEEKS SO I CAN LOOK UP IN THERE."

That's what the cops say when they suspect you holding.

Things are changing. Getting tighter, stricter, meaner. Lean times means you gotta get smarter. Ain't like back in the day when the shit was loose. Game's getting rougher.

But I'm playing. I'm schooling my boys. I'm telling them, "Be cool. Be smart. Not only will these motherfuckers crack your ass and look up your hole, they'll look up under your balls to see if you hiding rock there. So learn the hood, know who lives here and who don't, study every goddamn car cruising through, pay attention, niggas, and don't make no stupid mistakes."

My niggas had to be steely, steady, and ready to step. They had to have their heads on straight. If they were too nervous, they'd scatter when they didn't need to. If they were too spacey, they'd stay when it was time to scatter.

I trained 'em. I said, "Watch my eyes. Watch my eyes watching the street. I don't give out no expressions. My eyes ain't saying that I'm happy or sad or tired or wired. My eyes are dead set on the street. I can tell you exactly how many people passed by in the last thirty minutes, and I can tell you the color of their clothes. Damn near tell you the color of their eyes. You gotta be a hawk, niggas. You gotta be a goddamn hawk to get through this mess out here."

I was flying high. I was flying low. I was flying the right speed and the right distance. I was flying under the radar. Once in a while they might nab me for loitering, but I was in and out in a hot minute. Nothing was sticking on me. Nothing holding me back.

Broke up with that old girlfriend and found me another. Thought it might be serious but it turned out she was cheating. Girl she was cheating with was a bitch who looked like the Predator. I ain't kidding. But it was no big deal. What I thought was real romance wasn't real at all.

Cool.

I could find a girlfriend when I wanted one.

Besides, what I really wanted was to keep my shops poppin'.

I wanted to get bigger at the game.

That was my fate, my life, my only way of surviving.

I'd been in and I'd been out. Up and down. And even sideways. I knew which way was right for me.

Don't argue with me.

Don't tell me any different.

Don't give me no attitude.

If you wanna work for me, study the streets.

Maybe I'll give you a corner. Maybe I'll keep you around, look around to see how you do under fire.

You get one chance, but not two. If you fuck up the first time, that second chance could land me back at Grandma's House.

Ain't going back.

Going forward.

Don't get in my way.

"NO, NIGGA. I HIT THE BLOCK."

It was a Sunday night. Not much happening. Just hanging with a friend.

We were at a bar called Club One. Straight bar. Everything was cool.

I noticed this guy mad-dogging at me. He looked like a crime-type dude, so I looked the other way. But he kept staring.

"Who is that motherfucker?" I asked my friend.

"Michael K. Williams. He plays the gay gangsta on *The Wire*.

"What's *The Wire*?" I wanted to know.

My friend told me it was a TV show about Baltimore.

A little later Michael came over asked me, "You act or rap?"

"No, nigga," I said. "I hit the block."

"Well, come down to the set of *The Wire.* There some folks you should meet."

Next day I asked people I knew who watched the show what it was all about.

"People like you," they said.

"What does that mean?" I asked.

"Real people."

I wasn't thinking all that much about it, but figured I didn't have anything to lose.

So I went down to the show. When I got there, with all the trailers and shit, it didn't look like much to me.

"Please wait," they said.

"Wait for what?" I asked.

"Your screen test."

Well, I didn't know nothing about no screen test.

"What *is* a screen test?" I asked.

"We'll show you in a minute."

It was more than a minute. It was a long goddamn time. I was sitting in there, doing nothing but making calls to make sure my shops were running smooth.

Two hours later, I'd had it. I was about to get up and leave—fuck this shit—when they said they was ready.

Took me in a room, sat me down, and said, "You don't need to speak. Just look in the camera."

I looked in the camera for a couple of minutes.

I got paid $150.

"That's it?" I asked.

"That's it," they said.

"What's next?"

"We'll call you."

They did. They actually called the next day wanting another screen test. They said they'd pay another $150.

But I was thinking that's bullshit.

While I was getting $150 for a screen test I could be making many stacks on the block. In my business, time is money.

But on second thought, everyone thinks about being on TV, and I was no different. I started watching the show. *The Wire* had street characters running around every episode. I related. I liked the show. It was real.

"Okay," I said. "I'll take another test."

Second test happened. And a third.

Then someone came up and said, "You're a natural. We want you on the show."

I was a little shocked.

I didn't really believe it.

"No acting lessons?" I asked.

"No acting lessons," they said. "The directors will help you out."

I was feeling weird. I was feeling happy but I was also feeling like I was dreaming. They actually wanted to put me on TV.

"How 'bout my look?" I asked.

"We like your look," they said.

"I don't need to change it?"

"We don't want you to change it."

"How 'bout the way I talk?" I talk with this heavy Baltimore accent.

"We like the way you talk."

"It's all good?" I asked.

"All good," they said.

It's too good, I thought to myself. *My life don't work this way. It's too fuckin' good.*

FLIPPING THE SCRIPT

I knew *The Wire* was an HBO show for American TV, but I didn't know it was poppin' all over the world.

I didn't know, at the end of the third season of the series, when I started appearing, that I'd be so relaxed around the camera.

I had no idea that I'd take to it the way I did.

Strange, but I didn't look at it like acting.

It was being.

I just had to be.

On the show I had to be me: someone who hits the block.

They wanted me to keep my walk and my talk and even my name. They wanted me to be Snoop.

The other thing was this: Whenever and wherever we shot, I found myself in the middle of a family that loved me. All the actors, writers, and producers treated me like a long-lost daughter or sister or friend.

So there I was, doing what I'd always done: being a thug, only being a thug in front of the cameras.

What kind of crazy shit is that?

Suddenly I'm being recognized in restaurants. I'm being asked to act in other movies.

Real is pretend, and pretend is real.

Snoop is real-life me and Snoop is a pretend-life character on TV.

The script is flipped.

I wake up in the morning, get dressed, leave my work on the block to walk into a world about make-believe work on the block.

But because I ain't that sure the make-believe work is real, I keep my real-life work. My shops stay open.

"How long can you do that, Snoop?" asks my godmother, Denise. "How long can you keep selling dope?"

So Denise starts convicting me, and my conscience starts convicting me. My brain's spinning around and I'm getting confused all over again, just like when I was down in the Cut and learned that Uncle had been killed.

Back then I'd decided to go straight.

I'd seen the light.

But then when I got out and kept getting canned from straight jobs, the light went out.

I was drawn back into the darkness because the darkness was where I belonged. I was sure that the light was for others, not for me. I'd live and die in darkness. I'd even get rich in darkness. Darkness was all I knew. Darkness was my reality.

Now here comes all this *Wire* business.

TV cats talking about, "We want real people on this show. We want to show your reality."

But by showing my reality, these motherfuckers are changing my reality.

The shit's confusing.

By showing who I really am, they're changing who I really am.

I'm seeing that light again.

I'm feeling that love.

I'm thinking about closing down my shops. I'm thinking about not hitting the block anymore.

If I keep hitting the block, I'll fuck up this acting business. I'll fuck up everything. Getting other niggas killed or locked up. I'll get sent back to jail or I'll be killed.

Ain't no way around it.

The only way to leave my fucked-up reality is to throw myself into the pretend version of my fucked-up reality.

If I move toward the light—the light of the cameras, the light of the beautiful people who are running *The Wire* and acting on *The Wire*—then I escape the darkness.

The Wire is throwing light on that darkness.

That's what the show's about.

That's what I'm about.

My new life.

My new direction.

New light.

New hope.

New everything.

NEW SNOOP

New Snoop—the Snoop that's finally closed down her shops—is trying to make sense of this scene about a nail gun.

But the scene don't make sense and New Snoop's feeling stupid.

That's how it went in the beginning. I'd get some scripts that didn't make sense to me. I had trouble with the script supervisor, the gal who helps you with your lines. She was getting on my nerves and it took me a while to get used to her. Fact is, I never forgot my lines. I memorized them cold and never missed a beat.

I was still a little uneasy, though. Other than down at the courthouse, I'd never been around so many white people. It was a new experience. I didn't know what half of them did. I didn't understand how film works. I was nervous.

The thing about me, though—the thing I learned from

the streets—is not to show it. Keep my cool. Make it seem like I got my shit together.

That's what Snoop the Character is all about. And that's what Snoop the Actor has to be about too.

So I followed the directions I was given. I bonded with a couple of the actors. Michael K. Williams plays Omar. He's the one who got me through the door. Jamie Hector plays Marlo, the gangsta who hires me to kill niggas. Sometimes Omar, Hector, and I would hang out after the show. Sometimes they'd give me little pieces of advice about how to read and interpret a script.

The directors were cool. If I thought a line didn't flow right or read real, they let me change it up. If I said, "This ain't something Snoop would say," they'd say, "Well, how *would* she say it?" I'd say it my way, and my way almost always won out.

There's a character on *The Wire* called Proposition Joe. His real-life name is Robert Chew, and he's also a drama teacher. During the shoots, the producer suggested that some of the younger actors, including me, go to Robert for a few tips. He's a beautiful man who talks about emotions and instincts and relaxing in front of the camera until you're in the moment of the action. He talks about acting with your heart. My heart was open to Robert because I wanted to learn.

My heart was beating fast that day I read the nail gun scene. I didn't get it. I called in Ed Burns, one of the writers, and told him plain, "I got no fuckin' clue what's happening here."

He explained that Snoop had been sent on a job to find the best nail gun out there. "You ever been in a hardware store?" he asked me.

"Sure," I said. "When Pop was alive, I went all the time. Him and me lived in hardware stores."

"Well, that's all it is. You're walking through the door, inspecting all the merchandise. You come up to the clerk and ask his advice. He sells you on the biggest nail gun in the store. You're happy. You buy it for cash and tip him extravagantly. You've scored."

"So it's kinda like I'm going on an errand for Pop," I said.

"Exactly. This is a big scene because the nail gun you buy will board up deserted houses filled with the bodies of people you've killed. It might sound like a routine errand, but it's not. It's sinister, but you play it matter-of-factly."

Next morning I was ready to be sinister. When we rolled, I was feeling it. Everyone said the scene came out good. I don't wanna sound stuck on myself, but I nailed that sucker.

The other truth is when I started appearing on the show, I'd watch myself at home and liked what I saw. Again, I don't mean to be egotistical, but I thought I looked better on TV than in real life. That made me excited. And kept me excited.

I ain't ever seen myself that way before. I had to respect myself 'cause I'd become a professional actor. Being a pro actor made me act differently in my nonacting life.

Before *The Wire*, I was already a little star in the hood. Everyone knew me. But the more I was on *The Wire*, the more it seemed I was a little star all over the country. That amazed me. And it also gave me a different feeling when strangers came up to me and said, "I love your work."

When I dealt dope, no one came up and said, "I love you work." No one looked at me with eyes of appreciation.

"You doing a good job," an older lady told me in a restaurant. "We're proud of you."

Proud of me? Man, that made me feel ten feet tall.

"You're treating this role very responsibly," someone at work said.

Pride, responsibility—man, these were new concepts.

I liked feeling proud. I liked feeling responsible.

I wanted to act responsibly.

The responsible thing was to close down all my shops.

And I did.

Got out of the drug-running business.

Got more and more serious about acting.

Started feeling more positive vibes from David Simon, the guy who created the show and still writes lots of them. Started feeling the love from writers like Ed Burns and the other people who were turning out those great scripts. They was showing Baltimore for how it really is.

I started feeling—period.

Ain't saying I'm the best actor out here. I know I'm not. But I also know that acting, by showing me how to feel, also showed me I hadn't been feeling at all.

You can't sell dope all day and still feel.

You can't kill niggas and still feel.

You just can't.

When I acted out the part of Snoop, I saw that to do the things she does—the murders she commits—she had to shut herself down.

That's an awful thing. That's a fuckin' brutal thing.

***

Now there's this new thing.

This new Snoop.

I realize the newness is due to good luck or good fate or those good angels who came from Mama's prayers for protection. I realize I'm blessed. Being blessed is a new feeling that takes getting used to.

I'm believing we're all blessed—blessed to be alive. I had that blessing from the beginning but I blocked it. I hid from it. I threw off the blessing. I threw it away chasing some shit I had no business chasing.

The old Snoop messed up that blessing that came from being cared for by good people—Mama, Pop, my godmother. Uncle and Father, though they were caught up in their own bullshit, blessed me by trying to set me straight. They blessed me by loving me. But I flipped off the blessing.

I've come to believe that you gotta believe in the blessing. Ignore it and it ignores you. Embrace it and it powers you.

The old Snoop felt powerful, but it was a power that came from a gun or a bad-ass reputation. The new Snoop feels powerful, but the power is different; it's coming from a spirit I can't explain.

At first, I felt like I had to explain it. Now I don't. I just accept it. I breathe in the spirit just like I breathe in air. I feel the spirit. It keeps me up. It keeps me clear. Keeps me where I wanna be.

I wake up in the morning, yawn, stretch, get up, and look out the window. If the sun is shining, fine. If it ain't, that's fine too.

I'm saying a little two-word prayer. "Thank you."

That's the whole prayer.

I keep saying it during the day. Saying it out loud and saying it to myself.

I say thank you for a new point of view. Say thank you because I'm seeing everything differently.

I'm seeing that the point of this life we've been given is to not shut ourselves down, but open ourselves up.

Open up our hearts. Open up the part of our souls where hope lives. Open up our creativity and open up our minds.

Let light pour in.

Let light grow bright, not dim.

Let love come in and take over.

Let love direct us to where we need to go.

All this is new for me.

All this is amazing for me.

But now that it's happening, now that I've been saved by forces that I still don't really understand, all I can do is look back with sadness and look ahead with hope.

The sadness is for all the people I've fucked up. I'm truly sorry for that. I can't give back lives and I can't undo what I've done, but I can say that I regret it in the worst possible way.

Regret pulls me in one direction; hope pulls me in another.

Hope is for all the good I wanna do.

The people I wanna touch.

The light I wanna give, just as the light has been given to me.

The light has come back, the same light that came down on me in the Cut when I recovered from Uncle's death.

Where does the light come from? And what do you call it?

You can call it God. You call it Jesus. These names are good names.

But I call it the miracle of love.

I call it Grace after Midnight.